Sleep Disorders: Evaluation and Treatment

Sleep Disorders: Evaluation and Treatment

Editor: Destiny Lockhart

AMERICAN
MEDICAL PUBLISHERS
www.americanmedicalpublishers.com

AMERICAN
MEDICAL PUBLISHERS
www.americanmedicalpublishers.com

Cataloging-in-Publication Data

Sleep disorders : evaluation and treatment / edited by Destiny Lockhart.
p. cm.
Includes bibliographical references and index.
ISBN 978-1-63927-096-5
1. Sleep disorders. 2. Nervous system--Diseases. 3. Sleep disorders--Diagnosis.
4. Sleep disorders--Treatment. I. Lockhart, Destiny.
RC547 .S54 2022
616.849 8--dc23

American Medical Publishers,
41 Flatbush Avenue,
1st Floor, New York,
NY 11217, USA

ISBN 978-1-63927-096-5 (Hardback)

Contents

Preface

The medical disorder which affects the sleep patterns of a person is referred to as a sleep disorder. It can often interfere with the normal physical, social and emotional functioning of a person. It is commonly diagnosed with the help of tests such as polysomnography and actigraphy. Sleep disorders are classified into various categories namely dyssomnias, parasomnias and circadian rhythm sleep disorders. The condition where a person has difficulty falling asleep or staying asleep without any visible cause is known as insomnia. It is the most common sleep disorder and falls under the category of dyssomnia. It is often caused by psychological stress, hyperthyroidism, heartburn, heart failure, and other drugs such as caffeine, nicotine and alcohol. A few other common sleep disorders include sleep apnea, narcolepsy, hypersomnia, sleepwalking, and night terrors. Treatments of sleep disorders are grouped into four classes, namely, behavioral and psychotherapeutic treatment, medication, rehabilitation and management, and somatic treatment. This book provides comprehensive insights into sleep disorders. It consists of contributions made by international experts. Those in search of information to further their knowledge will be greatly assisted by this book.

This book unites the global concepts and researches in an organized manner for a comprehensive understanding of the subject. It is a ripe text for all researchers, students, scientists or anyone else who is interested in acquiring a better knowledge of this dynamic field.

I extend my sincere thanks to the contributors for such eloquent research chapters. Finally, I thank my family for being a source of support and help.

Editor

1

Changes of Procedural Memory in the Patients with Primary Insomnia

Yi-jun Ge[1], Lan Xia[2], Fang Wang[3] and Gui-hai Chen[1]*

[1]*Department of Neurology, the First People's Hospital of Chenzhou, China*
[2]*Department of Neurology, the Second Affiliated Hospital of Anhui Medical University, China*
[3]*Department of Neurology, the First Affiliated Hospital of Anhui Medical University, China*

Abstract

Objective: To explore changes of procedural memory in the patients with primary insomnia (PI) and its characteristics.

Methods: Thirty-six PI patients and 36 controls were enrolled. The procedural memory was respectively detected by category exemplar generation and motor sequence tasks respectively, and the declarative memory was assessed by free word task.

Results: Compared to the controls, the PI patients showed few correct numbers in the category exemplar generation (7.7 ± 2.1 vs. 9.9 ± 1.0, z = 5.247, P<0.001), motion sequence task (8.1 ± 3.3 vs 12.0 ± 3.0, z = 4.676, P<0.001) and the phases of immediate recall (3.3 ± 1.1 vs 6.0 ± 1.2, z=6.634, P<0.001), delayed recall (9.0 ± 2.2 vs. 11.2 ± 1.1, z=4.718, P<0.001) and delayed recognition (14.2 ± 1.0 vs. 15.0 ±0.0, z = 4.637, P<0.001) of the free word task. For the different subtypes of PI, the early morning awakening group had significantly worse performance in the motor sequence task compared to the difficulty initiating sleep (z=–2.768, P=0.006) and difficulty maintaining sleep (z=–2.502, P=0.012) groups, and less correct numbers of the word-delayed recognition compared to the difficulty maintaining sleep group too (z=–2.707, P=0.007).

Conclusion: The procedural and declarative memories are impaired in the PI patients, especially the early morning awakening insomniacs.

Keywords: Primary insomnia; Procedural memory; Declarative memory

Introduction

Insomnia refers to the difficulty in the sleep initiating maintaining of patients with adequate hours, good sleep environment and opportunities to sleep. As a result, the patients have a subjective experience of dissatisfied sleep time and/or quality, and daytime dysfunction, such as anxiety, depression, mental activity and cognitive (e.g. learning and memory) impairment in certain degree [1-4].

The imaging studies show that the insomnia patients had cerebral hypoper fusion of blood compared to the normal controls, and this change in the basal ganglia was more obvious than those in the frontal, occipital and parietal cortexes [5]. It is found by mean of magnetic resonance imaging that patients with insomnia had significantly reduced volume in the bilateral hippocampus [6]. In accordance with sleep deprivation experiments in animals, it is suggested that sleep deprivation leaded to decline of cognitive function in humans. Studies on memory with sleep deprivation model have shown that depriving different periods of sleep in the general population would make different impacts on learning and memory. For example, total sleep deprivation impairs semantic memory; slow wave sleep (SWS) deprivation without reducing total sleep time significantly affects declarative memory (DM) and coding related hippocampal activities; rapid eye movement sleep (REMS) deprivation influences the procedural memory (PM) rather than DM [7]. Polysomnography application has revealed some sleep characteristics of insomnia patients, such as the shortened total sleep time, extended sleep onset latency, decreased sleep efficiency, reductive SWS and incremental percentage of first-phase sleep [8]. The underlying mechanism of insomnia-related cognitive changes might be due to some kinds of sleep structure disorders or a specific SWS (0.5~2.0 Hz) defect, which is harmful to the brain protein synthesis, the establishment and consolidation of new synaptic connections and the recovery of synaptic homeostasis.

However, in the early stage of chronic insomnia patients, because of the mild condition, the body tends to have sufficient time to complete any compensation. So that, cognitive function changes between insomnia of the natural course and sleep deprivation are different. So far, memory impairment in patients with primary insomnia (PI) remains to be identified. A meta-analysis showed that patients with PI existed mild to moderate damage in working memory, episodic memory and certain aspects of attention, but there was no significant difference in perceptual processing, PM, speech and executive function [9,10]. PM impairment and its characteristics of patients with PI are inconclusive, which may be owing to different evaluation methods and sample sources. In the present, we observed the changes in PM and DM with three tasks (category exemplar generation, motor sequence tasks and free word task) in the patients whose symptoms met to the PI diagnostic criteria in the Diagnostic and Statistical Manual of Mental Disorders, Fourth Edition (DSM-IV) [11].

Materials and Methods

Study objects

PI group: Thirty-six patients were included, who went to the Sleep and Memory Disorders Clinic of the First Affiliated Hospital, Anhui

***Corresponding author:** Gui-hai Chen, Department of Neurology, the First People's Hospital of Chenzhou, Chenzhou, Hunan Province, PR 423000, China, E-mail: chenguihai1964@163.com

Medical University from September 2010 to May 2011 due to sleep difficulties. Their mean age was 37.0 ± 11.5 years, the illness duration ≥ 1 month and all of them met PI diagnostic criteria in the DSM-IV. All of them were right-handed, and were accepted high school education or above. Meanwhile, the Athens Insomnia Scale (AIS) [12] score was >6 and Montreal cognitive test scale (MoCA) [13] score was ≥ 26. Additionally, the following conditions were excluded: taking drugs (such as antidepressants, benzodiazepines, antiepileptics or other drugs/substances) possibly impacting on cognitive function past two weeks; suffering from other sleep disorders (such as sleep apnea syndrome, restless legs syndrome), medicine conditions (such as chronic obstructive pulmonary disease, chronic pain, or severe liver disease) and neuropsychiatric disorders (such as stroke, epilepsy, Parkinson's disease, dementia, depression and anxiety disorders, specifically, when 17-terms Hamilton Depression Rating Scale (HAMD-17) [14] score being ≥ 17); unable to complete the experiment; impaired visual acuity and audition. Furthermore, the patients were divided into several subgroups according to the type of insomnia: the difficultly initiating sleep group [7 males / 5 females; mean age 35.6 ± 13.2 years; education 12.5 ± 2.2 years], the early morning awakening group [6 males / 6 females; mean age 36.6 ± 10.2 years; education 12.7 ± 1.7 years] and the difficulty maintaining sleep group [5 males / 7 females; mean age 37.3 ± 11.0 years; education 13.2 ± 2.5 years]. There were no statistical differences among subgroups in gender, age and years of education (*Ps* > 0.05).

Healthy control group: A total of 30 cases consist of healthy adults who were subjected to health examination during the same period. The mean age was 37.3 ± 11.4 years. They were right-handed, and come from the comparable cities or countries with the similar habits, education, economics and other factors, in order to roughly match with the PI patients. Besides, they were required have no previous history of neuropsychiatric disorders and hypomnesis, and no obvious physical illness, with AIS score ≤ 4, MoCA score ≥ 26 and HAMD-17 score < 7.

This research was approved by the First Affiliated Hospital of Anhui Medical University Ethics Committee, and all participants signed informed consent.

Methods

Background information assessment: Background information, including AIS, Epworth Sleepiness Scale (ESS) [15], MoCA and HAMD-17, were completed by trained clinicians.

PM

Category exemplar generation task: Firstly, every subject was shown 10 randomized pictures of vegetables and household appliances, and then was required to name them. After 15 minutes, the subject was required to enumerate the name of vegetables and household appliances shown before as many as possible within 1 min successively, and the total correct numbers were recorded [16].

Motion sequence task: Subjects put their left fingers successively on the number keys of 1234 on the keyboard from little to index finger, and then entered a set of random sequences (such as 4-2-3-1-4) displayed on the computer screen as fast and accurate as possible within a certain period of time. After resting 24s, they would enter into the next round. They were required to complete 12 rounds in total consecutively. The average numbers of correct sequences in the last 3 rounds were counted [17].

DM

Words free recall task: Fifteen high-frequency Chinese notional words were selected in the test. Subjects were asked to read the words five times and recall them after reading immediately within 2 min. The correct number of first time recalling was defined as the immediate recall score. Then subjects recalled the free words after 15 min. The correct number of words was called the delayed recall score. After given another 15 new notional words, subjects were required to tell the word from old to new, the correct numbers of judgment of old words was called the delayed recognition score [18].

Statistical analysis

All statistical analyses were conducted by the SPSS 13.0. The data were expressed as mean ± standard deviation. The normal distribution data were analyzed by independent samples t test or ANOVA, and the non-normal distribution data were analyzed by Manne-Whitney U or Kruskal-Wallis H test.

Results

Background information

U or *t* test showed that there was no statistically difference in sex, age and years of education between the PI group and the control group (Table 1). There were no significantly difference in MoCA (z=1.781, P =0.075) and ESS (t=0.879, P=0.379) scores between the two groups, but the PI group had significantly higher scores of the AIS and HAMD-17 than the control group (z=7.345, P < 0.001; z=7.161, P < 0.001), indicating that the sample quality met requirement of the study (Table 1).

Memory testing

The U test showed that compared to the controls, the PI patients had worse performances in all measures of the immediate recall, delayed recall, delayed recognition, category generation and the motion sequence (z=6.634, 4.718, 4.637, 5.247 and 4.676, respectively, *Ps* <0.001) (Table 2).

Memories in the patients with different insomnia subtypes

The ANOVA or H test showed that there were significant or marginal differences among the three subgroups of difficultly initiating sleep, early morning awakening and difficultly maintaining sleep in the delay recall (F=3.264, P=0.051), delayed recognition (H=8.871, P=0.012) and exercise sequence (H=9.766, P=0.008) scores, but there were no significant differences in the immediate recall (H=0.840, P=0.657) and class generation (H=0.399, P=0.819) scores. Furthermore,

Groups	Gender (male/female)	Age (years)	Education Levels (years)	AIS	ESS	HAMD-17	MoCA
Insomnia	18/18	37.0 ± 11.5	13.0 ± 1.9	13.9 ± 3.1*	7.4 ± 3 .5	11.7 ± 3.9*	26.8 ± 1.2
Controls	14/16	37.3 ± 11.4	12.1 ± 2.7	2.5 ± 1.2	6.7 ± 2.1	2.6 ± 1.8	27.3 ± 1.5
Statistic	χ^2=0.073	t=0.378	z=1.262	z=7.345	z=0.879	z=7.161	z=1.781
P values	0.787	0.706	0.207	< 0.001	0.379	< 0.001	0.075

*Compare to the control group P<0.001

AIS: Athens Insomnia Scale; ESS: Epworth Sleepiness Scale; HAMD-17: 17-terms Hamilton Depression Rating Scale; MoCA: Montreal Cognitive Assessment

Table 1: Background information of the subjects (mean ± standard deviation).

Groups	Declarative memory			Procedural memory	
	Immediate recall	Delayed recall	Delayed recognition	Category generation	Motion sequence
Primary insomnia	3.3 ± 1.1*	9.0 ± 2.2*	14.2 ± 1.0*	7.7 ± 2.1*	8.1 ± 3.3*
Controls	6.0 ± 1.2	11.2 ± 1.1	15.0 ± 0.0	9.9 ± 1.0	12.0 ± 3.0
z	6.634	4.718	4.637	5.247	4.676
P values	<0.001	<0.001	<0.001	<0.001	<0.001

*Compare to the control group, *P*<0.001

Table 2: Memory test results of the subjects (the number of correct, mean ± standard deviation).

Groups	Declarative memory			Procedural memory	
	Immediate recall	Delayed recall	Delayed recognition	Category generation	Motion sequence
Difficultly initiating sleep	3.3 ± 1.1	9.3 ± 2.6	14.4 ± 0.8	7.9 ± 2.2	9.0 ± 2.7
Early morning awakening	3.2 ± 1.2	8.8 ± 2.0	13.4 ± 1.2#	7.2 ± 1.2	6.6 ± 2.6 *#
Difficultly maintaining sleep	3.4 ± 0.9	9.0 ± 2.2	14.7 ± 0.7	8.0 ± 2.7	8.6 ± 4.1
Statistic	*H* = 0.840	*F* = 0.101	*H* = 8.871	*H* = 0.399	*H* = 9.766
P values	0.657	0.904	0.012	0.819	0.008

*Compare to the difficultly initiating sleep group, *P*<0.017, # Compare to the difficulty maintaining sleep group, *P*<0.017

Table 3: Memory in the patients with different insomnia subtypes (correct number, mean ± standard deviation).

the U test for pair wise comparison (corrected size of the test: α=0.05 / 3=0.017) showed the early morning awakening patients got worse scores in motion sequences and delay recall task than the difficulty maintaining sleep patients (z=−2.502, P=0.012 and z=−2.707, P=0.007, respectively, both P values < 0.017). However, when compared to the difficultly initiating sleep group, the worse performance in the early morning awakening group only occurred in the motion sequences task (z=−2.768, P=0.006 < 0.017), but not in delay recall task (z = −2.157, P = 0.031> 0.017) (Table 3).

Discussion

One of the main functions of sleep is restoring brain synaptic plasticity and forming of new memories [19]. But previous studies have shown that patients with PI had generally no or slight damage in learning and memory [20], perhaps only in complex tasks memory [21]. An overview about the daytime function in PI patients has been exhibited i.e., no memory impairment was seen in simple tasks, such as audio verbal learning, Hopkins Verbal Learning, word matching, word recognition and visual recognition, however, the PI group had significantly worse performance than the control group in free word memory, the mirror image reading and phrase memory tasks [22]. Recent researches about mirror image reading (detecting PM) and visual verbal learning tasks (detecting DM) found that patients with PI showed decreased ability to complete these tasks [23]. In our study, the motion sequence and category generation tasks were respectively used to detect motor skill learning and priming effects on PM in the PI patients, while the free word recall task was used to detect DM. The results showed that compared to the control group, the motion sequence and category exemplar generation scores in the PI patients declined to certain degree, and three measures in the free word recall task were also damaged. Therefore, whether the PI patients have damaged PM or/and DM or not depended on a moderate difficulty of the tasks used.

Sleep plays an important role in the PM and DM, which is related to new memories and integration of existing knowledge [24]. Both REMS and SWS [25] would contribute to memory encoding, consolidation and neural plasticity. Studies on sleep deprivation have shown that the REMS deprivation only affected PM and SWS deprivation influenced DM [26]. However, the visual recognition task (a kind of DM) research found that the improved memory after sleep was only correlated to the amount of SWS in the first quarter of the night, but was also correlated to the amount of REMS in the last quarter. These results indicated that the consolidation of DM is connected with both SWS and REMS [27]. Actually, the data result from the PI patients indicated that PM also involved in the Stage 2 sleeps [28]. Relative to complex skills formation which relies more on REMS, the consolidation of existing skills and simple motor skills needs sleep spindles in Stage 2 [29]. Therefore, throughout the whole process of sleep, the memory consolidation of different types needs respectively unique pattern of sleep periods [28]. After comparison among diverse insomnia subtypes, the results showed that the early waking group had significantly impaired PM and DM when compared to the patients with difficultly maintenance sleep, and impaired PM when compared to ones with difficultly initiating sleep. We presumed that the reduction or changed percentage of REMS in early waking people may contribute to this result, because the patients with early waking mainly lose the sleep in the latter half of night, in which the REMS is predominant. Our results did not seem support the previous hypothesis that the SWS reduction in the difficultly initiating sleep patients should lead to DM damage. In fact, the difficultly initiating sleep patients often had earlier bedtime, but they don't always have reductive total sleep time or SWS. Furthermore, the changes of sleep architecture are not unitary in maintenance difficulties sleep patients, and some patients may be having a normal proportion of each phase. Without doubt, it is necessary to enlarge samples to certify our conclusion.

References

1. Schutte-Rodin S, Broch L, Buysse D, Dorsey C, Sateia M (2008) Clinical guideline for the evaluation and management of chronic insomnia in adults. J Clin Sleep Med 4: 487-504.
2. Pigeon WR (2010) Diagnosis, prevalence, pathways, consequences & treatment of insomnia. Indian J Med Res 131: 321-332.
3. Bastien CH (2011) Insomnia: Neurophysiological and neuropsychological approaches. Neuropsychol Rev 21: 22-40.
4. Varkevisser M, Kerkhof GA (2005) Chronic insomnia and performance in a 24-h constant routine study. J Sleep Res 14: 49-59.
5. Smith MT, Perlis ML, Chengazi VU, Pennington J, Soeffing J, et al. (2002) Neuroimaging of NREM sleep in primary insomnia: a Tc-99-HMPAO single photon emission computed tomography study. Sleep 25: 325-335.
6. Riemann D, Voderholzer U, Spiegelhalder K, Hornyak M, Buysse DJ, et al. (2007) Chronic insomnia and MRI-measured hippocampal volumes: a pilot study. Sleep 30: 955-958.

7. Roehrs T, Roth T (2000) Sleep-wake state and memory function. Sleep 23 Suppl 3: S64-68.

8. American Academy of Sleep Medicine (2005) The international classification of sleep disorders-Second edition (ICSD-2).

9. Li B (1999) The neural basis of learning and memory. World Sci Tech R & D 06: 47-50.

10. Fortier-Brochu E, Beaulieu-Bonneau S, Ivers H, Morin CM (2012) Insomnia and daytime cognitive performance: a meta-analysis. Sleep Med Rev 16: 83-94.

11. Ohayon MM, Reynolds CF 3rd (2009) Epidemiological and clinical relevance of insomnia diagnosis algorithms according to the DSM-IV and the International Classification of Sleep Disorders (ICSD). Sleep Med 10: 952-960.

12. Zhang ZJ (2005) Behavioral Medicine Scale Manual. Chinese Medical Multimedia Press.

13. Chen N, He L (2009) The research and application profiles of Montreal Cognitive Assessment. Chin J Nerv Ment Dis 35: 632-634.

14. Wang XD, Wang XL, Ma H (1990) Rating scales of mental health (Revised edition, in Chinese). Chin Ment Health J 13: 220-223.

15. Johns MW (1991) A new method for measuring daytime sleepiness: the Epworth sleepiness scale. Sleep 14: 540-545.

16. Fleischman DA, Wilson RS, Gabrieli JD, Schneider JA, Bienias JL, et al. (2005) Implicit memory and Alzheimer's disease neuropathology. Brain 128: 2006- 2015.

17. Walker MP, Stickgold R, Alsop D, Gaab N, Schlaug G (2005) Sleep-dependent motor memory plasticity in the human brain. Neuroscience 133: 911-917.

18. Cheng HD, Wang K, Gong L, Yin CL, Meng Y (2010) The disorder of prospective memory in patients with amnesia mild cognitive impairment. Chin J Neurol 43: 174-177.

19. Walker MP, Stickgold R (2004) Sleep-dependent learning and memory consolidation. Neuron 44: 121-133.

20. Riedel BW, Lichstein KL (2000) Insomnia and daytime functioning. Sleep Med Rev 4: 277-298.

21. Altena E, Van Der Werf YD, Strijers RL, Van Someren EJ (2008) Sleep loss affects vigilance: effects of chronic insomnia and sleep therapy. J Sleep Res 17: 335-343.

22. Shekleton JA, Rogers NL, Rajaratnam SM (2010) Searching for the daytime impairments of primary insomnia. Sleep Med Rev 14: 47-60.

23. Nissen C, Kloepfer C, Feige B, Piosczyk H, Spiegelhalder K, et al. (2011) Sleep-related memory consolidation in primary insomnia. J Sleep Res 20: 129-136.

24. Tamminen J, Payne JD, Stickgold R, Wamsley EJ, Gaskell MG (2010) Sleep spindle activity is associated with the integration of new memories and existing knowledge. J Neurosci 30: 14356-14360.

25. Walker MP (2008) Sleep-dependent memory processing. Harv Rev Psychiatry 16: 287-298.

26. Roehrs T, Roth T (2000) Sleep-wake state and memory function. Sleep 23 Suppl 3: S64-68.

27. Stickgold R, Whidbee D, Schirmer B, Patel V, Hobson JA (2000) Visual discrimination task improvement: A multi-step process occurring during sleep. J Cogn Neurosci 12: 246-254.

28. Fogel SM, Smith CT, Cote KA (2007) Dissociable learning-dependent changes in REM and non-REM sleep in declarative and procedural memory systems. Behav Brain Res 180: 48-61.

29. Morin A, Doyon J, Dostie V, Barakat M, Hadj Tahar A, et al. (2008) Motor sequence learning increases sleep spindles and fast frequencies in post-training sleep. Sleep 31: 1149-1156.

2

Comparison of Sleep Latency Measured by the Oxford Sleep Resistance Test and Simultaneous EEG in Japanese Patients

Keisuke Hosokawa, Tsuguo Nishijima*, Tetsuya Kizawa, Fumiyo Endo and Shigeru Sakurai

Division of Behavioral Sleep Medicine, Iwate Medical University, School of Medicine, Morioka, Japan

***Corresponding author:** Tsuguo Nishijima, Department of Sleep Medicine, Iwate Medical University, School of Medicine, 19-1 Uchimaru, Morioka City, Iwate Prefecture, Morioka, Japan, E-mail: tsuguo@iwate-med.ac.jp

Abstract

Excessive daytime sleepiness (EDS) is observed in various pathological conditions associated with sleep disorders. However, objective methods for the assessment of EDS rely on complex electroencephalographic (EEG) recording and are impractical for use in general clinical practice. To address this issue, the Oxford Sleep Resistance Test (OSLER) has been developed for use in clinical practice overseas, though few studies have examined the reliability of the OSLER test for measuring sleep latency in Japanese patients. Thus, in the present study, we aimed to determine whether sleep latency measured via the OSLER test (SL_{OSLER}) is consistent with that measured via EEG (SL_{EEG}) in Japanese patients with obstructive sleep apnea (OSA). Seventeen Japanese men with OSA (mean age: 51.5 ± 9.8 years) underwent simultaneous OSLER and EEG testing a total of four times on the day following polysomnography evaluation. SL_{OSLER} and SL_{EEG} were compared, and the reliability of the former was analysed using Bland-Altman plots. Mean SL_{OSLER} and SL_{EEG} for all patients were 26.9 ± 11.6 and 25.7 ± 12.2 minutes, respectively. A significant positive correlation was observed between these measurements ($p<0.0001$, $r=0.963$). Moreover, the Epworth Sleepiness Scale (ESS) scores were not significantly correlated with either SL_{OSLER} or SL_{EEG}. Bland-Altman plot analysis revealed that 94% of the plotted SL_{OSLER} or SL_{EEG} measurements converged within a range of mean ± 1.96 SD. Our findings thus demonstrated that SL_{OSLER} is consistent with SL_{EEG} in Japanese patients with OSA.

Keywords: Excessive daytime sleepiness; Oxford sleep resistance test; Sleep latency; Obstructive sleep apnea

Introduction

Excessive daytime sleepiness (EDS) presents a significant health and safety concern for individuals engaged in hazardous occupations-such as public transportation drivers, pilots, and heavy-equipment operators-as well as the general population. Obstructive sleep apnea (OSA) [1,2] is a prevalent disorder in which repetitive hypopnea or apnea during sleep induces frequent intermittent hypoxemia and electroencephalographic arousal, eventually resulting in EDS. The association between OSA and traffic accidents attributed to EDS has been highlighted as a serious social problem [3]. Sagaspe et al. reported that the frequency of lane departure during driving simulation was significantly higher in participants with a sleep latency of <20 minutes as measured using the Maintenance of Wakefulness Test (MWT) than in the with a sleep latency of ≥ 34 minutes [4]. Karimi et al. also reported that the incidence of motor vehicle accidents among patients with OSA decreases following initiation of continuous positive airway pressure (CPAP) therapy for ≥ 4 hours per night [5]. Thus, objective assessment of EDS is essential for the appropriate screening of patients and evaluation of outcomes following medical and social interventions.

Available methods for EDS assessment include both objective and subjective scales. The Epworth Sleepiness Scale (ESS) [6] and Stanford Sleepiness Scale (SSS) [7] are widely utilized for the subjective assessment of EDS in both daily clinical practice and clinical studies. Objective methods of EDS assessment include the Multiple Sleep Latency Test (MSLT) [8], which measures the time to sleep onset, and the MWT [9], which measures the duration of sustained wakefulness. In the MSLT and MWT, sleep latency and the duration of sustained wakefulness are repeatedly measured by recording electroencephalogram (EEG) activity four to five times per day under soporific conditions (e.g., in an examination room with low light) in the daytime, respectively. Not only are these tests time-consuming, but they also require the use of complex EEG equipment and constant observation by an EEG technologist. Due to the substantial human and economic burden of such tests, they are difficult to perform for many patients in general clinical practice. Moreover, previous studies have indicated that the results of subjective assessments do not always correlate well with those of objective scales such as the MWT [10]. Thus, simpler and more objective techniques for the assessment of EDS are required.

To address the aforementioned issues, researchers have proposed the Oxford Sleep Resistance Test (OSLER test), which measures the duration of sustained wakefulness via simple behavioural observation rather than EEG recording [11]. In the OSLER test, the examinee is required to operate a switch in response to a 1-s light-emitting diode (LED) stimulus presented in intervals of 3 s in a dimly lit examination room, and task performance is recorded to assess the state of wakefulness during the test.

Although the OSLER test has been compared to the MWT and used to evaluate clinical cases of EDS in Europe and the United States [11-13], no such studies have been conducted in Japanese populations. As such, whether the time to sleep onset measured using the OSLER test is comparable to that measured via EEG recording in Japanese individuals remains to be elucidated. Therefore, in the present study, we aimed to compare sleep latency measured via EEG (SL_{EEG}) and the OSLER test (SL_{OSLER}) in Japanese patients with OSA.

Materials and Methods

Participants

The present study was approved by the ethics committee of Iwate Medical University School of Medicine (permission number H26-51), and written informed consent was obtained from all participants following a thorough explanation of the study. The study included 17 Japanese men (mean age: 51.5 years ± 9.8 years) referred to the Division of Behavioural Sleep Medicine at Iwate Medical University Hospital for further evaluation of sleep-disordered breathing based on objective (e.g., snoring and/or apnea) or subjective symptoms (e.g., EDS and/or lethargy). The mean ESS score for all patients was 9.8 ± 5.4, and the mean Apnea/Hypopnea Index (AHI) was 61.4 ± 22.6 events/h (Table 1).

Variable	Value
Age (year)	51.5 ± 9.8
Gender (M:F)	17:00
BMI (kg/m^2)	30.3 ± 4.9
ESS (points)	9.8 ± 5.4
Sleep Study	
Total Sleep Time (min)	475.8 ± 47.6
Sleep efficiency (%)	80.7 ± 7.9
Sleep latency (min)	11.6 ± 8.6
%Stage N1 (%)	30.5 ± 10.7
%Stage N2 (%)	48.3 ± 9.6
%Stage N3 (%)	5.4 ± 4.6
%Stage R (%)	15.8 ± 5.7
Arousal index (events/h)	43.6 ± 16.5
Apnea/hypopnea events (events/h)	489.1 ± 179.9
Apnea/hypopnea index (events/h)	61.4 ± 22.6
Desaturation index (events/h)	55.6 ± 21.2
SpO_2 mean (%)	93.6 ± 2.0
SpO_2 minimum (%)	71.9 ± 10.8
Sleep Latency tests	
SL_{EEG} (min)	25.7 ± 12.2
SL_{OSLER} (min)	26.9 ± 11.6
Data are presented as the mean ± SD. BMI: Body mass index, ESS: Epworth Sleepiness Scale, SLEEG: Sleep Latency – Electroencephalogram, SLOSLER: Sleep Latency – OSLER test, % Stage N1: % non-stage	

Table 1: Patient characteristics (n=17).

Patients were prohibited from taking hypnotics, consuming caffeinated and alcoholic beverages, and smoking cigarettes over a 2-week period.

Subjective and objective assessment of EDS

At the initial outpatient visit, all patients were evaluated using the ESS questionnaire for the subjective assessment of EDS. Patients with a total ESS score of ≥ 11 were considered to have EDS [14]. On the day following completion of the PSG (hospital day 2), the OSLER test was performed simultaneously during EEG recording for the objective assessment of EDS. On hospital day 2, patients ate breakfast at 7:30 a.m. and lunch at 12:00 p.m. During the in-hospital tests, patients were strictly prohibited from consuming caffeinated drinks, smoking cigarettes, or taking a nap. Moreover, patients were instructed to remain awake as long as possible without moving the body, vocalizing, or applying any stimulus to the body during each test.

Overnight PSG

PSG was performed using an Alice 6^{TM} system (Philips Respironics Inc.; Murrysville, PA), and data were electronically recorded. All sleep studies were performed in a dedicated examination room with air conditioning (room temperature is between 24 to 26) at Iwate Medical University Hospital. PSG was initiated at 20:00 and completed at 6:00. Test conditions were kept as consistent as possible, and PSG was performed according to the performance standards indicated in the American Association of Sleep Medicine (AASM) guidelines version 2 [15]. Test results were displayed on a dedicated display device and visually assessed by laboratory technicians and physicians to determine the sleep and respiratory status of each patient.

Measurement of SL_{OSLER}

The OSLER test was performed using an OSLER device (Stowood Scientific Instruments, United Kingdom). All windows in the examination room were shaded, and the luminance in the room was set to 0.13 Lux. Patients were instructed to assume a comfortable Fowler position. An LED unit was placed in front of patients at eye level. Patients were instructed to hold the switch box in the dominant hand and gently place the index finger on the switch. In response to a 1-s LED stimulus presented every 3 s, patients were instructed to remove the index finger from the switch while the LED was illuminated, and to place the finger on the switch again when the LED was turned off. Based on the methodology described by Bennett et al. [11], each OSLER test session lasted up to 40 minutes, and a total of four sessions were performed every 2 h (9:00, 11:00, 13:00, and 15:00).

The session was terminated (1) when the patient failed to perform the switching task correctly seven times in a row (sleep onset) or (2) when 40 minutes had passed without seven consecutive failures (absence of sleep onset). SL_{OSLER} was defined as the time until termination of each OSLER test session. In case (2), SL_{OSLER} was expressed as a sleep latency of ≥ 40 minutes.

Measurement of SL_{EEG}

During each OSLER test session, EEG electrodes were placed based on the performance standards for PSG to assess the state of wakefulness for each participant. During EEG recording, patients were asked to remain awake and perform the OSLER task for as long as possible. Each EEG session lasted up to 40 minutes, and a total of four EEG sessions were performed every 2 hours (9:00, 11:00. 13:00, and 15:00). Sleep onset was defined as the first epoch of greater than 15 sec of cumulative sleep in a 30 sec epoch, whereas the absence of sleep onset was determined when 40 minutes had passed without sleep onset. SL_{EEG} was defined as the sleep latency measured via EEG during the OSLER test session. EEG sessions were terminated based on the same criteria used for OSLER test sessions. Moreover, patients were prohibited from sleeping for any length of time prior to PSG and between OSLER test sessions.

Statistical analysis

Statistical analysis was performed using StatView 5.0TM (Abacus Concepts, CA, and USA). The correlation between SL_{EEG} and SL_{OSLER} was analysed using Pearson's correlation coefficient, while the correlation between ESS scores and SL_{EEG} or SL_{OSLER} was analysed using Spearman's rank correlation coefficient. In addition, the consistency between SLEEG and SLOSLER was assessed using a Bland-Altman plot. A p value of <0.05 was considered to indicate a significant difference.

Results

Subjective and objective assessment of EDS

Patient characteristics and PSG data are presented in Table 1. The mean ESS score for all 17 patients was 9.8 ± 5.4. Six patients were considered to exhibit EDS, based on an ESS score ≥ 11. PSG yielded the following data: mean total sleep time (TST): 475.8 min ± 47.6 min; mean arousal index: 43.6 ± 16.5 events/h; mean AHI: 61.4 ± 22.6 events/h; mean desaturation index: 55.6 ± 21.2 events/h; mean peripheral artery oxygen saturation (SpO_2): 93.6% ± 2.0%; and minimum SpO_2: 71.9% ± 10.8%. The mean SL_{EEG} was 25.7 min ± 12.2 min, while the mean SL_{OSLER} was 26.9 min ± 11.6 min.

A significant positive correlation was observed between SL_{EEG} and SL_{OSLER}, which were obtained over four sessions per patient, for a total 68 sessions ($r=0.941$, $p<0.0001$) (Figure 1A).

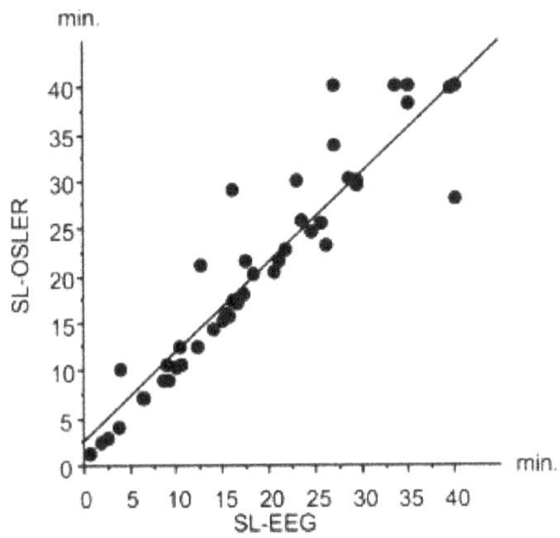

Figure 1A: Association between sleep latency as determined via the Oxford Sleep Resistance test (SL_{OSLER}) and electroencephalography (SL_{EEG}). A significant positive correlation was observed between SL_{OSLER} and SL_{EEG} across the 68 total sessions (*: $r=0.941$, $p<0.0001$). The correlation between SL_{OSLER} and SL_{EEG} was analysed using Pearson's correlation coefficient. A p value of <0.05 was considered to indicate a significant difference.

When the mean measurements obtained over the four sessions of each patient were analyzed, a significant positive correlation was again observed between SL_{EEG} and SL_{OSLER} ($r=0.963$, $p<0.0001$) (Figure 1B).

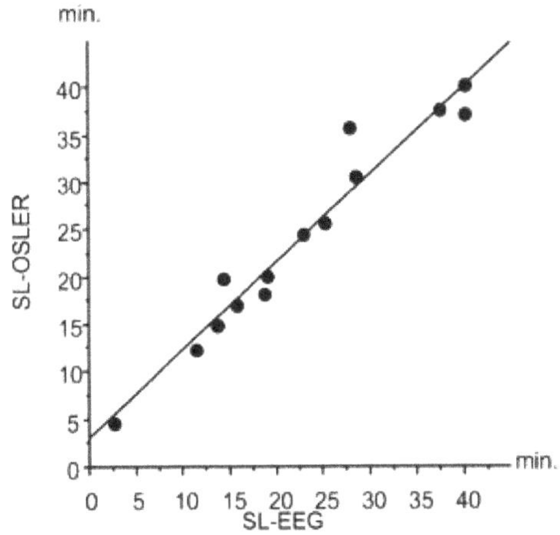

Figure 1B: When the mean measurements obtained over the four sessions of each patient were analyzed, a significant positive correlation was again observed between SLEEG and SLOSLER (#: $r=0.963$, $p<0.0001$).

However, SL_{EEG} and SL_{OSLER} tended to decrease as ESS scores increased, though no significant correlations were observed.

Bland-Altman plots revealed that the majority of SL_{EEG} and SL_{OSLER} measurements from all 68 sessions (94%) converged within a range of mean ± 1.96 SD (mean: 1.18; SD: 3.29; mean+1.96 SD: 7.62; mean −1.96 SD:−5.26) (Figure 2A).

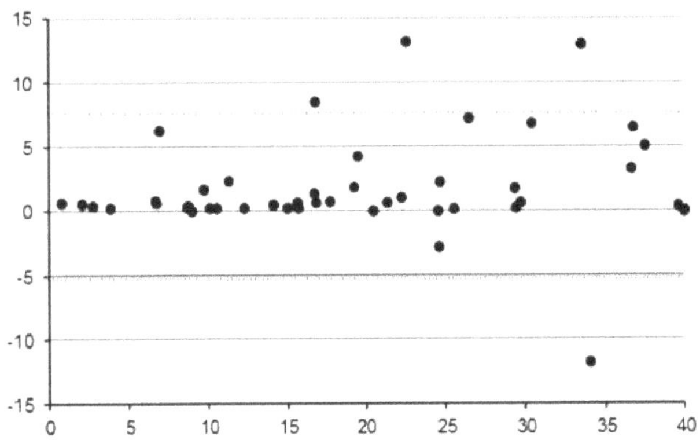

Figure 2A: Bland-Altman plots. Bland-Altman plot depicting the association between sleep latency as measured via the Oxford Sleep Resistance Test (SL_{OSLER}) and electroencephalography (SL_{EEG}) over all sessions (n=68; mean: 1.18; SD: 3.29; mean+1.96 SD: 7.62; mean−1.96 SD: −5.26).

Similarly, 94% of the plotted mean measurements for each of the 17 patients also converged within a range of mean ± 1.96 SD (Figure 2B).

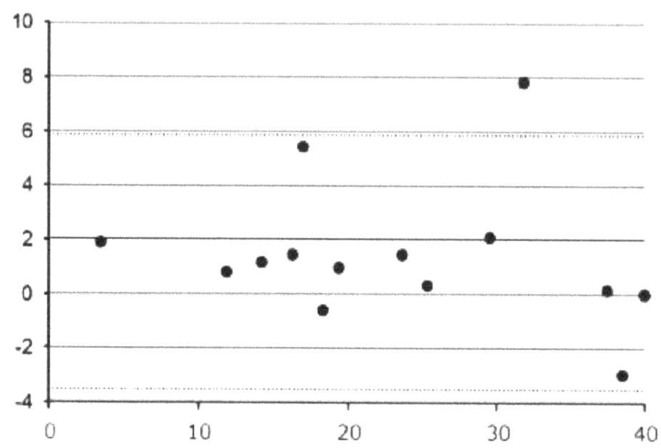

Figure 2B: Bland-Altman plots. Bland-Altman plot depicting the association between SL_{EEG} and SL_{OSLER} for each patient (n=17; mean: 1.18; SD: 2.39; mean+1.96 SD: 5.87; mean−1.96 SD: -3.51).

When a sleep latency of 20 minutes was set as the cut-off value for the "presence of sleepiness" based on the findings of a previous study by Sagaspe et al. [4], SL_{OSLER} was <20 minutes in seven patients (ESS=11.7 ± 5.5; three patients with ESS<11 [range, 3-10], four patients with ESS ≥ 11 [range, 12-18]) and ≥ 20 minutes in 10 patients (ESS=8.5 ± 5.1; eight patients with ESS<11 [range, 3-10], two patients with ESS ≥ 11 [range, 17-18]). Furthermore, an SL_{OSLER} cut-off of 20 minutes resulted in sensitivity and specificity values of 1.0, while an ESS cut-off of 11 resulted in a sensitivity of 0.57 and specificity of 0.8.

Discussion

The present study aimed to determine whether SL_{EEG} could be sufficiently estimated from SL_{OSLER} in Japanese patients with OSA. Our findings indicated that the duration of sustained wakefulness as determined by EEG could also be estimated using the results of the OSLER test when performed during EEG recording, consistent with the findings of Krieger et al. [12]. Thus, the present study is the first to demonstrate that assessment of EDS via the OSLER test is comparable to that via EEG in a Japanese population.

Although EDS is not inevitable in patients with OSA, it is nonetheless a clinically significant symptom. The ESS was developed by Johns et al. [6] for the evaluation of subjective sleepiness in soporific circumstances of daily life. Based on the findings of a previous study, which demonstrated that the ESS exhibits higher sensitivity and specificity for the diagnosis of narcolepsy than MSLT, a total ESS score of ≥ 11 is considered to indicate the presence of EDS [14]. While the mean ESS score of patients in the present study was 9.8 ± 5.4 (range: 3-18), six of the 17 patients had an ESS score ≥ 11. This result suggests that our study included patients without subjective EDS despite the presence of OSA, consistent with the findings of Mediano et al. [16]. As the ESS is subjective in nature, participants may provide inaccurate information regarding sleepiness and wakefulness [17]. Although we did not investigate the relative impact of under- or over-estimation in the present study, both factors may have influenced our findings.

Although objective methods for the assessment of EDS include the MSLT and MWT, AASM guidelines indicate that the MWT is more useful for determining therapeutic effects in patients with disorders associated with EDS [18]. In the present study, analysis of Bland-Altman plots revealed that 94% of SL_{OSLER} and SL_{EEG} measurements converged within a range of mean ± 2 SD. Bennett et al. [11] reported that sleep latency measured via the OSLER test correlated with that measured via the MWT. In the present study, we performed EEG recording and the OSLER test simultaneously to eliminate differences associated with performing the procedures in separate conditions. Our findings indicated that SL_{OSLER} was nearly identical to SL_{EEG}, demonstrating that the findings of Bennett et al. are applicable to Japanese patients as well.

Sangal et al. [10] performed Spearman's correlation analysis of sleepiness as assessed using the ESS and MWT in patients with OSA, reporting a weak correlation between the two techniques. Although comparison between SL_{EEG} and SL_{OSLER} in the present study revealed that sleep latency tended to decrease as ESS score increased, no statistically significant correlations were observed. Taken together, the findings of these studies suggest that the subjective results of the ESS are not as reliable as the objective results of the MWT or OSLER test.

Plante et al. [19] further reported that odds ratios for depression were higher in patients with high ESS scores, in contrast to findings obtained for MSLT scores, suggesting that subjective scale scores may be affected by events other than sleepiness. Moreover, Leclerc et al. [20] reported that pre-intervention ESS scores were significantly lower when measured prior to therapeutic interventions for OSA syndrome than when measured via recall following CPAP therapy. These findings suggest that, when OSA remains untreated for a long period of time, the ESS may underestimate EDS. Thus, it is likely that these subjective factors contributed to the lack of correlation between ESS scores and sleep latency in the present study.

In the present study, Bland-Altman plots were used to analyse SL_{EEG} and SL_{OSLER}. Although 94% of the plotted measurements converged within a range of mean ± 2 SD (1.96 SD), some patients exhibited longer SL_{OSLER} than SL_{EEG}. During EEG evaluation for the MSLT and MWT, sleep onset is determined by the appearance of sleep EEG patterns lasting for ≥ 50% of a 30-second epoch. In contrast, sleep EEG patterns must be observed for at least 21 seconds during the OSLER test, as sleep onset is determined when the examinee fails to correctly perform the switching task seven times in a row. Thus, when sleep EEG patterns appear for a total of ≥ 15 seconds in an EEG epoch, instead of 21 seconds, the examinee is determined to have fallen asleep, though he or she may continue to perform the OSLER task, which may explain the longer SL_{OSLER} than SL_{EEG} duration for some patients in the present study (3/68 sessions; 4.4%). Moreover, EEG may be unable to determine sleep onset when sleep EEG patterns appear for ≥ 21 seconds over two epochs but total <15 seconds in each epoch, resulting in a shorter SL_{OSLER} than SL_{EEG}. In addition, Priest et al. [21] examined the number of OSLER test failures and micro sleep patterns on EEG, reporting some cases with <7 failures in OSLER test despite sleep patterns lasting ≥ 15 to ≤ 23 seconds on EEG. These authors reported a sensitivity of 85% and specificity of 94% for the detection of micro sleep using the OSLER test.

The discrepancy between SL_{OSLER} and SL_{EEG} may also be attributable to variations in the manner in which examinees perform the task. For example, if an examinee moves only the tip of the thumb and keeps a part of it attached to the switch during the OSLER test, a failure may be recorded. Such failures can be avoided to some extent through careful monitoring by laboratory technicians.

In the present study, Bland-Altman analysis revealed that 94% of the plotted measurements converged within a range of mean ± 2 SD, indicating that SL_{OSLER} and SL_{EEG} were sufficiently consistent. When the presence of sleepiness was determined using an SL_{OSLER} cut-off of <20 minutes, the sensitivity and specificity were 1.0, suggesting that sleep latency measurements were comparable between the OSERL test and EEG recording.

The present study has some limitations. First, it is possible that the OSLER task itself may be a stimulus for wakefulness on EEG. Thus, it is difficult to strictly compare the test results with those of the MWT, during which no tasks are assigned. However, Krieger et al. [12] reported that the duration of sustained wakefulness measured by the OSLER test (referred to as SL_{OSLER} in the present study) was significantly correlated with the duration measured by simultaneously performed EEG recording (referred to as SL_{EEG} in the present study), as well as the duration measured by standard MWT performed on a separate day. Second, the sample size of the present study was relatively small (n=17). Future studies should evaluate the usefulness of the OSLER test using larger sample sizes in patients with various clinical presentations.

Conclusion

The findings of the present study demonstrated that SL_{OSLER} is consistent with SL_{EEG} in Japanese patients with OSA. Moreover, because a significant positive correlation was observed between SL_{OSLER} and SL_{EEG}, SL_{OSLER} may also be correlated with sleep latency measured by MWT. In order to determine whether the OSLER test is an appropriate substitute for the MWT, future studies should analyse the association between the duration of sustained wakefulness determined by each test. Overall, our findings indicate that the OSLER test may represent a simple method for the objective assessment of EDS and duration of sustained wakefulness on EEG.

Acknowledgment and Disclosures

Conflicts of interest

Financial support for the present study was provided by a grant from the Project for Development of Innovative Medical Devices. No other financial support was received. The authors declare no conflicts of interest that may have influenced the results of the study or their interpretation.

Author contributions

Keisuke Hosokawa had full access to all of the data in the study and takes responsibility for the integrity of the data and the accuracy of the data analysis. Keisuke Hosokawa, Tetsuya Kizawa, and Tsuguo Nishijima prepared the application to the ethics committee and performed data management. Tsuguo Nishijima contributed to the study design and revision of the manuscript, and Shigeru Sakurai contributed to the study concept and design, acquisition of funding, study supervision, and writing of the manuscript.

References

1. Goncalves MA, Paiva T, Ramos E, Guilleminault C (2004) Obstructive sleep apnea syndrome, sleepiness, and quality of life. Chest 125: 2091-2096.
2. Douglas NJ, Polo O (1994) Pathogenesis of obstructive sleep apnoea/hypopnoea syndrome. Lancet 344: 653-655.
3. Ward KL, Hillman DR, James A, Bremner AP, Simpson L, et al. (2013) Excessive daytime sleepiness increases the risk of motor vehicle crash in obstructive sleep apnea. J Clin Sleep Med 9: 1013-1021.
4. Sagaspe P, Taillard J, Chaumet G, Guilleminault C, Coste O, et al. (2007) Maintenance of wakefulness test as a predictor of driving performance in patients with untreated obstructive sleep apnea. Sleep 30: 327-330.
5. Karimi M, Hedner J, Häbel H, Grote L (2015) Sleep apnea-related risk of motor vehicle accidents is reduced by continuous positive airway pressure: Swedish Traffic Accident Registry data. Sleep 38: 341-349.
6. Johns MW (1991) A new method for measuring daytime sleepiness: The Epworth sleepiness scale. Sleep 540-545.
7. Hoddes E, Zarcone V, Smythe H, Phillips R, Dement WC (1973) Quantification of sleepiness: A new approach. Psychophysiology 10: 431-436.
8. Carskadon MA, Dement WC, Mitler MM, Roth T, Westbrook PR, et al. (1986) Guidelines for the multiple sleep latency test (MSLT): A standard measure of sleepiness. Sleep 9: 519-524.
9. Doghramji K, Mitler MM, Sangal RB, Shapiro C, Taylor S, et al. (1997) A normative study of the maintenance of wakefulness test (MWT). Electroencephalogr Clin Neurophysiol. 103: 554-562.
10. Sangal RB, Sangal JM, Belisle C (1999) Subjective and objective indices of sleepiness (ESS and MWT) are not equally useful in patients with sleep apnea. Clin Electro encephalo gr 30: 73-75.
11. Bennett LS, Stradling JR, Davies RJ (1997) A behavioural test to assess daytime sleepiness in obstructive sleep apnoea. J Sleep Res 6: 142-145.
12. Krieger AC, Ayappa I, Norman RG, Rapoport DM, Walsleben J (2004) Comparison of the maintenance of wakefulness test (MWT) to a modified behavioral test (OSLER) in the evaluation of daytime sleepiness. J Sleep Re 13: 407-411.
13. Alakuijala A, Maasilta P, Bachour A (2014) The oxford sleep resistance test (OSLER) and the multiple unprepared reaction time test (MURT) detect vigilance modifications in sleep apnea patients. J Clin Sleep Med 10: 1075-1082.
14. Johns MW (2000) Sensitivity and specificity of the multiple sleep latency test (MSLT), the maintenance of wakefulness test and the epworth sleepiness scale: failure of the MSLT as a gold standard. J Sleep Re 9: 5-11.
15. Berry RB, Brooks R, Gamald CE, Harding SM, Marcus CL, et al. (2014) The AASM Manual for the Scoring of Sleep and Associated events: Rules, Terminology and Technical Specification, Version 2.03.
16. Mediano O, Barceló A, de la Peña M, Gozal D, Agustí A, et al. (2007) Daytime sleepiness and polysomnographic variables in sleep apnoea patients. Eur Respir J 30: 110-113.
17. Arand D, Bonnet M, Hurwitz T, Mitler M, Rosa R, et al. (2005) The clinical use of the MSLT and MWT. Sleep 28: 123-144.
18. Littner MR, Kushida C, Wise M, Davila DG, Morgenthaler T, et al. (2005) Practice parameters for clinical use of the multiple sleep latency test and the maintenance of wakefulness test. Standards of Practice Committee of the American Academy of Sleep Medicine. Sleep 28: 113-121.
19. Plante DT, Finn LA, Hagen EW, Mignot E, Peppard PE (2016) Subjective and objective measures of hypersomnolence demonstrate divergent associations with depression among participants in the Wisconsin sleep cohort study. J Clin Sleep Med 12: 571-678.
20. Leclerc G, Lacasse Y, Page D, Sériès F (2014) Do obstructive sleep apnea syndrome patients underestimate their daytime symptoms before continuous positive airway pressure treatment? Can Respir J 21: 216-220.
21. Priest B, Brichard C, Aubert G, Liistro G, Rodenstein DO (2001) Microsleep during a simplified maintenance of wakefulness test. A validation study of the OSLER test. Am J Respir Crit Care Med 163: 1619-1625.

3

Computed Tomographic Evaluation of Degenerative Spine Changes in Patients with Obstructive Sleep Apnea Syndrome

Tulay Ozer[1*], **Gokhan Duygulu**[1], **Rabia Terzi**[2] **and Zahide Yilmaz**[3]

[1]*Kocaeli Derince Education and Research Hospital, Clinic of Radiology, Turkey*

[2]*Kocaeli Derince Education and Research Hospital, Clinic of Physical Medicine and Rehabilitation, Turkey*

[3]*Kocaeli Derince Education and Research Hospital, Clinic of Neurology, Turkey*

[*]**Corresponding author:** Tulay Ozer, Kocaeli Derince Education and Research Hospital, Clinic of Radiology, Turkey, E-mail: ozertulay@yahoo.com

Abstract

Objective: Recently few studies have described presence of cervical spine anomalies in obstructive sleep apnoea syndrome (OSAS) patients. It is also reported that some cases of cervical spine pathologies and osteophytes producing obstructive sleep apnea. We aim to investigate the prevalence of facet joint arthrosis and degenerative disc disease (DDD) in cervical spine using computed tomography (CT) in OSAS patients.

Materials and Methods: We studied on thirty patients with OSAS who had cervical spine CT. Facet joints were evaluated in four grades and scored in 1-4 points by using multiplanar CT images. Disc levels was evaluated by using two-point subjective scale for loss of height, posterior osteophytes, endplate sclerosis, and spinal canal stenosis to determinate DDD. Degeneration of anterior atlanto-odontoid joint (AAOJ) were classified into four grades. Tomographic findings were compared with those for thirty control subjects.

Results: The mean degeneration scores of C2-T1 facet joints and C2-C5, C7-T1 disc spaces were significantly higher in the cases of OSAS group than the cases of the control group. There were no significant differences in the mean degeneration scores for C5-6 and C6-7 cervical intervertebral disc levels between the groups. Degeneration scores of the facet and disc for whole cervical spine in the cases of the OSAS group was significantly higher than in cases of the control group ($P<0.001$ and $P=0.002$). AAOJ degeneration degrees showed differences between the groups. Statistically significant correlations were found between the OSAS degrees and the intervertebral disc degeneration ($R=0.338$, $P=0.007$) and facet joint degeneration ($R=0.543$, $P=0.000$) for all cervical vertebrae.

Conclusions: The cervical spine of the OSAS patients has more severe disc degeneration and facet joint and AAOJ arthrosis, compared to subjects without OSAS. This findings may contribute to clinic evaluation of OSAS patients with servical pain and limited movement.

Keywords: Cervical spine; Intervertebral disc degeneration; Facet joint; Multidetector computed tomography; Sleep apnea; Obstructive

Introduction

Obstructive sleep apnea syndrome (OSAS) is a variety of sleep-disordered breathing characterized by repetitive episodes of upper airway obstruction during sleep. These episodes are associated with recurrent oxyhemoglobin desaturations, and they give rise to intermittent hypoxemia, hypercapnia, acidosis, sympathetic nervous system activation and arousals from sleep [1]. It has been shown that the frequency of repeated apnea episodes is correlated with the cardiovascular and cerebrovascular complications in patients with OSAS [1-4]. The pathophysiology of the disease has not been fully identified yet. However, obesity and upper airway tissue abnormalities decreasing width of the upper respiratory tract may increase the predisposition to OSAS [5,6]. It has been described some craniofacial abnormalities such as thicker soft palate, bigger neck circumference, more inferior localization of the hyoid bone, large cranio-cervical angle and more extended head posture in OSAS patients [1,3,6,7]. Recently, presence of cervical spine anomalies including posterior arch deficiency and fusion anomalies in OSAS patients have been reported in some studies [8-10]. Additionally, it has been observed that OSAS patients with block fusion in the cervical vertebrae differ significantly in craniofacial profiles (such as larger anterior face height, greater mandibular length) from the other OSAS patients [9]. It is also reviewed that some cases of cervical osteophyte may predispose patients to OSAS [11]. On the other hand, to our knowledge, there is no information about the frequency and distribution of cervical spine degeneration in OSAS patients. Therefore, the aims of the present study were to investigate the prevalence of facet joint arthrosis and degenerative disc disease in cervical spine using multidetector computed tomography (CT) in adult patients with OSAS and to compare those of the cervical spine in a group of adult subjects with no history of OSAS.

Material and Methods

This study protocol was approved by our institutional ethics committee (registration number: KOÜ KAEK 2015/60). We performed a retrospective study of adult OSAS patients who had apnea/ hypopnea index (AHI) ≥ 5 per h according to overnight polysomnography in sleep center of our hospital, Kocaeli (Turkey).

After providing their informed consent, subjects with OSAS underwent overnight polysomnographic recording (Embla N 7000). The polysomnography included electroencephalogram, electrooculogram, chin and leg electromyography, electrocardiography, snoring, oronasal thermistor, nasal pressure transducer, finger pulse oximeter, thoracic and abdominal respiratory movements, and body position. Apnea was defined as ≥ 90% decrease from baseline in the oronasal thermistor signal amplitude for at least 10 seconds, and hypopnea was defined as ≥ 50% decrease from baseline in the nasal cannula signal amplitude at least for 10 seconds. The apnea/hypopnea index (AHI) was defined as the number of occurrences of apnea/hypopneas per hour (/h) during sleep. Patients with AHI of 5-15 per h was considered mild, AHI of 15-30 per h was considered moderate, and AHI ≥ 30 per h was considered severe OSAS.

The controls were diagnosed as non-OSA subjects based on clinical criteria, which means they did not present a medical history of snoring or sleep apnea symptoms. The control subjects also did not have any sleep testing or complete questionnaires regarding sleepiness.

Both of the groups were selected from patients who underwent cervical CT because of neck pain without neurologic deficits. Subjects with congenital spinal disease, scoliosis, inflammatory arthropathy, history of trauma or fracture or spinal surgery, severe obesity (BMI>30), severe diabetes mellitus, and history of metabolic disease were excluded from both OSAS and control groups. All cervical spine images were taken with a 16-multidetector computed tomography device (Activion 16; Toshiba Medical Systems). All of the OSAS patients and control subjects were in the supine position. Continuous axial sections with 2 mm thickness were obtained from the base of the cranium to the first thoracic vertebrae (T1) level. Coronal and sagittal reformatted images were created by using bone algorithm. Images were evaluated by two radiologists to assess interobserver reliability. The second radiologist had no prior knowledge about patients' clinical information. All the images were examined in three categories in terms of cervical spine degenerative changes. 1) Degenerative arthrosis of bilateral facet joints between the C1-T1 vertebrae; 2) findings of degenerative disc disease in C2-T1 intervertebral disc spaces; and 3) degeneration findings in anterior atlanto-odontoid joint (AAOJ).

Facet joints were evaluated in four categories according to the grading system which was suggested by Park et al. [12]: Grade I, normal; Grade II, degenerative changes including joint space narrowing, cyst formation, small osteophytes without joint hypertrophy; Grade III, joint hypertrophy secondary to large osteophytes without fusion; Grade IV, bony fusion of the joint. Then, the facet joints in each intervertebral level was scored with the following scoring system: grade I: 1 point, grade II: 2 points, grade III: 3 points, grade IV: 4 points. When each facet joint in the same disc level had different degeneration grades, the grade value, which showed the higher degeneration of facet joint, was taken into consideration for disc level. Facet joint degeneration score for whole cervical spine was created by adding the facet degeneration scores at seven intervertebral disc levels (C1-C2, C2-3, C3-4, C4-5, C5-6, C6-7, and C7-T1).

To evaluate degenerative disc disease, we used a scoring system described by Walraevens et al. [13] on lateral cervical graphies with a simplified version of its. On sagittal CT images, each intervertebral disc space (C2-3, C3-4, C4-5, C5-6, C6-7, and C7-T1) was evaluated for a 'loss of height', 'posterior osteophytes', 'endplate sclerosis', and 'spinal canal stenosis due to posterior osteophytes' (anterio-posterior diameter of the spinal canal was <12 mm in the midsagittal images) by using a two-point subjective scale (0 point: absent; 1 point: present). At last, each intervertebral disc had degeneration score ranging between 0 and 4. Total score of degenerative disc disease for whole cervical spine was created by adding the disc degeneration scores at six intervertebral disc levels (C2-3, C3-4, C4-5, C5-6, C6-7, and C7-T1).

The degeneration of the AAOJ were evaluated according to Lakshmanan et al. [14] by using axial and sagittal CT images. The degenerative changes were graded as: none (Grade 0), normal joint space with no osteophyte formation; mild (Grade 1), narrowed joint space or normal joint space with osteophyte formation; moderate (Grade 2), obliterated joint space with or without osteophyte formation; and severe (Grade 3), ankyloses of the joint with excrescences either in the joint or transverse ligament calcification, or both.

SPSS v.20.0 statistical software was used for statistical analysis (IBM; Chicago). The level of statistical significance was $P<0.05$. The Mann - Whitney U -test and Pearson's chi-square test were used to analyze the variables. Pearson's r correlation coefficients were used to investigate the linear correlation between OSAS degrees and facet joint degenerations, and between OSAS degrees and cervical disc degenerations. The effect of gender on severity of disc degeneration was assessed by univariate analysis, adjusting for men and women. Kappa statistics were used to compare interobserver reliability. Kappa values<0 were interpreted as poor agreement, between 0.0-0.20 as slight agreement, between 0.21-0.40 as fair agreement, between 0.41-0.60 as moderate agreement, between 0.61-0.80 as substantial agreement, and between 0.81-1.00 as almost perfect agreement.

Results

A total of 30 patients (18 male and 12 female) with fulfilling the criteria for OSAS and 30 control subjects (14 male and 16 female) were included in the study (P=0.12). There were more women in the control group and gender was not a statistically important demographic factor associated with disc degeneration. The mean age was 52.43 years ± 11.55 years (34 years - 77 years, median: 52) in OSAS group, and 57.13 years ± 11.27 years (34 years - 73 years, median: 57) in control subjects (P=0.72). The mean BMI was not statistically different between the groups (P=0.46) (Table 1). As we not studied in obese patients (BMI>30), our findings may not be applicable to patients with high BMI. According to AHI scores, nine patients had mild, four patients had moderate and seventeen patients had severe OSAS.

Variable	OSAS (Mean ± S.D; n = 30)	Group C (Mean ± S.D; n = 30)	P value
Age (years)	52.43 ± 11.55	57.13 ± 11.27	0.72
BMI (m/kg^2)	22.33 ± 3.91	21.57 ± 4.15	0.46
Gender	18 M, 12 F	14 M, 16 F	0.12
M: male, F: female, Group C: control subjects			

Table 1: Parameters of OSAS and control group.

The numbers of facet joints with degeneration grades at the seven cervical intervertebral levels which are consisting of OSAS and control cases are shown in Table 2. We evaluated totally 210 bilateral facet joints of seven intervertebral levels in thirty subjects of each group (Figures 1 and 2). The mean degeneration scores of facet joints at C2-3, C3-4, C4-5, C5-6, C6-7, C7-T1 cervical intervertebral disc levels were significantly higher in the cases of OSAS group than in the cases of the control group (P=0.000, P=0.050, P=0.001, P=0.000, P=0.000, P=0.000, respectively). There was no significant difference between the groups in terms of the mean degeneration scores of the facet joints at C1-2 intervertebral disc levels (P=0.078). The total score of facet degeneration in all cervical vertebrae was significantly higher in the OSAS group, compared to the control group (P=0.000) (Table 3).

	OSAS	Group C
Grade	n (%)	n (%)
I	79 (37.6)	175 (83.3)
II	78 (37.2)	24 (11.5)
III	34 (16.2)	11 (5.2)
IV	19 (9.0)	0 (0)

Group C: Control subjects

Table 2: The total number of bilateral facet joints in seven cervical intervertebral levels according to degeneration grades.

	OSAS; Mean ± S.D	Group C; Mean ± S.D	P value
C1-2	1.10 ± 0.30	1.00 ± 0.00	0.078
C2-3	1.90 ± 0.84	1.17 ± 0.46	0.000*
C3-4	1.83 ± 0.95	1.40 ± 0.72	0.050*
C4-5	2.03 ± 0.96	1.30 ± 0.65	0.001*
C5-6	2.20 ± 0.92	1.27 ± 0.58	0.000*
C6-7	2.30 ± 0.83	1.20 ± 0.48	0.000*
C7-T1	2.27 ± 0.90	1.20 ± 0.40	0.000*
Total facet joint degeneration score for whole cervical spine	13.63 ± 4.52	8.56 ± 1.85	0.000*

S.D: Standard deviation, Group C: Control subjects, P values: Between two groups by Mann-Whitney U-test, *P: Value of statistically significant

Table 3: Comparison of degeneration grading scores for cervical intervertebral facet joints and total facet joint degeneration score for whole cervical spine between OSAS and control subjects.

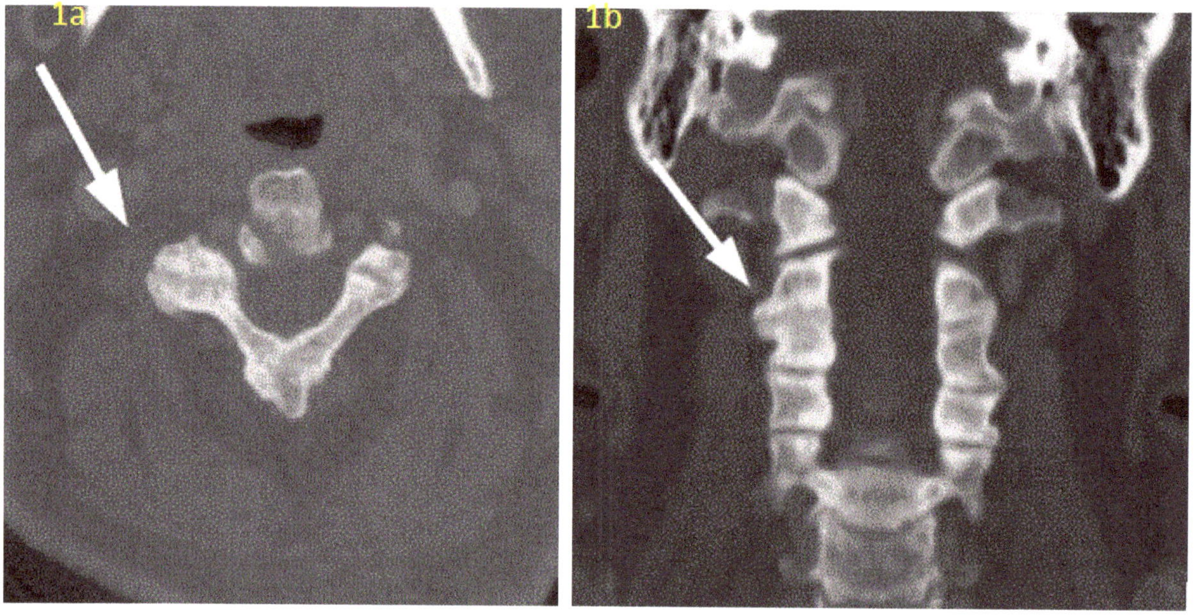

Figure 1: Axial (a) and coronal (b) CT images of cervical vertebra showing hypertrophy and obliteration of the joint space in right facet joint at C3-4 intervertebral disc level (arrow) (Grade III).

When degenerative disc disease of the cervical spine was analyzed, the mean degeneration scores for C2-3, C3-4, C4-5, C7-T1 intervertebral disc levels were significantly higher in cases of the OSAS group than in cases of the control group (P=0.023, P=0.001, P=0.049, P=0.005, respectively).

There were no significant differences in the mean degeneration scores for C5-6 and C6-7 cervical intervertebral disc levels between the groups (P=0.230, P=0.176, respectively).

On the other hand, the total mean disc degeneration score for whole cervical spine in the cases of the OSAS group was significantly higher than in cases of the control group (P=0.002). The comparison of mean scores at the C2-3, C3-4, C4-5, C5-6, C6-7 cervical intervertebral disc levels and mean total scores for whole cervical spine between the groups is shown in Table 4.

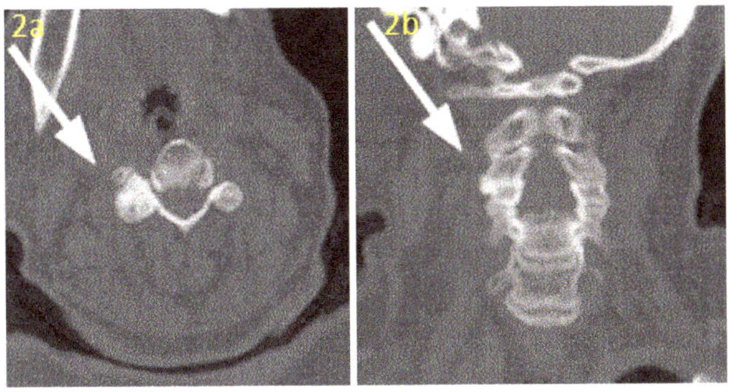

Figure 2: Axial (a) and coronal (b) CT images of cervical vertebra of a patient with severe OSAS, showing ankyloses in the right facet joint at C3-4 intervertebral disc level (arrow) (Grade IV).

	OSAS	Group C	P value
	Mean ± S.D	Mean ± S.D	
C2-3	0.63 ± 1.12	0.10 ± 0.54	0.023*
C3-4	1.67 ± 1.57	0.50 ± 0.93	0.001*
C4-5	2.23 ± 1.40	1.47 ± 1.54	0.049*
C5-6	3.00 ± 1.39	2.50 ± 1.77	0.230
C6-7	2.00 ± 1.57	1.40 ± 1.81	0.176
C7-T1	1.40 ± 1.49	0.40 ± 1.10	0.005*
Total disc degeneration score for whole cervical spine	10.93 ± 6.22	6.36 ± 4.39	0.002*

S.D: Standard deviation, Group C: Control subjects, P values: Between two groups by Mann-Whitney U test, *P: Value of statistically significant.

Table 4: Comparison of mean scores for each cervical intervertebral disc levels and total disc degeneration score for whole cervical spine between OSAS group and control subjects.

When the degeneration of AAOJ were analyzed, twenty-five cases (83.3%) had grade 1 and five cases (16.7%) had grade 2 degeneration in OSAS group (Figure 3). Neither grade 0 nor grade 3 degeneration of AAOJ was observed in OSAS group. In the control group, eleven subjects (36.7%) had grade 0, eighteen subjects (60.0%) had grade 1, one subject (3.3%) had grade 2 degeneration of AAOJ. None of the subjects in the control group had grade 3 degeneration of AAOJ. There was a significant difference in AAOJ degeneration percentages between the OSAS group and the control group (P=0.001). The comparison of AAOJ degeneration percentages between both groups is shown in Table 5.

Atlanto-odontoid joints	OSAS n (%)	Group C n (%)
Grade 0	0 (0.0)	11 (36.7)
Grade 1	25 (83.3)	18 (60.0)
Grade 2	5 (16.7)	1 (3.3)
Grade 3	0 (0.0)	0 (0.0)

Group C: control subjects, Grade 0 (None): Normal joint space with no osteophyte formation, Grade 1 (Mild): Narrowed joint space or normal joint space with osteophyte formation, Grade 2 (Moderate): Obliterated joint space with or without osteophyte formation, Grade 3 (Severe): Ankyloses of the joint with excrescences either in the joint or transverse ligament calcification, or both; Pearson's chi-square test P=0.006

Table 5: Comparison of grading of degenerative changes in AAOJ between OSAS group and control subjects.

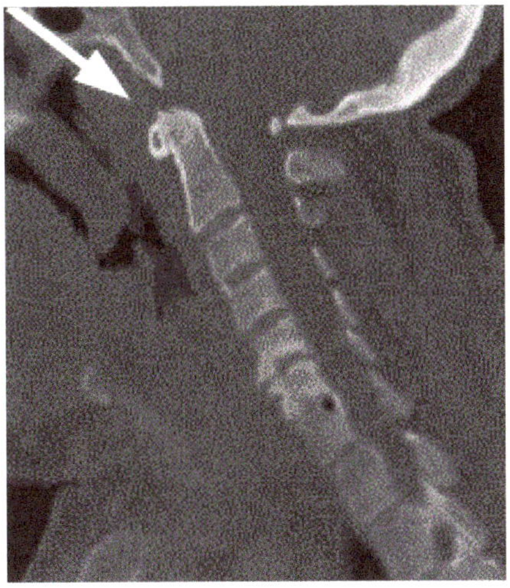

Figure 3: Obliterated view of the AAOJ space (arrow) (Grade 2). Additionally, degeneration findings at C5-6 and C6-7 intervertebral disc spaces are present.

We investigated the correlation between the degree of OSAS and intervertebral disc degeneration or facet joint degeneration values for all cervical vertebrae. Statistically significant correlations were found for the OSAS degrees with the intervertebral disc degeneration of all cervical vertebrae (R=0.338 P=0.007). Statistically significant correlations were also found for the OSAS degrees with facet joint degeneration levels of all cervical vertebrae (R=0.543, P=0.000). To evaluate the AAOJ, the kappa value for interobserver reliability test was 0.973, which corresponds to almost perfect agreement. To evaluate cervical vertebra disc degeneration and facet joint degeneration, the kappa values for interobserver reliability test were 0.827 and 0.812, respectively, which correspond to almost perfect agreement again.

Discussion

In the present study, we showed that facet joint arthrosis and intervertebral disc degeneration of the cervical spine existed in more severe grades in patients with OSAS, compared to control subjects. In addition, AAOJ degeneration was more advanced in OSAS group, compared to control subjects.

To our knowledge, there is only a few studies described the morphology of the cervical spine in patients with OSAS in the previous literature [8-10]. In these studies, the authors examined the morphological characteristics in the cervical spine into two categories: 'posterior arch deficiency' and 'fusion anomalies'. Posterior arch deficiency was consisted of partial cleft and dehiscence and fusion anomalies were consisted of fusion, block fusion, and occipitalization. Fusion is defined as fusion of one unit with another at the articulation facets, neural arch or transverse processes in that studies. The prevalence of fusion anomalies in patients with OSAS taken with standardized lateral skull radiography was found out 46% and 43% in the two studies [8,9]. They showed that the fusion anomalies occurred as fusions between C2 and C3, C3 and C4, or C4 and C5 and as block fusions between C2, C3, and C4, C2, C3, C4, and C5, or C3, C4, and C5. They also exposed that the craniofacial profile of OSAS patients with block fusions in the cervical vertebrae and fusion of two vertebrae differed significantly from the craniofacial profile of other OSAS patients [9]. Then, the researchers suggested the associations between craniofacial morphology including the cranial base and fusion of the cervical vertebral column, and they also have explained these relations with the early embryogenesis. In the early embriyogenetic period, when the notochord determinates the development of the vertebral bodies and the basilar part of the occipital bone in the cranial base, it also induces the formation of the para-axial mesoderm forming the vertebral arches. Before the notochord is surrounded by bone tissue and disappears, by means of a kind of signalling from the notochord to the neural crest, bilateral neural crest cells migrate to the craniofacial area to create the mandible, maxilla and lastly the nasofrontal region [15]. Then, in a later study, Sonnesen et al. [15] reported the incidence of fusion anomalies as 21.1% (fusion 10.5%, block fusion 8.8%, and occipitalization 1.8%) in the OSAS patients, when used cone beam CT to overcome the superposition of structures in the cervical vertebrae. In our study, we defined fusion of the facet joint as bony fusion of the joint, seen in grade IV facet degeneration on coronal and axial images. We found that the prevalence of the grade IV degeneration was 9% in OSAS patients, our result is consistent with the findings of Sonnesen et al. [10]. Moreover, we also found that the degeneration grading scores of facet joints in C2-3, C3-4, C4-5, C5-6, C6-7, C7-T1 cervical levels was higher in OSA patients, compared to control subjects. There was a positive correlation between facet joint degeneration and the degree of OSAS. Having evaluated the images, we detected more or less the classic radiographic hallmarks of facets arthrosis, including osteophyte formation and hypertrophy of the articular process, in addition to fusion in grade IV degeneration. Therefore, we suggest that fusions anomalies itselfs or its leading to biomechanical alterations can be a contributing factor for increasing in the degeneration grades for facet joints in OSAS patients.

It is well known that prevalence of cervical facet joint degeneration is associated with aging. Pathological studies on fresh frozen cervical spine specimens, as well as tomographic studies, have shown that the prevalence of cervical facet joint degeneration increases with age [12,16,17]. In the literature, the rate of facet joint degeneration for C2-C7 intervertebral levels have been reported 91.3% in Grade I, 2.9% in Grade II, 5.2% in Grade III, and 0.6% in Grade IV in normal subjects between 40-79 years old [12]. The prevalence of facet joint degeneration in our control group were consistent with values reported in the literature. Our results suggest that the aging process does not contribute significantly to the elevated the rates of facet joint degeneration in patients with OSAS.

In this study, we chose multislice CT imaging to examine degenerative changes of the cervical spine. Because reformatted CT images of the spine with bone algorithms is excellent to demonstrate degenerative changes such as reduced height of the intervertebral space, osteophytes, sclerosis of the adjacent cartilaginous endplates, facet joint arthrosis, calcifications and narrowing of the spinal canal [18,19]. Although the grading system for the cervical facet joint arthrosis on CT images were defined in the literature before, in this study we could not find a appropriate grading and scoring system for tomography to compare findings of disc degeneration in both groups. Therefore, we used a scoring system based on three criteria-i.e. disc height loss, posterior osteophytes and endplate sclerosis, which was defined by Walverens et al. [13] on lateral roentgenograms. We however created a new version of this scoring system by adding the fourth scoring criteria, 'spinal canal stenosis due to posterior osteophytes', and then applied its simplified version on the sagittal tomography images.

Cervical intervertebral disc degeneration initially starts in the nucleus pulposus. Once, nucleus pulposus undergoes progressive dehydration with resulting loss of height of the disc space, disc becomes brittle and fibrotic and is unable to provide the necessary elasticity for the maximum loadcarrying capacity, and then apophyseal joints start to grow osteophytes [20]. Osteophytic projections rarely can cause compression of the pharynx, esophagus or upper airway [11]. Some cases with anterior osteophytes have reported that causing obstruction in the retropharyngeal area and lead to sleep disorders [21,22]. On the other hand, airway obstruction due to pressure by large osteophytes and dysphagia has been reported in a few patients with diffuse idiopathic skeletal hyperostosis, who were previously diagnosed with OSAS [23]. In our study, we did not determine too large osteophytes to narrow or pressure on airway in the images of the all subjects. However, degeneration scores at the C2-3, C3-4, C4-5 and C7-T1 intervertebral disc levels and total degeneration score of whole cervical spine were significantly higher in patients with OSAS, compared to the control group. Additionally, there was a positive correlation between disc degeneration grades and severity of OSAS grades. On the other hand, we did not observe statiscally difference for the scores of degeneration at C5-6 and C6-7 cervical intervertebral disc levels between two groups. Previous studies have represented that C5-6 intervertebral disc space has the highest prevalence of disc degeneration and the C6-7 disc space has the second highest prevalence in the cervical spine in a population aged between 21 and 97 years old [24]. These findings of the present study indicated that different mechanisms can have effects on the increase of degenerative changes in upper and lower intervertebral disc levels except the degenerative effects due to aging in OSAS patients. As it is known during sleep, repetitive episodes of airway occlusion, with consequent hypoxemia and hypercapnia and dramatic changes in intrathoracic pressure, elicit a wide variety of autonomic, hemodynamic, humoral, and neuroendocrine responses patients with OSAS [25]. Accordingly, we can suppose that the increase in facet joint degeneration gives rise to abnormal loading to intervertebral disc spaces, or changes in metabolic status in OSAS patient may play a role in increased cervical disc degeneration scores in the OSAS group. Interestingly, the electrophysiological studies of OSAS patients using motor evoked potentials by Transcranial Magnetic Stimulation (TMS) have found a global hypoexcitability of the stimulated motor cortex and a decrease in cortico-spinal conductivity [26,27]. Lanza et al. [27] offered TMS can be considered an additional tool for the understanding of clinical and pathophysiological aspects of sleep disorders, and possibly for the evaluation of the effect of therapy. As the descending motor pathways run primarily in the lateral columns of the spinal cord, coexistence of cervical disc degeneration and decrease in motor evoked potentials in OSAS patients, requires an understanding to differentiate clinically important signal changes.

Our findings showed considerably amounts of Grade 0 (0%), 1 (83.3%) and Grade 2 (16.7%) AAOJ degeneration in patients with OSAS whereas 36.7%, 60% and 3.3% consecutive Grade 0, 1 and 2 degenerative changes determined in control subjects. This article demonstrated that the prevelance of AAOJ degeneration was significantly higher in OSAS group. Previous studies have shown that degenerative changes of AAOJ may contribute to pain and limitation in motion [14,28]. Furthermore, besides the growing effect of age on degeneration, degeneration of the AAOJ may have an effect on potentiating injury in OSAS.

There are some limitations of our study. First, the community evaluated in present study consisted of patients who sustained a neck pain that required a cervical spine CT. This population does not necessarily reflect a general OSAS population and could bias our findings. However, the subjects of the control group also have a neck pain. Since we must take into account the radiation dose for the subjects with minimum level, we designed this study retrospectively. Prospective studies may be investigated for evaluation of the early degenerative changes and spinal cord lesion in randomly selected subjects from OSAS patients using magnetic resonance imaging. Second, the control subjects did not undergo polysomnography. According to their retrospective clinical histories, these subjects did not report sleep disorders.

In conclusion, this study indicates that patients with OSAS have higher degeneration of cervical spine in terms of degeneration in disc spaces, AAOJ and facet joints when compared to normal subjects. To our knowledge, this is the first study to document degenerative changes of cervical spine of OSAS patients.

We would like to emphasize that the presence of cervical vertebrae degeneration has to be considered when evaluating the clinical findings of patients with OSAS. We also think that the symptoms of disc and facet joint degeneration should be investigated prospectively in larger populations of patients with OSAS.

References

1. Prisant LM, Dillard TA, Blanchard AR (2006) Obstructive sleep apnea syndrome. J Clin Hypertens 8: 746-750.
2. Young T, Palta M, Dempsey J, Skatrud J, Weber S, et al. (1993) The occurrence of sleep-disordered breathing among middle-aged adults. N Engl J Med 328: 1230-1235.
3. Bonsignore MR, Marrone O, Insalaco G, Bonsignore G (1994) The cardiovascular effects of obstructive sleep apnoeas: analysis of pathogenic mechanisms. Eur Respir J 7: 786-805.
4. Altin R, Ozdemir H, MahmutyazicioÄŸlu K, Kart L, Uzun L, et al. (2005) Evaluation of carotid artery wall thickness with high-resolution sonography in obstructive sleep apnea syndrome. J Clin Ultrasound 33: 80-86.
5. Bonsignore MR, McNicholas WT, Montserrat JM, Eckel J (2012) Adipose tissue in obesity and obstructive sleep apnoea. Eur Respir J 39: 746-767.
6. Yucel A, Unlu M, Haktanir A, Acar M, Fidan F (2005) Evaluation of the upper airway cross-sectional area changes in different degrees of severity of obstructive sleep apnea syndrome: cephalometric and dynamic CT study. AJNR Am J Neuroradiol 26: 2624-2629.
7. Solow B, Skov S, Ovesen J, Norup PW, Wildschiødtz G (1996) Airway dimensions and head posture in obstructive sleep apnoea. Eur J Orthod 18: 571-579.
8. Sonnesen L, Petri N, Kjaer I, Svanholt P (2008) Cervical column morphology in adult patients with obstructive sleep apnoea. Eur J Orthod 30: 521-526.
9. Svanholt P, Petri N, Wildschiødtz G, Sonnesen L, Kjaer I (2009) Associations between craniofacial morphology, head posture, and cervical vertebral body fusions in men with sleep apnea. Am J Orthod Dentofacial Orthop 135: 702.
10. Sonnesen L, Jensen KE, Petersson AR, Petri N, Berg S, et al. (2013) Cervical vertebral column morphology in patients with obstructive sleep apnoea assessed using lateral cephalograms and cone beam CT. A comparative study. Dentomaxillofac Radiol 42: 20130060.
11. Khan A, Than KD, Chen KS, Wang AC, La Marca F, et al. (2014) Sleep apnea and cervical spine pathology. Eur Spine J 23: 641-647.
12. Park MS, Lee YB, Moon SH, Lee HM, Kim TH, et al. (2014) Facet joint degeneration of the cervical spine: a computed tomographic analysis of 320 patients. Spine 39: 713-718.
13. Walraevens J, Liu B, Meersschaert J, Demaerel P, Delye H, et al. (2009) Qualitative and quantitative assessment of degeneration of cervical intervertebral discs and facet joints. Eur Spine J 18: 358-369.
14. Lakshmanan P, Jones A, Howes J, Lyons K (2005) CT evaluation of the pattern of odontoid fractures in the elderly--relationship to upper cervical spine osteoarthritis. Eur Spine J 14: 78-83.
15. Sonnesen L (2010) Associations between the cervical vertebral column and craniofacial morphology. Int J Dent 2010: 295728.
16. Gellhorn AC, Katz JN, Suri P (2013) Osteoarthritis of the spine: the facet joints. Nat Rev Rheumatol 9: 216-224.
17. Kettler A, Werner K, Wilke HJ (2007) Morphological changes of cervical facet joints in elderly individuals. Eur Spine J 16: 987-992.
18. Siemund R, Thurnher M, Sundgren PC (2015) How to image patients with spine pain. Eur J Radiol 84: 757-764.
19. Xu C, Ding ZH, Xu YK (2014) Comparison of computed tomography and magnetic resonance imaging in the evaluation of facet tropism and facet arthrosis in degenerative cervical spondylolisthesis. Genet Mol Res 13: 4102-4109.
20. Cs-Szabo G, Ragasa-San Juan D, Turumella V, Masuda K, Thonar EJ, et al. (2002) Changes in mRNA and protein levels of proteoglycans of the anulus fibrosus and nucleus pulposus during intervertebral disc degeneration. Spine (Phila Pa 1976) 27: 2212-2219.
21. Eyigor H, Selcuk OT, Osma U, Koca R, Yilmaz MD (2012) Cervical osteophytes: a rare cause of obstructive sleep apnea. J Craniofac Surg 23: e444-e446.
22. Ando E, Ogawa T, Shigeta Y, Hirai S, Ikawa T, et al. (2009) A case of obstructive sleep apnoea with anterior cervical osteophytes. J Oral Rehabil 36: 776-780.
23. Fuerderer S, Eysel-Gosepath K, Schröder U, Delank KS, Eysel P (2004) Retro-pharyngeal obstruction in association with osteophytes of the cervical spine. J Bone Joint Surg Br 86: 837-840.
24. Teraguchi M, Yoshimura N, Hashizume H, Muraki S, Yamada H, et al. (2014) Prevalence and distribution of intervertebral disc degeneration over the entire spine in a population-based cohort: the Wakayama Spine Study. Osteoarth Cart 22: 104-110.
25. Lanfranchi P, Somers VK (2001) Obstructive sleep apnea and vascular disease. Respir Res 2: 315-319.
26. Lanza G, Cantone M, Lanuzza B, Pennisi M, Bella R, et al. (2015) Distinctive patterns of cortical excitability to transcranial magnetic stimulation in obstructive sleep apnea syndrome, restless legs syndrome, insomnia, and sleep deprivation. Sleep Med Rev 19: 39-50.
27. Lanza G, Lanuzza B, Aricò D, Cantone M, Cosentino FI, et al. (2015) Direct comparison of cortical excitability to transcranial magnetic stimulation in obstructive sleep apnea syndrome and restless legs syndrome. Sleep Med 16: 138-142.
28. Betsch MW, Blizzard SR, Shinseki MS, Yoo JU (2015) Prevalence of degenerative changes of the atlanto-axial joints. Spine J 15: 275-280.

Day Care Office Procedures for Management of Simple Palatal Snoring

Zafarullah Beigh[1,*], Raja Salman Khursheed[2], Omar Mohammad Shafi[1] and Rafiq Ahmad Pampori[1,3]

[1]*Department of Otorhinolaryngology, Government Medical College, Srinagar, India*

[2]*Department of Otorhinolaryngology, Zain and Alsabah Hospital, Kuwait*

[3]*Government Medical College, Srinagar, India*

***Corresponding author:** Dr. Zafarullah Beigh MBBS, MS, 90 feet road Bachapora Srinagar, Jammu and Kashmir-190001, India, E-mail: beighzafarullah@yahoo.com

Abstract

Introduction: Snoring is the production of sound by the upper aero digestive tract during sleep. Snoring is commonly regarded as a laughable circumstance or a source of irritation to the observer, about which little can be done but to awaken the unwitting culprit habitual loud snoring may be socially unacceptable, and may constitute a reason for sleeping apart, marital disharmony, divorce, aggression and homicide. There are various treatments for snoring, both medical and surgical depending upon severity of snoring and site of snoring sound production. Aim of this study was to compare three surgical treatments for palatal snoring done under local anesthesia, sling Snorplasty, modified sling snorplasty and injection snorplasty.

Material and method: This study was conducted in the department of Otorhinolaryngology Head and Neck Surgery, Government Medical College Srinagar and includes 48 patients who presented in our OPD with complaints of snoring or are referred from some other specialty or institution for the complaints of snoring. After thorough history and examination, all patients were evaluated with Mullers maneuver, overnight polysomnography and intensity of snoring sound measured with the help of sound level meter. All patients with Mullers maneuver documented soft palatal obstruction and PSG documented simple snoring were randomly distributed using random number table into three different treatment groups, Sling Snorplasty, modified Sling Snorplasty and injection Snorplasty.

Results: This study showed that there were Statistically significant ($P<0.05$) improvement in percentage of snoring and intensity of snoring after 3 weeks, 3 months and 6 months of treatment in sling snorplasty and modified sling snorplasty treatment groups. Patients in injection snorplasty treatment group showed improvement in percentage of snoring and intensity of snoring after 3 weeks of treatment but that improvement was not statistically significant ($P>0.05$) and no improvement was seen after 3 months and 6 months of treatment.

Conclusion: The present study suggested that modified sling snorplasty and sling snorplasty are day care procedures of choice for treatment of simple palatal snoring and should be offered to all patients with simple palatal snoring.

Keywords: Snoring; Mullers maneuver; Snorplasty

Introduction

According to the American Heritage Dictionary of the English Language it snoring is "to breathe during sleep with harsh, snorting noises caused by vibration of the soft palate" [1]. Naturally occurring or drug-induced sleep is a requirement for its appearance. Snoring is a breathing noise that appears during the inspiratory and sometimes also the expiratory phase of the respiratory cycle [2]. The source of the sound is the pharyngeal segment of the upper airway. Relative atonia of the upper airway dilator muscles during sleep induces narrowing and increased resistance at this level [3]. As a consequence, airflow becomes turbulent and the pharyngeal tissues vibrate as the air passes through. More specifically, snoring is characterized by oscillations of the soft palate, pharyngeal walls, epiglottis and tongue [4,5].

Snoring is commonly associated with abnormalities of the soft palate or uvula. An overly long or floppy soft palate may vibrate irregularly with airflow. This abnormal vibration makes a sound snoring. It may be that simple snoring does not exist because when the sleep of a bed partner is disturbed snoring constitutes a social nuisance [6]. The sleep disturbance to a bed partner has been linked to chronic insomnia and its consequences. Previous research also suggests that snoring constitutes excessive bedroom noise exposure and may cause hearing problems [7].

It is known to be an important clinical hallmark of Obstructive Sleep apnea (OSA) [8] and, as such, may be a useful and an easily accessible marker to screen for obstructive sleep disordered breathing (SDB).

Materials and Methods

This study was conducted in the department of Otorhinolaryngology Head and Neck Surgery, Government Medical College Srinagar and includes 48 patients who presented in our OPD themselves with complaints of snoring or are referred from some other specialty or Institution. After thorough history and examination all patients were evaluated with mullers maneuver, overnight polysomnography and intensity of snoring sound measured with the help of sound level meter.

The Muller's Maneuver was performed with the patient in the sitting position after topical nasal anesthesia was achieved with 4% lidocaine and 0.5% ephedrine spray. A flexible nasopharyngoscope was inserted through the anesthetized nasal cavity to the lower oropharynx. Collapse of the lateral pharyngeal walls (LPWs) and the base of tongue (BOT) were assessed during a maximal inspiratory effort against a closed mouth and sealed nose ("reverse Valsalva"). The nasopharyngoscope was withdrawn to a level just cephalad to Passavant's ridge. Collapse of the soft palate (PAL) was assessed, again during a maximal inspiratory effort against a closed mouth and sealed nose.

Full night sleep study (PSG) that included the determination of sleep stages (electroencephalogram), nasal airflow with nasal thermisters. SpO_2, with a pulse oximeter and thoracoabdominal movements by respiratory inductive plethysmography calibrated by the isovolume method. Snoring percentage during sleep was calculated in addition to number of apnea and hypopnea episodes during sleep. During PSG Net Intensity of snoring sound was measured with the help of sound level meter. Net snoring intensity was calculated by subtracting intensity of background sound in sleep lab room when patient was not present from intensity of snoring sound with patient snoring in sleep lab room.

All patients with mullers maneuver documented soft palatal obstruction and PSG documented simple snoring were randomly distributed using random number table into three different treatment groups, Sling Snorplasty, modified Sling Snorplasty and injection Snorplasty.

Results

Results of treatment were documented on the basis of PSG findings and intensity of snoring sound measurement done after 3 weeks, 3 months and 6 months of treatment (Tables 1-4).

Age (year)	N	%age
20-30	07	14.58
31 to 40	15	31.24
41 to 50	22	45.83
>50	4	8.33
mean ± SD	43.4 ± 7.2 (20, 60)	

Table 1: Age wise distribution of patients (n=48).

Sex	No. of patients	Percentage
Males	31	64.58
Females	17	35.41
Total	48	100

Table 2: Sex wise distribution of patients.

Percentage of Snoring Procedure	Before treatment	3 weeks after treatment	3 months after treatment	6 months after treatment	P value
Modified sling snorplasty (n=15)	72%	21%	17%	17%	<0.05*
Sling snorplasty (n=17)	70%	19%	17%	17%	<0.05*
Injection snorplasty (n=16)	71%	60%	71%	71%	>0.05**

Table 3: Percentage of snoring before and after 3 weeks, 3 months and 6 months of treatment in various treatment groups (*Statistically significant, **Statistically non-significant).

Mean net Intensity of Snoring in dB Procedure	Before treatment	3 weeks after treatment	3 months after treatment	6 months after treatment	P value
Modified sling snorplasty (n=15)	42 dB	17 dB	11 dB	11 dB	< 0.05*
Sling snorplasty (n=17)	43 dB	21 dB	11 dB	11 dB	<0.05*
Injection snorplasty (n=16)	41 dB	33 dB	41 dB	41 dB	>0.05**

Table 4: Net snoring intensity before and after 3 weeks, 3 months and 6 months of treatment in various treatment groups (*Statistically significant, **Statistically non-significant).

Discussion

This study was conducted in the department of Otorhinolaryngology Head and Neck Surgery, Government Medical College Srinagar from September 2012 to august 2013 and includes 48 patients who presented in our OPD themselves with complaints of snoring or are referred from some other specialty or institution. In our study majority of patients were (45%) in age group 41 to 50 years, majority of patients in our study were male (64. 84 5). Marianne J Davey [9] studied 1075 patients, the principle finding of this study was that from the 1075 participants who were not pre-selected from any one homogenous group 41.5% reported, or were reported to be, snorers. Of those snorers, 69% were male, 31% were female (2.2:1). Olsen et al. objectively studied 441 subjects aged 35-69 years with a population bias towards snorers and those with subjective sleep complaints. 56% of them were men. Results of our study are in accordance with these studies.

All 48 patients were examined thoroughly and diagnosed as having obstruction at soft palate level by muller's maneuver. Weitzman et al. [10] and hill et al. [11] were the first to report the use of fiber-optic endoscopy in awake state in order to investigate pharyngeal collapse in patients with snoring and sleep apnea.

In our study 15 patients of simple palatal snoring undergo modified sling snorplasty procedure, 17 patients undergo sling snorplasty procedure and 16 patients undergo treatment by injection snorplasty method.

Sling Snoreplasty with a permanent thread [12] is performed under local anesthesia and in the sitting position. The instrument requirements include a nylon no. 4 suture, two needle-holders (or one needle-holder and a straight kelly), and a tongue depressor. Sling snoreplasty with a permanent thread is a retention suture technique applied to three portions of redundant soft palate in a triangular, tetragonal or pentagonal shape.

Sling snoreplasty could be called a three-dimensional retention suture technique to shorten, conglomerate, and tense the soft palate. It also elevates the soft palate forward and upward, and widens the oral cavity and nasopharyngeal space. The suture not only provides a sling effect in the soft palate but also incorporates into the soft palate musculature, imparting rigidity to the airway like tongue suspension suture. Patients have only a little pain and normal diet on the day after surgery. There are minimal postoperative complications.

Modified sling snoreplasty [13] is Double triangle shaped suture uvulopalatopexy can lead to anterosuperior repositioning of the soft palate by giving tonus. The final knot is embedded into soft palate via a horizontal incision after the completion of suturing. The retropalatal airway is enlarged and palatal collapse is reduced with this technique

Injection Snoreplasty [14]; is a nonsurgical treatment for snoring that involves the injection of a hardening agent (sodium tetradecoyl sulphate) into the soft palate. Injection snoreplasty is performed on an outpatient basis under local anesthesia. After numbing the soft palate with topical anesthetic, a hardening agent is injected just under the skin on the top of the mouth in front of the uvula (soft palate), creating a small blister. Within a couple of days the blister hardens, forms scar tissue, and pulls the floppy uvula forward to eliminate or reduce the palatal flutter that causes snoring.

patients who were treated by modified sling snorplasty and sling snorplasty showed statistically significant ($p<0.05$) improvement in percentage of snoring and intensity of snoring after 3 weeks, 3 months and 6 months of treatment. Patients who were treated by injection snorplasty showed improvement in percentage of snoring and intensity of snoring after 3 weeks, but that improvement was not statistically significant ($P>0.05$) and no improvement was seen after 3 months and 6 months of treatment.

Conclusion

Large randomized controlled studies are needed to compare different types of treatment for simple snoring but this study showed that modified sling snorplasty and sling snorplasty are day care procedures of choice done under local anesthesia.

References

1. The American Heritage dictionary of the English language (2000) Boston, Houghton Mifflin Company.
2. Guilleminault C, Stoohs R, Duncan S (1991) Snoring (I). Daytime sleepiness in regular heavy snorers. Chest 99: 40-48.
3. Skatrud JB, Dempsey JA (1985) Airway resistance and respiratory muscle function in snorers during NREM sleep. J Appl Physiol (1985) 59: 328-335.
4. Liistro G, Stănescu DC, Veriter C, Rodenstein DO, Aubert-Tulkens G (1991) Pattern of snoring in obstructive sleep apnea patients and in heavy snorers. Sleep 14: 517-525.
5. Lugaresi E, Cirignotta F, Montagna P (1988) Pathogenic aspects of snoring and obstructive apnea syndrome. Schweiz Med Wochenschr 118: 1333-1337.
6. Hoffstein V, Mateika S, Anderson D (1994) Snoring: is it in the ear of the beholder? Sleep 17: 522-526.
7. Prazić M (1973) Snoring and presbyacusis. Acta Otolaryngol 75: 216-219.
8. The international classification of sleep disorders (2005) (2ndedn). Westchester: American Academy of Sleep Medicine.
9. Marianne J Davey, Epidemiological study of snoring from a random survey of 1075 participants, British Snoring & Sleep Apnoea Association.
10. Weitzman ED, Pollak C, Borowiecki B, Burack B, Shprintzen R, et al. (1977) The Hypersomnia Sleep-Apnea Syndrome: site and mechanism of upper airway obstruction. Trans Am Neurol Assoc 102: 150-153.
11. Hill MW, Guilleminault C, Simmons FB (1978) Fiber-optic and EMG studies in hypersomnia-sleep apnea syndrome. Sleep apnea syndromes new york: Alan r. liss inc 249-58.
12. Hur J (2008) A new treatment for snoring: sling snoreplasty with a permanent thread. Acta Otolaryngol 128: 1381-1384.
13. Enöz M, Lapeña JF, İnançlı HM, Hafız G (2010) Modified sling snoreplasty: Double triangle shaped suture uvulopalatopexy. Kulak Burun Bogaz Ihtis Derg 20: 51-55.
14. Brietzke SE, Mair EA (2001) Injection snoreplasty: how to treat snoring without all the pain and expense. Otolaryngol Head Neck Surg 124: 503-510.

5

Effect of Maladaptive Beliefs and Attitudes about Sleep among Community-dwelling African American Men at Risk for Obstructive Sleep Apnea

Natasha J Williams[1]*, Girardin Jean-Louis[1], Mirnova E Ceïde[2], Abishek Pandey[3], Ricardo Osorio[4], Mary Mittelman[5] and Samy I McFarlane[6]

[1]*Center for Healthful Behavior Change, Division of Health and Behavior, Department of Population Health NYU School of Medicine, New York, USA*

[2]*Montefiore Medical Center, Department of Psychiatry and Behavioral Science, Bronx, New York*

[3]*Department of Medicine, State University of New York-Downstate Medical Center, Brooklyn, New York, USA*

[4]*Department of Psychiatry NYU School of Medicine, New York, New York, USA*

[5]*Department of Psychiatry and Department of Rehailitation Medicine, NYU School of Medicine, New York, USA*

[6]*Department of Medicine, Division of Endocrinology State University of New York-Downstate Medical Center, Brooklyn, New York, USA*

***Corresponding author:** Natasha J Williams, Center for Healthful Behavior Change, Division of Health and Behavior, Department of Population Health NYU School of Medicine, New York, E-mail: Natasha.williams2@nyumc.org

Abstract

This study compared differences in both maladaptive beliefs and attitudes about sleep between African American (heareafter referred to as black) men at risk for obstructive sleep apnea (OSA) and those without OSA risk.

Methods: A convenience sample of 120 community-dwelling men provided sociodemographic, health and sleep data. A validated questionnaire was used to identify men at high risk for OSA and the Dysfunctional Beliefs and Attitudes about Sleep (DBAS-16) scale was used to measure endorsed attitudes and beliefs about sleep.

Results: The mean age of the sample was 42 ± 15 years. Men reported difficulty falling asleep (23%), difficulty maintaining sleep (23%), early morning awakening (35%), and use of sleep medicine (6%). 27% were at high risk for OSA. Men at high OSA risk had greater DBAS scores [F1, 92=13.68, p<0.001]; OSA risk was related to greater rate of sleep dissatisfaction overall [46% *vs.* 13%, X2=24.52, p<0.001].

Conclusion: The findings suggest that maladaptive beliefs and attitudes about sleep are important characteristics of black men at risk for OSA, and potential screenings around sleep difficulties should also consider these factors.

Keywords: Beliefs about sleep; Obstructive sleep apnea; Black; African american; Race, Men; Insufficient sleep

Introduction

Obstructive sleep apnea (OSA) is a debilitating chronic condition characterized by snoring and repetitive partial or complete obstruction of the upper airway. It is estimated to affect approximately 18 million adults in the US. Risk factors for OSA include habitual snoring, older age, craniofacial abnormalities, alcohol consumption, and obesity [1]. Men are at greater risk for OSA and the ratio of OSA in men to women in the general population is estimated to be 5 to 1 [2].

Black race is also reported to be a risk factor for OSA [3,4] with reports of higher prevalence of OSA among Blacks. However, this finding is not consistent across all age groups. Moreover, there is some evidence to suggest that blacks are underdiagnosed [5] and because of the limited population level data 1, the prevalence of OSA in this population is poorly characterized.

A few studies have also examined the severity of OSA by race/ethnicity. Pranathiageswaran et al. [6] showed that black men younger than 39 years of age and those between 50-59 years of age had higher odds of an increased apnea hypopnea index compared to white men after controlling for body mass index. Similarly, Meetze et al. [7] compared four groups to assess if OSA severity differed by race/ethnicity. Among black men, adjusted analysis for body mass index and age, resulted in a higher mean respiratory disturbance index and lower mean oxygen saturation rate, suggesting that black men have more severe OSA compared to white men.

Absent from this body of evidence, however, is an assessment of the attitudes and beliefs toward sleep in this high-risk population. There is growing evidence that attitudes, perceptions, and beliefs about an individual's illness are linked to health outcomes [8]. For instance, dysfunctions and rigidly-held beliefs about sleep are used to discriminate between good and poor sleepers [9].

Thus, it is also plausible that dysfunctional attitudes and maladaptive beliefs toward sleep could be related to risk perceptions of OSA and the optimal amount of sleep needed. Therefore, identifying attitudes and maladaptive beliefs about sleep could have important clinical implications for identifying black men at risk for OSA.

The present study recruited a sample of black men from barbershops in a large metropolitan area in Brookly, NY, to assess the maladaptive beliefs and attitudes about sleep. We hypothesized that maladaptive beliefs would be associated with men at high risk for OSA compared to men with low risk for OSA.

Methods

Participants were a convenience sample of black adult men age 18 years or older (n=120) recruited from barbershops in Brooklyn, NY. Recruitment was conducted weekdays and weekends including evening hours. After introduction by the shop owner, research assistants introduced the study to customers on site to solicit participation. Once informed about the study, consenting participants completed self-administered questionnaires and provided socio-demographic and health data. Body mass index was based on self-reported height and weight, and was calculated as weight (kg)/height (m^2).

To assess risk for OSA, we administered the Apnea Risk Evaluation System^{TM} questionnaire (ARESTM), which includes questions on sleep patterns, daytime functioning, sleep apnea-related factors, and diseases associated with risk for sleep apnea (e.g., hypertension, diabetes mellitus).

ARESTM questionnaire data was used to identify men at high OSA risk (cut-off: >5). The questionnaire has a sensitivity of 0.94, specificity of 0.79 (based on a clinical cut-off of apnea-hypopnea index AHI>5), positive predictive value of 0.91, and negative predictive value of 0.86 [10]. Although there are other widely used tools including the STOP-Bang [11], we have used the ARESTM questionnaire to screen over 1,000 black patients in primary-care settings and 150 blacks in the community without documented refusals by participants, suggesting that it is feasible to administer this questionnaire in this population [12,13].

Participants completed the Dysfunctional Beliefs and Attitudes about Sleep scale-16 (DBAS-16) [14]. The scale assesses insomnia-related misconceptions. DBAS-16 is a Likert-type scale in which participants indicate a number ranging from 0 (strongly disagree) to 10 (strongly agree) in response to questions about beliefs and attitude toward sleep; the total score is an average of ratings on each of the 16 items.

A high score on the DBAS-16 indicates a high endorsement of dysfunctional beliefs and attitudes about sleep. The DBAS-16 has adequate internal consistency (Cronbach's alpha 0.79) and temporal stability [14]. People who receive treatment for OSA who score high on the DBAS scale are more likely to have insomnia than people treated for OSA who score low on the DBAS scale [15].

Insomnia complaints were assessed by using the three commonly used questions in the field: "Do you have difficulty falling asleep?" (difficulty falling asleep); "Do you have difficulty staying asleep?" (difficulty maintaining sleep); and "Do you wake up earlier in the morning than you mean to?" (early morning awakening). Other sleep related measures included sleep duration, sleep medicine use, and naps during the day.

The study was approved by the Institutional Review Board at SUNY Downstate Medical Center.

Analysis

We used frequency and measures of central tendency to describe the study sample. Contingency tables yielding Fisher's exact tests were used to compare characteristics of participants with high and low OSA risk scores (Table 1). A one-way Analysis of Covariance (ANCOVA) was conducted to determine whether there were significant differences between insufficient (≤ 6 h) and healthy sleep (7-8 hours) in DBAS scores. In the ANCOVA model, we adjusted for the effects of age, body mass index, self-reported diagnosis of hypertension, diabetes mellitus, and mood and sleep variables. All statistical analyses were performed using SPSS version 18.

Variable	OSA Low Risk	OSA High Risk
Body Mass Index		
Overweight/obese (%)	63	81*
Hypertension (%)	17	43*
Diabetes mellitus (%)	9	18
Heart disease (%)	1	9
Caffeine (%)	21	24
Alcohol (%)	27	32
Naps (%)	27	56*
Employed (%)	13	26
Difficulty falling asleep (%)	17	38*
Difficulty staying asleep (%)	39	24
Early wakening (%)	29	50*
*Indicates significant differences using Fisher's Exact test at alpha=0.05		

Table 1. Relationship between socio-demographic and health risk data based and OSA risk

Results

The mean age of the sample was 42 ± 15 years. Participants experienced high unemployment and had a history of several chronic diseases. Specifically, 83% were unemployed, 68% were overweight or obese (BMI>25), 25% reported hypertension, 11% reported diabetes, and 3% reported heart disease. Regarding rates of self-reported sleep-related problems, 23% reported difficulty falling asleep, 23% reported difficulty maintaining sleep, 35% reported early morning awakening, and 6% reported the use of sleep medicine (Figure 1).

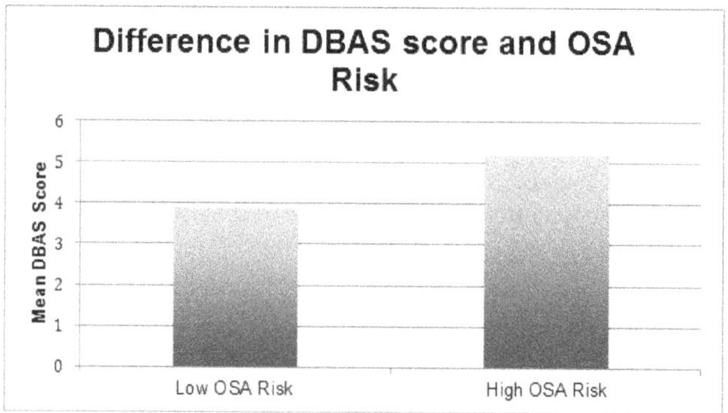

Figure 1: Difference in mean DBAS score between men with low OSA risk and high OSA risk adjusted for age, hypertension, heart disease, diabetes, body mass index, and hours of sleep.

Whereas 57% reported insufficient sleep (≤ 6 h), 34% were satisfied with their sleep, 36% reported daytime napping, and 27% were at high OSA risk.

Table 1 provides sociodemographic and health data comparing men by OSA risk status. Compared with those at low OSA risk, black men at high risk of OSA were significantly more likely to be overweight/obese, to report a physician-rendered diagnosis of hypertension, to report taking naps, and to report any one of the insomnia symptoms The mean DBAS score was 4.27 ± 1.99.

Figure 1 illustrates the difference in the mean DBAS score, of men with low and high OSA risk adjusted for sociodemographic and health variables. In the ANCOVA results indicated that men at high OSA risk had greater DBAS scores [$F1,129=7.73$, $p<0.001$] and tended to report a greater rate of sleep dissatisfaction [46% *vs.* 13%, $X2=24.52$, $p<0.001$]. Participants who reported insufficient sleep did not have greater DBAS scores than healthy sleepers [$F1,92=0.89$, NS].

Discussion

The main finding of our study is that participants at high risk for OSA endorsed maladaptive beliefs toward sleep and they also reported dissatisfaction with sleep. Previously reported results from focus groups with black men and women revealed sleep quality was not synonymous with or reflected in their overall health and wellbeing [16]. Therefore, it is plausible that maladaptive beliefs and lack of knowledge about the significance of sleep to overall health could contribute to poor symptom recognition. There is also evidence that blacks respond differently to the Epworth Sleepiness Scale, a commonly used measure in sleep clinics to assess symptoms of OSA [17]. Similarly, in a study among a sample of black patients exploring factors related to OSA assessment and referral, patients who communicated their sleep behaviors and practices with their physician were more likely to express a desire to undergo a sleep assessment [5].

A handful of studies have examined perceptions of OSA risk, but these studies largely focus on adherence to treatment for OSA [18-20]. None, to our knowledge, have focused on general perceptions about sleep. This is particularly important, as several studies have demonstrated that individuals who perceive that they are at risk of illness are more likely to engage in health-promoting behaviors [21]. Therefore, greater emphasis should be placed on cognitive factors that are likely to influence black men's health-promoting behavior about healthy sleep practices.

Our findings are similar to another study that used DBAS and found that sleep-related cognitions occur across a wide-spectrum of sleep disorders including OSA and restless leg syndrome [22], In that study, patients diagnosed with sleep disorders other than insomnia scored high on the DBAS suggesting that dysfunctional beliefs about sleep present themselves in the context of sleep problems in general. This is an important finding as DBAS was developed used to discriminate between good and poor sleepers in a sample of insomniacs [23]. It remains a widely used tool in patients with insomnia and relatively underutilized with other sleep disorders. A few studies have used the DBAS in other patient populations, including patients with fibromyalgia [24] and patients with comorbid insomnia and mood disorders [25]. These studies also found high levels of maladaptive beliefs. In future studies, it would have been interesting to correlate self-reported symptoms with objective measures for OSA and insufficient sleep such as actigraphy measurements and maladaptive beliefs.

The second observation is that over half of participants in our study (51%) reported insufficient sleep, a consistent finding in the literature on sleep duration among blacks [26-28]. Moreover, 36% reported daytime napping and napping is associated with OSA [29]. Based on the ARESTM score, 27% were at high risk for OSA. Given that black men may experience symptoms of OSA at a younger age compared with White men [30], primary physicians could play an important role in communicating risk and encouraging objective screenings for OSA including referrals for home sleep testing and polysomnography.

The ARESTM was well accepted in this setting, but one must exercise caution as the US Preventive Task Force recently stated that there is insufficient evidence to recommend population level screening for OSA in asymptomatic patients [31]. In addition, the DBAS is not a clinical or screening tool, but may be very useful for understanding maladaptive beliefs toward sleep in the clinical setting.

The fact that sleep data in this study was self-reported, rather than measured with actigraph or other objective assessment could be considered as a limitation. However, self-reported data proved to be most acceptable to minority individuals in community-based samples that we studied [12,32]. Given that the study design was cross-sectional and used a convenience sample, causality could not be determined. It is also unclear whether these findings would be generalizable to other populations. In this study, confirming an OSA diagnosis with the use of home-based testing or polysomnography was not feasible. Despite these limitations, the study makes an important contribution to the sleep literature, as it provided data from black men, a population that is at high-risk for OSA, but is underrepresented in sleep health research in particular as well as the conduct of the research in a community-based setting. The setting for the study was successful in reaching black men and could be used effectively in future sleep health services research. Future studies should also consider further evaluation of sleep-related beliefs and practices among black men. It is plausible that black men may be more likely to endorse incorrect beleifs about sleep such as using alcohol for improved sleep quality or under-recognition of symptoms such as loud and habitual snoring.

The study sample was recruited exclusively from barbershops, and our results indicatat this is useful strategy for recruiting black men from a community-based setting. Additionally, it contributes further understanding regarding the relationships of OSA with both health status and sleep beliefs, which have not been previously examined.

Acknowledgement

This research was supported by funding from the NIH. Dr. Williams ws supported by funding from NIH/NHLBI, K23HL125939.

References

1. Young T, Peppard PE, Gottlieb DJ (2002) Epidemiology of obstructive sleep apnea - A population health perspective. Am J Respir Crit Care Med 165: 1217-1239.
2. Lin CM, Davidson TM, Ancoli-Israel S (2008) Gender differences in obstructive sleep apnea and treatment implications. Sleep Med Rev 12: 481-496.
3. Redline S, Tishler P, Hans M, Tosteson T, Strohl K, et al. (1997) Racial differences in sleep-disordered breathing in African-Americans and Caucasians. Am J Respir Crit Care Med 155: 186-192.
4. Ruiter ME, DeCoster J, Jacobs L, Lichstein KL (2010) Sleep disorders in African Americans and Caucasian Americans: a meta-analysis. Behav Sleep Med 8: 246-259.

5. Jean LG, Zizi F, Clark L, Brown C, McFarlane S (2008) Evaluation of sleep apnea in a sample of black patients. J Clin Sleep Med 4: 421-425.
6. Pranathiageswaran S, Badr MS, Severson R, Rowley JA (2013) The Influence of Race on the Severity of Sleep Disordered Breathing. J Clin Sleep Med 9: 303-309.
7. Meetze K, Gillespie MB, Lee FS (2002) Obstructive sleep apnea: A comparison of black and white subjects. Laryngoscope 112: 1271-1274.
8. Ajzen I (2011) The theory of planned behaviour: Reactions and reflections. Psychol Health 26: 1113-1127.
9. Carney CE, Edinger JD (2006) Identifying critical beliefs about sleep in primary insomnia. Sleep 29: 444-453.
10. Levendowski DJ, Morgan TD, Patrickus JE, Westbrook PR, Berka C, et al. (2007) In-home evaluation of efficacy and titration of a mandibular advancement device for obstructive sleep apnea. Sleep Breath 11: 139-147.
11. Chung F, Yegneswaran B, Liao P, Chung SA, Vairavanathan S, et al. (2008) STOP questionnaire - A tool to screen patients for obstructive sleep apnea. Anesthesiology 108: 812-821.
12. Benoit J, Pandey A, Racine C (2012) Differences in sleep measures between caribbean- and us-born blacks with metabolic syndrome. Sleep 35: 305-305.
13. Demede M, Pandey A, Zizi F, Bachmann R, Donat M, et al. (2011) Resistant hypertension and obstructive sleep apnea in the primary-care setting. Int Journal of Hypertens 2011: 340929-340929.
14. Morin CM, Vallieres A, Ivers H (2007) Dysfunctional beliefs and attitudes about sleep (DBAS): Validation of a brief version (DBAS-16). Sleep 30: 1547-1554.
15. Yang CM, Chou CP, Hsiao FC (2011) The association of dysfunctional beliefs about sleep with vulnerability to stress-related sleep disturbance in young adults. Behav Sleep Med 9: 86-91.
16. Shaw R, McKenzie S, Taylor T, Olafiranye O, Boutin-Foster C, et al. (2012) Beliefs and attitudes toward obstructive sleep apnea evaluation and treatment among blacks. J Natl Med Assoc 104: 510-519.
17. Hayes AL, Spilsbury JC, Patel SR (2009) The Epworth Score in African American Populations. J Clin Sleep Med ine 5: 344-348.
18. Weaver TE, Maislin G, Dinges DF, Younger J, Cantor C, et al. (2003) Self-efficacy in sleep apnea: Instrument development and patient perceptions of obstructive sleep apnea risk, treatment benefit, and volition to use continuous positive airway pressure. Sleep 26: 727-732.
19. Olsen S, Smith S, Oei TPS (2008) Adherence to continuous positive airway pressure therapy in obstructive sleep apnoea sufferers: A theoretical approach to treatment adherence and intervention. Clin Psychol Rev 28: 1355-1371.
20. Balachandran JS, Yu X, Wroblewski K, Mokhlesi B (2013) A brief survey of patients' first impression after cpap titration predicts future cpap adherence: A pilot study. J Clin Sleep Med 9: 199-205.
21. Brewer NT, Chapman GB, Gibbons FX, Gerrard M, McCaul KD, et al. (2007) Meta-analysis of the relationship between risk perception and health behavior: The example of vaccination. Health Psychol 26: 136-145.
22. Cronlein T, Wagner S, Langguth B, Geisler P, Eichhammer P, et al. (2014) Are dysfunctional attitudes and beliefs about sleep unique to primary insomnia? Sleep Med 15: 1463-1467.
23. Morin CM, Stone J, Trinkle D, Mercer J, Remsberg S (1993) Dysfunctional beliefs and attitudes about sleep among older adults with and without insomnia complaints. Psychol Aging 8: 463-467.
24. Theadom A, Cropley M (2008) Dysfunctional beliefs, stress and sleep disturbance in fibromyalgia. Sleep Med 9: 376-381.
25. Carney CE, Edinger JD, Manber R, Garson C, Segal ZV (2007) Beliefs about sleep in disorders characterized by sleep and mood disturbance. J Psychosom Res 62: 179-188.
26. Hale L and Do DP (2007) Racial differences in self-reports of sleep duration in a population-based study. Sleep 30: 1096-1103.
27. Patel NP, Grandner MA, Xie D, Branas CC, Gooneratne N (2010) "Sleep disparity" in the population: poor sleep quality is strongly associated with poverty and ethnicity. Bmc Public Health 10: 474.
28. Nunes J, Jean-Louis G, Zizi F, Casimir GJ, Gizycki HV et al. (2008) Sleep duration among black and white Americans: results of the National Health Interview Survey. J Natl Med Assoc 100: 317-322.
29. Masa JF, Rubio M, Perez P, Mota M, de Cos JS (2006) Association between habitual naps and sleep apnea. Sleep 29: 1463-1468.
30. O'Connor GT, Lind BK, Lee ET, Nieto FJ, Redline S, et al. (2003) Variation in symptoms of sleep-disordered breathing with race and ethnicity: The sleep heart health study. Sleep 26: 74-79.
31. Bibbings-Domingo K, Grossman DC, Curry SJ, Davidson KW, John W, et al. (2017) screening for obstructive sleep apnea in adults US preventive services task force recommendation statement. J Am Med Assoc 317: 407-414.
32. Demede M, Pandey A, Innasimuthu L, Jean-Louis G, McFarlane SI, et al. (2011) Management of hypertension in high-risk ethnic minority with heart failure. Int Journal of Hypertens 2011: 417594-417594.

6

Effect of Weight and Obstructive Sleep Apnea Severity on Sleep Surgery Outcomes in Children with Down Syndrome

Xue Zhao[1], Woravipa Ayudhaya[2], Fauziya Hassan[3] and Jeffrey J Stanley[4*]

[1]*Department of Otolaryngology-Head and Neck Surgery, University of Michigan, Ann Arbor, MI, USA*

[2]*Department of Neurology, Sleep Disorders Center, University of Michigan, Ann Arbor, MI, USA*

[3]*Department of Pediatrics and Communicable Diseases, Sleep Disorders Center, University of Michigan, Ann Arbor, MI, USA*

[4]*Department of Neurology and Otolaryngology-Head and Neck Surgery, Sleep Disorders Center, University of Michigan, Ann Arbor, MI, USA*

[*]**Corresponding author:** Jeffrey J. Stanley, Department of Neurology and Otolaryngology-Head and Neck Surgery, Sleep Disorders Center, University of Michigan, Ann Arbor, MI, USA, 1500 E. Medical Center Drive, Ann Arbor, MI 48109, USA, E-mail: jjst@med.umich.edu

Abstract

Objectives: To assess the effect of weight status and obstructive sleep apnea (OSA) severity on polysomnographic (PSG) outcomes following sleep surgery inclusive of adenotonsillectomy (AT) in children with Trisomy 21.

Methods: A retrospective chart review was completed on thirty-six children ages 1-13 years with Trisomy 21 and OSA who underwent at a tertiary care academic hospital between 2005 to 2015 and had both preoperative and postoperative PSGs. Postoperative changes in apnea hypopnea index (AHI) and other PSG parameters, including percentage of various sleep stages, were compared between children who were normal weight, overweight and obese.

Results: The mean preoperative AHIs for normal weight, overweight and obese children were 15.6, 12.2 and 15.0, respectively while the mean postoperative AHIs were 10.6, 9.4 and 10.2, respectively. Improvement in AHI was significant only among children with severe OSA (AHI >10), but not among children with mild (AHI 1.5 to 5) or moderate OSA (AHI 5 to 10), both with and without controlling for weight status (p=0.01, p=0.009). There were no significant differences in postoperative PSG parameters comparing obese vs. non-obese and overweight vs. normal weight children.

Conclusion: Weight status does not appear to affect sleep surgery outcomes in children with Trisomy 21. This subset of children was found to have persistent OSA following sleep surgery regardless of weight. Other factors associated with Trisomy 21, such as macroglossia, glossoptosis and hypotonia, may play a greater role in the pathogenesis of OSA in this patient population. Only those children with severe OSA were found to have a significant improvement in AHI after sleep surgery, inclusive of AT.

Keywords: Down syndrome; Sleep surgery; Adenotonsillectomy; Obstructive sleep apnea

Introduction

The incidence of obstructive sleep apnea (OSA) in the general pediatric population is 1-4% [1,2]. OSA is characterized by recurrent episodes of prolonged partial or complete upper airway obstruction associated with arousals and/or oxyhemoglobin desaturations during sleep. Sequelae of untreated OSA include failure to thrive, endothelial dysfunction, systemic inflammation, systemic and pulmonary hypertension, cor pulmonale, developmental delay and hematologic changes including a significantly higher red cell distribution width, neutrophil-to-lymphocyte and platelet-to-lymphocyte ratios [3]. In addition, untreated OSA has been associated with excessive daytime sleepiness, hyperactivity, cognitive dysfunction, and poor school performance. The most common source of airway obstruction among children with OSA is adeno-tonsillar hypertrophy. Other factors associated with upper airway obstruction include obesity, craniofacial anomalies, retrognathia and neuromuscular disorders with associated hypotonia of upper airway musculature.

Trisomy 21 (Down's syndrome) is a genetic disorder caused by a trisomy of all, or part of, chromosome 21 and is observed in 1 in 650 to 1000 live births in the United States [4-6]. There is a high prevalence of OSA (30-70%) among children with Trisomy 21 [7-9]. Characteristics of children with Trisomy 21 that predispose to this high prevalence include hypotonia, macroglossia, midface hypoplasia, a narrowed pharyngeal inlet and increased incidence of upper respiratory tract anomalies, such as laryngomalacia [10-13].

During the past few decades, a significant increase in the prevalence of childhood obesity has been observed in the United States [14]. Obese children are at higher risk for persistent OSA following adeno-tonsillectomy (AT). Children with Trisomy 21 have a higher body mass index (BMI) in comparison to the general pediatric population, which may account, in part, for the higher prevalence of OSA in this population [15-17].

The initial step in treatment of OSA among children with or without Trisomy 21 is sleep surgery, inclusive of AT. The success rate of AT is higher among children who do not have co-morbidities and are of normal weight. There is a higher incidence of persistent OSA after AT among obese children and children with Trisomy 21 [18,19]. This study was designed to evaluate the relative efficacy of sleep surgery, inclusive of AT among children with Trisomy 21 and OSA as a function of their weight status and OSA severity. Specifically, changes in polysomnographic parameters including apnea hypopnea index (AHI), percentage of sleep stages and extent of oxygen desaturation were assessed.

Methods

Study design

The retrospective chart review was approved by the Institutional Review Board (IRB) at University of Michigan Health System (UMHS). The electronic medical record was reviewed for all children aged 1-13 years with Trisomy 21 and a diagnosis of OSA based on in-lab diagnostic PSG conducted between January 2005 and December 2015.

Only children who underwent AT at UMHS and had a post-operative in-lab PSG at the same institution were included in the study. Children who did not have both preoperative and postoperative PSGs were excluded.

Data recorded included patients' demographic information, BMI, as well as pre- and postoperative PSG measures. Data analyzed included changes in AHI and changes in sleep architecture including percent of N1, N2, N3 and REM sleep stages, arousal index, end tidal CO_2 ($ETCO_2$) or transcutaneous CO_2 (TCO_2) and the degree of oxygen desaturation. Changes in PSG parameters were compared between children of varying weight categories.

Weight status determinations (normal weight, overweight, and obese) were made using age and gender specific norms from the Centers for Disease Control and Prevention (CDC) growth charts.

BMI percentiles were used for children two years of age or older, while weight-for-length (WFL) percentiles were used for children under two years of age. According to the CDC's definitions, obesity was defined as BMI or WFL ≥ 95th percentile, overweight as BMI or WFL ≥ 85th percentile but <95th percentile, and normal weight as BMI or WFL>5th and <85th percentiles.

Polysomnography

All subjects underwent standard clinical overnight PSG using Profusion Sleep software (Compumedics, USA) and the electrodes were placed according to the 10-20 international system. This included six channel electroencephalogram (F3-A2, F4-A1, C3-A2, C4-A1, O1-A2, O2-A1), left and right electro-oculograms, chin electromyogram, left and right leg electromyograms, electrocardiogram, thoracic and abdominal wall movement (piezoelectric strain gauges), oronasal airflow (thermocouple and nasal pressure), carbon dioxide ($ETCO_2$ or TCO_2) and pulse oximetry.

Sleep architecture and associated events were scored by standard techniques based on the American Academy of Sleep Medicine scoring manual (AASM) for pediatric patients [20].

Measurements included total sleep time (TST), percentage of sleep time in N1, N2, N3 and REM stage, arousal index, $ETCO_2$ or TCO_2, AHI, obstructive apnea index (OAI), central apnea index (CAI), and oxygen saturation nadir. Using both the previous and current AASM scoring guidelines, hypopneas were defined as events lasting ≥ 2 respiratory cycles with at least 50% decrease in oronasal flow with ≥ 3% oxyhemoglobin desaturation or associated arousal, and events lasting ≥ 2 respiratory cycles with ≥ 30% drop of peak signal excursions from the baseline and 4% oxygen desaturation or arousal, respectively. The criteria used for diagnosis of OSA was an OAI>1 event/hour or AHI>1.5 events/hour, further delineating the OSA severity as mild (AHI between 1.5-5 events/hour), moderate (AHI between 5-10 events/h, or severe (AHI>10 events/h). We defined a successful outcome of surgery as postoperative AHI<1.5 events/hour or OAI<1.0 events/h. Postoperative PSGs were obtained between 2 and 4 months following surgery.

Statistical analysis

Absolute change in sleep parameters was calculated by subtracting the preoperative value from the postoperative value.

Repeated measures ANOVA were used to test for changes in sleep parameters over time (preoperative vs. postoperative) and to examine whether weight status or severity of OSA moderated the impact of surgery.

To test for the potential moderation of surgery's impact by weight status, we tested an interaction term of weight status x time period (pre- or postoperative). To test for the potential moderation of surgery's impact by severity of OSA, we tested an interaction term of OSA severity x time period (pre- or postoperative).

When the interaction term was significant, we performed subgroup analysis to examine the effect of surgery within specific groups of interest.

All analyses were performed using SAS 9.4 (SAS Institute Inc., Cary, NC). A 2-tailed α level of ≤ 0.05 was considered statistically significant.

Results

Demographics

Thirty-six children, 14 boys and 22 girls with a mean age of 44.36 months (range 6-118 months), with Trisomy 21 and OSA who underwent sleep surgery, inclusive of AT and had both preoperative and postoperative PSGs were included in the study. The preoperative and postoperative mean BMI were not significantly different at 18.2 (range, 14.5-24.6) and 18.6 kg/m^2 (range 14.1-26.2), respectively.

Among the 36 children included in the study, 47% (n=17) were normal weight, 28% (n=17) were overweight and 25% (n=9) were obese. There were a higher proportion of children with severe OSA (53%) than moderate (22%) or mild OSA (25%). Of the 36 children who underwent AT, 11 had additional concurrent surgery at the discretion of the operative surgeon:Eight underwent uvulopalatopharyngoplasty (UPPP), one underwent UPPP with supraglottoplasty, one underwent lingual tonsillectomy and one underwent supraglottoplasty.

The median hospital length of stay was 1 day, although 1 subject had a prolonged hospitalization lasting 76 days due to aspiration pneumonia and resultant respiratory failure (Table 1).

Variables	n
Total	36
Males	14
Females	22
Normal weight	17
Overweight	10
Obese	9
Mild OSA	9
Moderate OSA	8
Severe OSA	19

Table 1: Patient demographics.

Polysomnographic parameters

Mean preoperative and postoperative PSG parameters are shown in Table 2. There were high percentages of N3 sleep both pre- and postoperatively, at 40.0% and 47.8%, respectively, with an increase in percentage of N3 sleep following surgery. An increase in the percentage of REM sleep and a decrease in percentage of stage N1 and N2 sleep was also observed postoperatively, but was not found to be statistically significant. Comparisons were made between obese *vs.* non-obese (n=9 *vs.* 27) and normal weight *vs.* non-normal weight (overweight and obese) children (n=17 *vs.* 19). There were no significant differences in absolute change of sleep parameters (Figures 1a and 1b) or relative change of sleep parameters, including AHI, OAI, arousal index, percentage of N3 and percentage of REM, in both obese *vs.* non-obese and normal weight *vs.* non-normal weight groups.

PSG Parameters	Pre-operative	Post-operative
TST, min	420.4	435.8
W, min	68.1	61.8
N1, %	5.2	3.5
N2, %	40	29
N3, %	40	47.8
REM, %	14.4	19.5
Arousal Index	13.1	13.2
OAI	1.8	0.7
AHI	13.8	10
CAI	1.3	1.2
Mean SpO_2 (%)	96.2	95

TST: Total Sleep Time; W: Wake Stage; N1, N2, N3, Non-REM Sleep Stages 1, 2 And 3; REM: Rapid Eye Movement Sleep Stage; OAI: Obstructive Apnea Index; AHI: Apnea-Hypopnea Index; CAI: Central Apnea Index; SpO_2: Oxygen Saturation.

Table 2: Comparison of mean pre-operative and post-operative polysomnographic parameters.

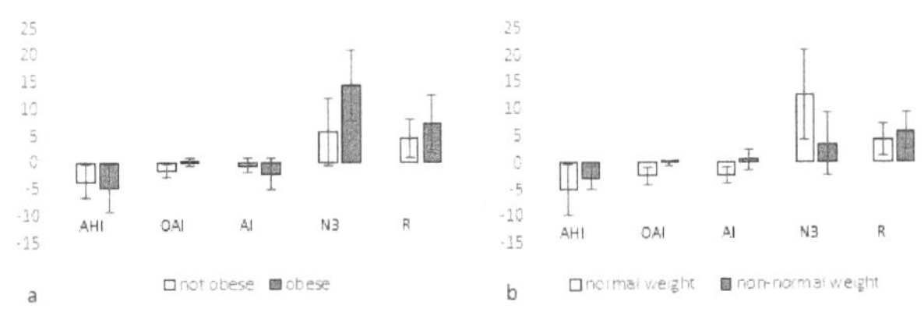

Figure 1: Absolute changes in sleep parameters after surgery in obese vs. non-obese (a) and normal weight vs. non-normal weight (overweight and obese) children (b).

Mean AHI and OAI values prior to and after surgery in both normal weight *vs.* non-normal weight (overweight and obese) and non-obese (normal and overweight) *vs.* obese are shown in Table 3. The mean pre- and postoperative AHI were 12.2 and 9.4, respectively, for non-normal weight (overweight and obese) children and 15.0 and 10.2 for obese children. There was no significant improvement in AHI and OAI following surgery among either non-normal weight or normal weight children (p>0.05) and there were no significant differences in the change in AHI and OAI in normal weight children compared to non-normal weight children (p>0.05). Similarly, AHI and OAI were not improved significantly after surgery in either obese or non-obese children (p>0.05) and there were no significant differences in the change of AHI and OAI following surgery when comparing obese to non-obese children (p>0.05).

	Normal Weight		Non-Normal Weight		p-value	Non-obese		Obese		p-value
	Pre-	Post-	Pre-	Post-	Pre-	Post-	Pre-	Post-		
AHI (SD)	15.6 (14.2)	10.6 (11.6)	12.2 (10.1)	9.4 (9.0)	NS	13.4 (12.2)	9.9 (10.0)	15.0 (12.6)	10.2 (11.5)	NS
OAI (SD)	2.9 (6.8)	0.5 (0.9)	0.9 (1.1)	0.5 (0.9)	NS	2.0 (5.5)	0.5 (0.9)	1.2 (1.4)	1.3 (3.4)	NS
AHI: Apnea-Hypopnea Index; OAI: Obstructive Sleep Apnea; NS: Not Significant P>0.05.										

Table 3: Comparison of mean pre-operative and post-operative AHI and OAI in normal weight vs. non-normal weight (overweight and obese) and obese vs. non-obese.

Comparisons between the preoperative and postoperative AHI and OAI respiratory parameters based on OSA severity both with and without controlling for weight status are shown in Table 4. When children are not categorized by OSA severity, there were no statistically significant changes in AHI and OAI following surgery with or without controlling for weight status. When the children were classified by OSA severity, there were no statistically significant changes in respiratory parameters among children with mild and moderate OSA ($p>0.05$). In children with severe OSA, the mean preoperative AHI was 21.6 while their mean postoperative AHI was 11.5. Children with severe OSA were found to have a significant improvement in AHI, both with and without controlling for overweight status ($p=0.01$ and $p=0.009$, respectively). There was also a significant difference between pre- and postoperative AHI comparing severe *vs.* mild/moderate OSA patients ($p=0.006$) indicating that the change in AHI following AT depended on the initial severity of OSA.

Preoperative (SD)		Postoperative (SD)	p-Value not controlling for weight	p-value, controlling overweight *vs.* normal weight
All severities				
AHI	13.8 (12.2)	10.0 (10.2)	0.15	0.15
OAI	1.8 (4.8)	0.7 (1.9)	0.20	0.2
Mild OSA				
AHI	3.3 (1.4)	8.8 (15.5)	0.33	0.32
OAI	0.2 (0.2)	0.5 (1.1)	0.43	0.42
Moderate OSA				
AHI	7.1 (1.0)	7.8 (4.9)	0.70	0.72
OAI	0.2 (0.3)	0.7 (1.2)	0.26	0.26
Severe OSA				
AHI	21.6 (12.1)	11.5 (9.0)	0.009	0.01
OAI	3.3 (6.3)	0.8 (2.4)	0.12	0.12
AHI: Apnea-Hypopnea Index; OAI: Obstructive Apnea Index.				

Table 4: Respiratory parameter changes based on severity of OSA and weight control.

Discussion

This is the first study to evaluate the effect of weight status on the efficacy of sleep surgery inclusive of AT for treatment of OSA in children with Trisomy 21. The first line treatment among healthy children with OSA is AT. However, a high proportion of obese children have residual OSA following AT [21,22]. Mitchell et al. demonstrated that obese children had higher AHI than normal weight children and that 76% of obese children had residual OSA after AT compared to only 28% of normal weight children [23] Similarly, children with Trisomy 21 have a high likelihood of persistent OSA following AT. In 2007, Merrell et al. showed that only one third of children with Trisomy 21 had a normal postoperative AHI on PSG following AT.21 A recent systematic review of AT outcomes in children with Trisomy 21 confirmed that the majority of these patients do not have resolution of OSA (defined as AHI<1) after AT [22] It may be expected then, that children with Trisomy 21 who are also obese would be even less likely to benefit from sleep surgery. However, the results of the current study did not support this premise as no significant difference in surgical outcomes ware identified between obese vs. non-obese and normal *vs.* non-normal weight children with Trisomy 21.

In addition, no significant change in OSA severity was observed following sleep surgery, with or without controlling for weight status, in Trisomy 21 children with mild and moderate OSA. Only children with severe OSA demonstrated a statistically significant improvement in AHI following sleep surgery. However, there was still significant residual disease, as measured by AHI, in this subset of patients.

Besides weight status, there are several other potential factors that may contribute to persistent OSA following sleep surgery for children with Trisomy 21 including the presence of upper airway abnormalities such as macroglossia, midface hypoplasia, increased upper airway fat distribution and hypotonia [10,12]. Donelly et al. found that of Trisomy 21 patients with persistent OSA following AT 74% had macroglossia, 63% had glossoptosis and 30% had enlarged lingual tonsils [24]. Scott et al. proposed a mechanism to explain how pubertal changes modify determinants of OSA severity between childhood and adolescence, since BMI becomes a more important predictor of severe OSA in older children [25]. OSA severity in younger children has been linked to increased lymphoid hyperplasia, instead of parapharyngeal fat pad size. However, among children with Trisomy 21, studies have noted fatty infiltration in the muscular portion of the tongue on T1-weighted signal magnetic resonance imaging (MRI), as well as fat deposits in the lateral pharyngeal wall and uvula, similar to the fat distribution that increases the risk of OSA among adults [6,25,26]. These factors may also help explain the current study findings of no significant change in AHI and OAI following sleep surgery in both obese *vs.* non-obese and overweight vs. normal weight children.

Both the Muller's maneuver (MM) and drug induced sleep endoscopy (DISE) have been utilized to help identify potential site (s) of obstruction in patients diagnosed with OSA. This information is useful in determining which procedure (s) should be recommended for each individual patient. Although there is a reasonable concordance between the results of MM and DISE for the pattern of collapse at the velum (73-92%), there is a poor concordance between the results of the two examinations at the base of the tongue (24%) [27-38]. Therefore, DISE is a potentially invaluable tool for determining the need for additional surgery directed at the base of tongue in children with Trisomy 21 and OSA [27].

The current study demonstrates that sleep surgery inclusive of AT as primary treatment for children with Trisomy 21 and OSA is, at best, partially effective. Marcus et al. has suggested using CPAP as first line management among children with OSA and complex diagnoses [3]. However, achieving high levels of CPAP compliance among children, with or without developmental disabilities, can be challenging and may make this treatment option impractical for some. Prosser et al. recently found that lingual tonsillectomy significantly improved AHI and sleep outcomes in Trisomy 21 patients with persistent OSA after AT. Only one of the 36 children in the current study underwent concurrent lingual tonsillectomy [28].

When considering surgical treatment options including AT and additional procedures such as UPPP, lingual tonsillectomy, genioglossus muscle advancement, and supraglottoplasty, one must consider that these procedures may still not address the underlying hypotonia associated with Trisomy 21. Hypoglossal nerve stimulation therapy has recently been shown to have a significant impact on upper airway patency by increasing both the retropalatal and retrolingual air space [29-31]. At present, there is only one published report on the use of hypoglossal nerve stimulation therapy in an adolescent with Trisomy 21 and OSA who had significant improvement in AHI from 48.5 to 3.4 [32].

Previous studies have reported an increase in stage N3 sleep after AT in children with OSA and Trisomy 21 [33-36]. These findings are similar to the results of the current study. An increase in the percentage of REM sleep and decrease in percentages of N1 and N2 sleep were also observed in the current study, although these changes were not found to be statistically significant.

There are several limitations to the current study. First, this was a retrospective study. The sample size is relatively small because only children who had both pre- and postoperative PSGs were included in the study, which risks inclusion bias. One possible explanation for the limited improvement in AHI found in our study is that only those with severe or clinically persistent disease underwent postoperative PSG, as patients' families may have forgone additional testing if symptomatic improvement was achieved. In addition, PSG data was collected over a 10-year period so two different PSG scoring methods were used in accordance with the American Academy of Sleep Medicine Scoring Guidelines. Finally, children included in this study were evaluated and treated by more than Otolaryngologist, who elected to perform AT with or without additional surgery based on their clinical impression regarding the likely additional site (s) of obstruction.

Conclusion

Weight status does not appear to affect sleep surgery outcomes in children with Trisomy 21. This subset of children was found to have persistent OSA following sleep surgery regardless of weight. Other factors associated with Trisomy 21, such as macroglossia, glossoptosis and hypotonia, may play a greater role in the pathogenesis of OSA in this patient population. Only those children with severe OSA were found to have a significant improvement in AHI after sleep surgery, inclusive of adenotonsillecomty [37,38].

References

1. Lumeng JC, Chervin RD (2008) Epidemiology of pediatric obstructive sleep apnea. Proc Am Thorac Soc 15: 242-252.
2. Sinha D, Guilleminault C (2010) Sleep disordered breathing in children. Indian J Med Res 131: 311-320.
3. Marcus CL, Brooks LJ, Draper KA, Gozal D, Halbower AC, et al. (2012) Diagnosis and management of childhood obstructive sleep apnea syndrome. Pediatrics 130: e714-55.
4. Presson AP, Partyka G, Jensen KM, Devine OJ, Rasmussen SA, et al. (2013) Current estimate of Down syndrome population prevalence in the United States. J Pediatr 163: 1163-1168.
5. Goffinski A, Stanley MA, Shepherd N, Duvall N, Jenkinson SB, et al. (2015) Obstructive sleep apnea in young infants with Down syndrome evaluated in a Down syndrome specialty clinic. Am J Med Genet A 167: 324-330.
6. Bassell JL, Phan H, Leu R, Kronk R, Visootsak J (2015) Sleep profiles in children with Down syndrome. Am J Med Genet A 167: 1830-1835.
7. Ng DK, Hui HN, Chan CH, Kwok KL, Chow PY, et al. (2006) Obstructive sleep apnea in children with Down syndrome. Singapore Med J 47: 774-779.
8. Shott SR, Amin R, Chini B, Heubi C (2006) Obstructive sleep apnea: Should all children with Down syndrome be tested? Arch Otolaryngol Head Neck Surg 132: 432-436.
9. Lam DJ, Jensen CC, Mueller BA, Starr JR, Cunningham ML, et al. (2010) Pediatric sleep apnea and craniofacial anomalies: A population-based case-control study. Laryngoscope 120: 2098-2105.
10. Marcus CL, Keens TG, Bautista DB, Von Pechmann WS, Ward SL (1991) Obstructive sleep apnea in children with Down syndrome. Pediatrics 88: 132-139.
11. Nisbet LC, Phillips NN, Hoban TF, O'Brien LM (2015) Characterization of a sleep architectural phenotype in children with Down syndrome. Sleep Breath 19: 1065-1071.

12. Lin SC, Davey MJ, Horne RS, Nixon GM (2014) Screening for obstructive sleep apnea in children with Down syndrome. J Pediatr 165: 117-122.
13. Hoffmire CA, Magyar CI, Connolly HV, Fernandez ID, Van Wijngaarden E (2014) High prevalence of sleep disorders and associated comorbidities in a community sample of children with Down syndrome. J Clin Sleep Med 10: 411-419.
14. May AL, Freedman D, Sherry B, Blanck HM (2013) Obesity-United States, 1999-2010. CDC, MMWR Suppl 62: 120-128.
15. Lal C, White DR, Joseph JE, Van Bakergem K, La Rosa A (2015) Sleep-disordered breathing in Down syndrome. Chest 147: 570-579.
16. Murray J, Ryan-Krause P (2010) Obesity in children with Down syndrome: Background and recommendations for management. Pediatr Nurs 36: 314-319.
17. Basil JS, Santoro SL, Martin LJ, Healy KW, Chini BA, et al. (2016) Retrospective study of obesity in children with Down syndrome. J Pediatr 173: 143-148.
18. Com G, Carroll JL, Tang X, Melguizo MS, Bower C, et al. (2015) Characteristics and surgical and clinical outcomes of severely obese children with obstructive sleep apnea. J Clin Sleep Med 11: 467-474.
19. Rosen D (2011) Management of obstructive sleep apnea associated with Down syndrome and other craniofacial dysmorphologies. Curr Opin Pulm Med 17: 431-436.
20. Berry RB, Budhiraja R, Gottlieb DJ, Gozal D, Iber C, et al. (2012) Rules for scoring respiratory events in sleep: Update of the 2007 AASM Manual for the Scoring of sleep and associated Events. Deliberations of the sleep apnea definitions task force of the American academy of sleep medicine. J Clin Sleep Med 8: 597-619.
21. Merrell JA, Shott SR (2007) OSAS in Down syndrome: T&A versus T&A plus lateral pharyngoplasty. Int J Pediatr Otorhinolaryngol 71: 1197-1203.
22. Farhood Z, Isley JW, Ong AA, Nguyen SA, Camilon TJ, et al. (2017) Adenotonsillectomy outcomes in patients with Down syndrome and obstructive sleep apnea. Laryngoscope 127: 1465-1470.
23. Mitchell RB, Kelly J (2007) Outcome of adenotonsillectomy for obstructive sleep apnea in obese and normal-weight children. Otolaryngol Head Neck Surg 137: 43-48.
24. Donnelly LF, Shott SR, LaRose CR, Chini BA, Amin RS (2004) Causes of persistent obstructive sleep apnea despite previous tonsillectomy and adenoidectomy in children with Down syndrome as depicted on static and dynamic cine MRI. AJR Am J Roentgenol 183: 175-181.
25. Scott B, Johnson RF, Mitchell Md RB (2016) Obstructive sleep apnea: Differences between normal-weight, overweight, obese, and morbidly obese children. Otolaryngol Head Neck Surg 154: 936-943.
26. Schwab RJ, Pasirstein M, Pierson R, Mackley A, Hachadoorian R, et al. (2003) Identification of upper airway anatomic risk factors for obstructive sleep apnea with volumetric magnetic resonance imaging. Am J Respir Crit Care Med 168: 522-530.
27. Propst EJ, Amin R, Talwar N, Zaman M, Zweerink A, et al. (2017) Midline posterior glossectomy and lingual tonsillectomy in obese and nonobese children with down syndrome: Biomarkers for success. Laryngoscope 127: 757-763.
28. Prosser JD, Shott SR, Rodriguez O, Simakajornboon N, Meinzen-Derr J, et al. (2017) Polysomnographyic outcomes following lingual tonsillectomy for persistent obstructive sleep apnea in down syndrome. Laryngoscope 127: 520-524.
29. Soose RJ (2016) Novel surgical approaches for the treatment of obstructive sleep apnea. Sleep Med Clin 11: 189-202.
30. Certal VF, Zaghi S, Riaz M, Vieira AS, Pinheiro CT, et al. (2015) Hypoglossal nerve stimulation in the treatment of obstructive sleep apnea: A systematic review and meta-analysis. Laryngoscope 125: 1254-1264.
31. Woodson BT, Soose RJ, Gillespie MB, Strohl KP, Maurer JT, et al. (2016) Three-year outcomes of cranial nerve stimulation for obstructive sleep apnea: The STAR trial. Otolaryngol Head Neck Surg 154: 181-188.
32. Diercks GR, Keamy D, Kinane TB, Skotko B, Schwartz A, et al. (2016) Hypoglossal nerve stimulator implantation in an adolescent with down syndrome and sleep apnea. Pediatrics 137: e1-7.
33. Miano S, Bruni O, Elia M, Scifo L, Smerieri A, et al. (2008) Sleep phenotypes of intellectual disability: A polysomnographic evaluation in subjects with Down syndrome and Fragile-X syndrome. Clin Neurophysiol 119: 1242-1247.
34. Shete MM, Stocks RM, Sebelik ME, Schoumacher RA (2010) Effects of adeno-tonsillectomy on polysomnography patterns in Down syndrome children with obstructive sleep apnea: A comparative study with children without Down syndrome. Int J Pediatr Otorhinolaryngol 74: 241-244.
35. Trois MS, Capone GT, Lutz JA, Melendres MC, Schwartz AR, et al. (2009) Obstructive sleep apnea in adults with Down syndrome. J Clin Sleep Med 5: 317-323.
36. Mims M, Thottam PJ, Kitsko D, Shaffer A, Choi S (2017) Characterization of sleep architecture in Down syndrome patients pre and post airway surgery. Cureus 9: e983.
37. Erdim, Erdur O, Oghan F, Mete F, Celik M (2017) Blood count values and ratios for predicting sleep apnea in obese children. Int J Pediatr Otorhinolaryngol 98: 85-90.
38. Yegïn Y, Çelik M, Kaya KH, Koç AK, Kayhan FT (2017) Comparison of drug-induced sleep endoscopy and Müller's maneuver in diagnosing obstructive sleep apnea using the VOTE classification system. Braz J Otorhinolaryngol 83: 445-450.

7

Effects of the CPAP Treatment on the NON-REM Sleep Microstructures in Patients with Severe Apnea-Hypoapnea Syndrome

Marcela Smurra[1], Susana Blanco[2]*, Veronica Eguiguren[1] and Cecilia DiRisio[3]

[1]*Hospital Tornú, Argentina*
[2]*Faculty of Engineering, University of Belgrano-CONICET, Argentina*
[3]*Dosimetry Laboratory and Medical Technology, Faculty of Engineering, University of Belgrano, Argentina*

Abstract

Sleep quality is affected in patients with sleep apnea- hypopnea syndrome (SAHS) with nocturnal and diurnal consequences. Most of these patients who are treated with positive airway pressure (CPAP) return to normal sleep patterns. We could consider good sleepers those patients who present more sleep spindles in stage II, and slower wave sleep as a good sign of better sleep quality.

The objective in this research study was to compare the microstructure of stage II using the number of spindles and the increase of slow wave sleep before and after CPAP night titration.

We developed a wavelet filter using a spline cubic function from a wavelet mother, which was appropriate to be used over electroencephalographic signal. By means of this filter in a multi-resolution mode, the spindles were detected from the increase of the IV band power; the sampling rate of the device determined the filter characteristics. The staging of polysomnographic studies was made by an expert according AASM (American Academy of Sleep Medicine) and then processed by the filter to get the index of sleep spindles before-and-after CPAP during stage II as well as the relationship between fast and slow powers from the EEG signal. An increase in the power of the slow waves vs. fast activity was observed in all the cases as a feature of better sleep. The neuroprotective effect described in previous research works regarding the density of the sleep spindles seems to be detected in patients improving their sleep quality after the correction of the apnea-hypopnea syndrome using CPAP.

Keywords: Sleep spindles; Polisomnographic; Wavelets analysis; Slow wave sleep; CPAP

Introduction

The Sleep Apnea-Hypopnea Syndrome (SAHS) is a disorder characterized by recurrent episodes of either a partial or complete collapse of the upper airway during sleep. The resulting reduction of the airflow leads to alterations in gas exchange as well as recurrent arousals causing sleep fragmentation.

The prevalence rate is 3-7% and 2-5% in men and women respectively [1-3]. Clinically, somnolence is the most important symptom and it depends on the sleep fragmentation caused by microarousals related to respiratory effort and intermittent hypoxemia or both. With CPAP treatment, it is possible to achieve shorter times of reaction in vigilance tests as well higher levels in talking, visual and spatial memory tasks. It is also possible to improve depression and anxiety scores.

Spindles are structures of sleep EEG with a frequency range between 12 and 15 Hz, and with a duration of more than 0.5 seconds and a minimum width of 15 mV [4,5]. In previous studies comparing frequency patterns of spindles in patients with sleep apnea vs. control subjects, there was less frequency of sleep spindles within the former group, with no increase of spindles towards the end of the night [6].

Accordingly, the aim of the present work was to study the increase of spindles in phase II and slow wave sleep power vs fast wave sleep power frequency in patients with severe sleep apnea syndrome, quantifying them by indexes, before and after modifying the breathing pattern with CPAP treatment, considering these changes features of stable sleep.

Materials and Methods

We have performed the analysis of the sleep structure in the polysomnographic studies of 10 patients at baseline situation and post-calibration of CPAP to score sleep according to AASM standards [7].

Records were taken through the following standard:

1. Three channels of EEG: Two central (C3 and C4) and one occipital (O1) referenced to the left and right mastoids (A2 and A1) (systems 10-20) with sampling frequency of 349 Hz.
2. Two EOG channels with left and right eyelid electrodes.
3. Three EMG channels, two of them in sub-chin position and the other one in tibial location with a sampling frequency of 349 Hz.
4. EKG recorded from two electrode derivations in the second right and left intercostals space in paraesternal location with a sampling frequency of 349 Hz.
5. Oronasal flow sensors. One of them, of a thermistor type, and a nasal cannula with a pressure transducer to detect flow limitation through nasal pressure measurement.

***Corresponding author:** Susana Blanco, Faculty of Engineering, University of Belgrano-CONICET, Villanueva 1324, Buenos Aires, Argentina; E-mail: susana.blanco2006@gmail.com

6. A thoracic and abdominal piezoelectric band to record breathing effort.
7. A body position sensor.
8. Pulse oxymetry.

All records were carried out with 18-channel ATI Praxis equipment specially designed for polysomnography. (Polysomnograph equipment, Praxis 18-Line AMP18P-Lermed s.r.l Trade Mark).

Visual assessment of the alpha band power behavior with respect to the marked micro-awakenings was performed with the software associated with the AMP 18P. The remaining algorithms required to calculate the synchronization between ECG and EEG channels were developed with the help of MatLab 7.0.

Polysomnographic tracings in NREM stage were chosen and read sequentially in order to avoid the bias produced by the simultaneous observation of EEG and breathing events. At first, the EEG scoring was performed according to AAMS standards [7]; arousals are defined as an abrupt shift of EEG frequency including alpha, theta and/or frequencies greater than 16 Hz (but not spindles) that last at least 3 seconds, with at least 10 seconds of stable sleep preceding the change. Scoring of arousal during REM requires a concurrent increase in sub mental EMG lasting at least 1 second.

The respiratory events were classified as follows:

Apneas: There is a drop in the peak signal excursion by ≥ 90% of pre-event baseline using an oronasal thermal sensor (diagnostic study), PAP device flow (titration study) or an alternative apnea sensor (diagnostic study), during ≥ 10 seconds. Score an apnea as obstructive if it meets apnea criteria and is associated with continued or increased inspiratory effort throughout the entire period of absent airflow, as central if it meets apnea criteria and is associated with absent inspiratory effort throughout the entire period of absent airflow, and an apnea as mixed if it meets apnea criteria and is associated with absent inspiratory effort in the initial portion of the event, followed by resumption of inspiratory effort in the second portion of the event.

Hypopnea: The peak signal excursions drop by ≥ 30% of pre-event baseline using nasal pressure (diagnostic study), PAP device flow (titration study), or an alternative hypopnea sensor (diagnostic study) during ≥ 10 seconds. There is a ≥ 3% oxygen desaturation from pre-event baseline or the event is associated with an arousal.

Respiratory effort-related arousals, score a respiratory event as a respiratory effort-related arousal (RERA) if there is a sequence of breaths lasting ≥ 10 seconds characterized by increasing respiratory effort or by flattening of the inspiratory portion of the nasal pressure (diagnostic study) or PAP device flow (titration study) waveform leading to arousal from sleep when the sequence of breaths does not meet criteria for an apnea or hypopnea.

We have scored the severity of the disease according to the RDI (respiratory disturbance index) calculated as: numbers of respiratory events/Total sleep time x 60. More than 15 events/hour are considered an index of severity to determine the application of CPAP.

To obtain an optimal CPAP titration, we have taken into account the elimination of respiratory events or their reduction to reach a residual respiratory disturbance index not exceeding 5/h.

An adequate oxygenation and the lack of arousals partially ensure some improvement of sleep quality.

As a measure of this improvement in phase II sleep, we defined in this work the index IS=spindles number /time (minutes) and the index IW=SWP/FWP as the relationship between the power of slow and rapid waves with independence of the spindle frequency.

Mathematical Detection of Sleep Spindles and Cuantification of Swp Y Fwp

The wavelet transform gives us a powerful tool to analyze, from a time-frequency point of view, very diverse problems in applied sciences or pure mathematics [8-12].

A wavelet is a smooth and quickly vanishing oscillating function with good localization in both frequency and time.

A wavelet family $\psi_{a,b}(t)$ is a set of elemental functions generated by dilations and translations of a unique admissible mother wavelet $\psi(t)$:

$$\psi_{a,b}(t) = |a|^{-1/2}\psi(t-b/a)$$

Where **a, b** $\mathcal{E}$ **R, a** $\neq$ **0** are the scale and translation parameters respectively and **t** is the time. As **a** increases, the wavelet becomes narrower. Thus we have a unique analytic pattern and its replicas at different scales and with variable localization in time.

Given a finite energy signal S(t), the different correlations $< S, \psi_{a,b}>$ indicate how precisely the wavelet function locally fits this signal at every scale **a.** This correlation operation defines the transformation that synthesizes the numerical information obtained in this way. From a different viewpoint, the wavelets of a family play the role of elemental functions, representing the functions as a superposition of wavelets correlated with the function for different scales (different **a's**). This makes it possible to organize the information in some particular structure to distinguish, for example, trends or the shape associated with long scales of the local details from corresponding short scales.

For the special selection of the function ψ and a discrete net of parameters $a_j = 2^{-j}$ and $b_{j,k} = 2^{-j}k$, with $j, k \,\mathcal{E}\, Z$ and the scale 2^{-j} give us the shift parameter.

The subfamily

$$\Psi_{j,k}(t) = 2^{j/2}\Psi(2^j(t-k))j, k \,\mathcal{E}\, Z$$

constitutes an orthonormal basis of the Hilbert space L^2 (R). In this way, we can obtain discrete transformations, and it is possible to expand the signal in series of wavelets.

The discrete wavelet transform associated with ψ is simply seen as a restriction of the continuous wavelet. In this case, as it is well known, the information given by the discrete wavelet transform can be organized according to a hierarchical scheme of nested subspaces called multi resolution analysis in L^2 (R).

In the present analysis, we used a multirresolution scheme based on cubic orthogonal spline functions as a mother wavelet, with a discretized version of the integral wavelet transform given by Unser (Unser, 1996 [8]). We selected this wavelet due to the fact that it forms a base in L^2 (R) with a very convenient characteristic of symmetry and simplicity:

$$S(t) = \sum_K S_O(k)\phi(t-k)$$

where $\Phi(t)$ is the cubic cardinal spline.

For any resolution level N<0 we can write the decomposition of the signal as:

$$S(t) = \sum_K SN(k)\phi(2^N t-k) + \sum_{j=-N}^{-1}\sum_K C_j(k)\psi_{j,k}(t)$$

where Cj(*k*)are the wavelet coefficients and the sequence {sN(k)} represents the coarser signal data at resolution level N.

The second term is the wavelet expansion.

Since the family $\{\psi_{j,k}(t)\}$ is an orthonormal basis for L^2 (R), the concept of energy is linked with the usual notions derived from the Fourier theory. The sum $E_j = \sum_K |C_j(k)|^2$ gives us the energy of the details of S(t) at level j; and the total energy is given by $Etot = |S|^2 = \sum_{j<0} E_j$.

The polysomnographic system used for this research study let us obtain the raw data of each biological signal. Accordingly, we were able to develop the wavelet algorithm in the MATLAB programming environment.

We divided the EEG signals into 5 wavelet levels and we calculated a filter involving the characteristic frequencies of the sleep spindles (a burst with a spindle shape with frequencies between 11 and 15 Hz).

According to the characteristics of the multi-resolution scheme and sample rate of our equipment (349 Hz), spindles can be correlated to level 4 of a multi-resolution scheme.

Using the condition that the cubic spline functions constitute a base, each octave in which the signal is unfolded is linearly independent.

This enables us to calculate the energy of each octave independently by squaring the coefficients of the decomposition.

Using the power of the filtered signal in the band between 11 and 15 Hz as a way of viewing the spindles is both practical and graphic since the presence of a spindle is viewed as an increase of the resulting signal power.

In this manner it is simple to count spindles either manually or with peak-counting software. The software used for the wavelet analysis of the EEG signal was developed in Delphi language in order to connect it to the commercial software, with the authorization of the manufacturers and using windows to display and compare the signals.

As this multiresolution scheme let us calculate the energy of each octave independently, by squaring the coefficients of the wavelet decomposition, we define SPW summing the wavelet levels since 0.5 Hz to 8.0 Hz, and FWP summing the levels since 8.0 Hz to 30 Hz.

Results

The one-way ANOVA test was used to evaluate the differences between the indexes RDI, IS and IW in pre and post CPAP conditions. In the same way, by using the two-way ANOVA test, we evaluated the behavior of pre and post CPAP IS during the three different periods in which we divided every night of study. In all cases, we considered a 95% confidence level ($p<0.05$).

Table 1 shows the demographic characteristics of the patients and the respiratory disturbance index (RDI) pre and post CPAP results of the index. Statistical differences were observed when we compared the RDI (respiratory disturbance index) before and after CPAP.

Table 2 shows, for every patient, the indexes IS and IW before and after use of CPAP for the hole night.

There was an average percentage growth of the spindle rate per minute (IS) in all cases and an increase in the IW too. The use of CPAP leads to an increase in IW which is much higher than the increase of the index IS.

Statistical analysis (with α= 0.05) showed significant differences between the indexes IS before and after CPAP.

The relationship between slow wave power vs. fast waves (IW) statistical analysis of the indices (with α=0.05) showed significant differences pre and post CPAP.

To make a more detailed analysis, the nights were divided into thirds and spindles were counted in each. Table 3 shows the results for the IS index in each third of the night. Figure 1 show, plotted for the three thirds, pre and post CPAP IS indexes for each patient.

In the sample used, no significant differences were observed in the three night-time periods, either with or without CPAP, using the statistical variance F to a 95% confidence level. Significative differences were found for each third, pre and post CPAP.

Conclusion

The new proposed indexes, IS and IW, show a coherent behavior with the traditional RDI. These new indexes represent physiological information instead only statistical. We centralized our analysis in phase II.

Both indexes represent an indication of the physiological response to the CPAP use. Both are a representation of sleep quality but as it is well known, both have different neurological sources. It is interesting that both have a coherent response.

In our study, we detected a significant increase of the spindles/time index in patients with sleep breathing disorders, before and after the night of CPAP titration. There were no significant differences in the rate of spindles/time when we took into account three different times

Patient	Age	Sex	Weight	Height	BMI	RDI PRE	RDI POST
P1	62	M	82	1,67	29,40	68	6,4
P2	70	F	51	1,55	21,23	24,3	4,67
P3	70	F	61	1,58	24,43	14,9	6
P4	66	F	118	1,58	47,27	36,5	5,2
P5	60	M	107	1,8	33,02	37,3	0,45
P6	75	M	128	1,76	41,32	56,6	24
P7	65	M	89	1,78	28,09	56	5,6
P8	47	F	85	1,69	29,76	25,8	2,5
P9	76	F	74	1,59	29,27	32,5	1,2
P10	69	M	82	1,63	30,86	20,6	2,7

Table 1: Patient data, BMI: body mass index, RDI: respiratory disturbance index pre and post CPAP.

Patient	ISPr	ISPo	IWpr	IWpo
1	1.2	1.5	3,5	13,1
2	1.2	1.9	1,8	25,2
3	0.87	1.6	2,5	15,7
4	1.18	1.30	2,7	20,6
5	1.61	1.74	2,1	15,4
6	1.18	2.14	3,5	5,2
7	2.	2.16	4,3	17,2
8	1.74	1.89	2,2	7,3
9	1.56	2.6	0,9	1,2
10	2.1	2.7	1	2,1

Table 2: ISPr :spindles number /time (minutes) pre CPAP, ISPospindles number / time (minutes) post CPAP. IWprand, IWporelationship between the power of slow and rapid waves pre and post CPAP.

	ISPo	ISPr
P1	1,72	1,3
	1	1,27
	0,94	2,14
P2	1,53	1,9
	1,4	1,96
	1,78	1,82
P3	0,73	1,51
	1,06	1,76
	0,85	1,67
P4	1,2	1,03
	1,12	1,39
	1,18	1,37
P5	1,54	1,75
	1,57	1,57
	1,72	1,88
P6	1,2	2,21
	0,8	1,73
	1,41	2,16
P7	2	2,78
	1,8	2,3
	2,18	1,86
P8	1,55	1,7
	2,02	1,75
	1,81	2,5
P9	1,55	3,28
	1,53	2,27
	1,61	2
P10	2,13	2,35
	2,16	2,75
	2,27	2,75

Table 3: ISPo/r are the ISP index with and without CPAP during each third of the sleep time, for each patient.

at night. In the same sense, the increase of slow wave power vs. fast frequencies in EEG in studies with CPAP supports the hypothesis of the sleep protecting function in the transition of stage II to SWS.

The automatic spindle analysis has been technically solved with enough accuracy to detect these structures with antecedents in literature published since 1979, showing a good correlation between automatic and manual analysis and achieving 90% accuracy [13,14]. However, automatic scoring cannot take into consideration the differences in type and frequency of spindles [15]. In our study, we reached be very good results in identifying sleep structures using manual and automatic models to read polysomnographic tracings.

Old reports related sleep spindles as inhibitors of arousals and sleep preserver function; Hongo et al. [16] and Gaillard respectively [16,17] associated them with arousal inhibition. Accordingly, considering the K-complex as a possible transitory activation reaction, there is a description of an antagonistic effect with respect to the spindles, in other words, the higher the number of spindles, the fewer K-complexes. K-complexes represent an organismic state leading towards activation reaction [5]. Gora et al. [18] describe a "blunted" response to occlusion stimulus to elicit K-Complex in mild OSAS patients. We cannot detect a typical pattern in K-Complex distribution in relationship to Sleep Breathing Disorder before and after CPAP titration.

However, spindles participate in an activating effect through different ways generating thalamic activation processes for inhibiting access during NREM intrusive sounds, protecting the stability of sleep [19]. They also participate in sensory-motor processes and memory information [20].

The transition from low to high delta activity (starting in phase II with the progression from 3 to 4), which may indicate the deepness of sleep, supports the hypothesis of the relationship "sleep spindles-sleep stabilization", and sleep protecting function [15].

Patients with SAHS showed a lower level of neurocognitive information processing, initially related to sleep fragmentation and, secondly, to hypoxia episodes [19,20]. Hence, we hypothesized that other mechanisms, like the structural alterations of sleep that we observed in this study, can act as co-factors adding to transient arousal and hypoxia.

There are special situations to consider; in children, lower levels of sleep disruption were observed. NREM 2 sleep decreases but slow wave sleep is fairly preserved [21,22]. Sleep quality in obese patients is affected independently of the presence of sleep-related respiratory disorders with increased superficial sleep stages and decreased efficiency [23,24]. Even in patients with mild SAHS, a lower rate of sleep spindles, deep slow-wave sleep (SWS) and a greater index of arousal were observed in comparison with controls [25].

Although the efficacy of positive pressure for the elimination of respiratory events is fairly acknowledged, few details about its effect on sleep structure have been evaluated.

The slow spindle frequencies in apnea patients could indicate disturbed sleep and altered neural mechanisms in the structures regulating sleep spindle activity [26].

Loredo et al. [27] studied the effect of CPAP treatment on sleep quality in patients using the device for a short term and found no differences in those compared with sham CPAP [27].

More recently, an evaluation in the long term after an average 9-month CPAP use, the increase of deep slow wave sleep observed in the patients treated was similar to the proportion of SWS seen in the control group [28]. There was more SWS in prefrontal areas both before and after CPAP treatment, and SWS increased significantly more in prefrontal than central areas during treatment; even using a central location of electrodes, significant changes were obtained in SWS proportion [29].

The decrease of the tendency to present arousals in deep slow wave sleep would be the explanation for the increased neuromechanical stability of the upper airway at this stage of sleep [30-32] even though the compensatory ventilation response in either deep slow wave sleep or stage II does not appear to be different when assessed through the use of dial-down techniques from therapeutic levels of CPAP. The only finding that establishes a difference is that in phase II, the arousal threshold is lower than in the slow sleep pattern [33].

As far as we know, there are no bibliographic references about structural changes in sleep in relation to the effect of nasal positive pressure during the titration process in the same patient. The choice of indexes of spindles/minute, or the relationship SWS/fast frequencies seems to illustrate more clearly, according to our criteria, the change of EEG frequencies rather than their absolute variations as dynamic indicators of the changes generated by the treatment, showing significant modifications in the sleep microstructure as a sign of therapeutic success in the same patient.

However, it should certainly be emphasized that in our study, we can add sleep structural modifications to sleep and oximetric stability

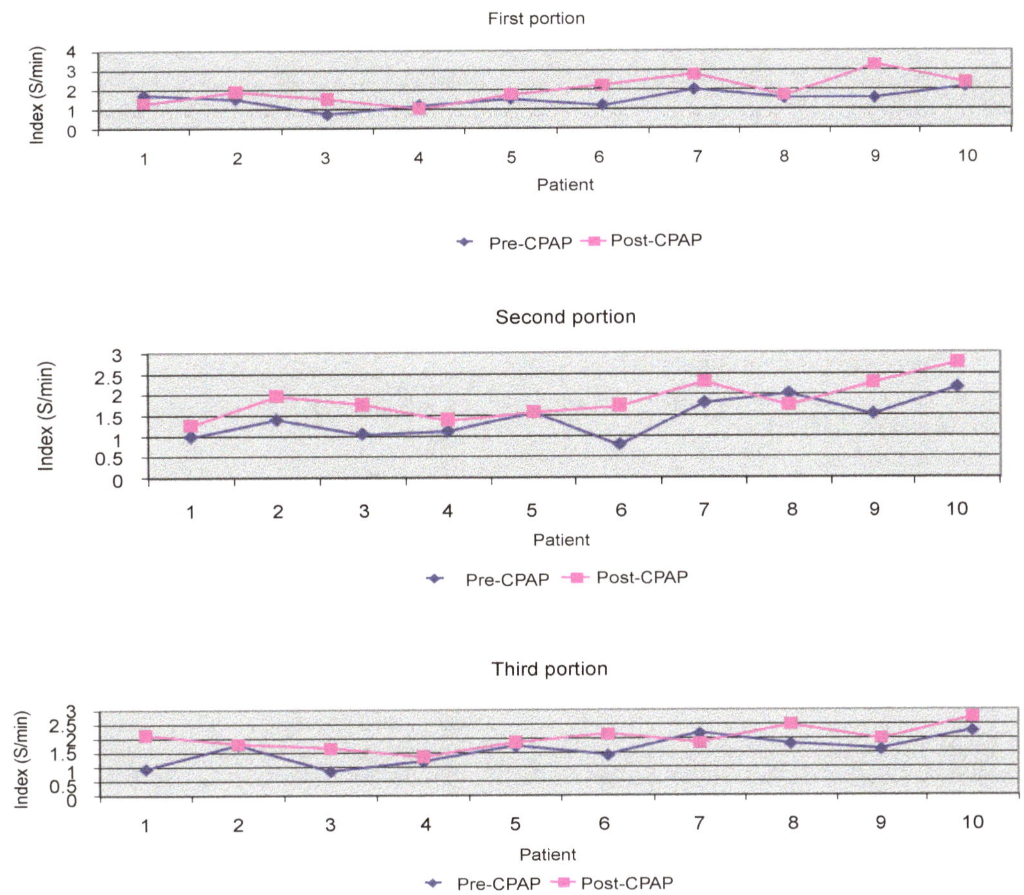

Figure 1: IS index for each patient and portion of sleep time.

to consider efficient CPAP titration, and with long term use of CPAP, the improvement in both the clinical and the neurocognitive courses can be achieved.

We think that a multirresolution scheme filter, using a mother wavelet cubic spline, is an appropriate tool to isolate sleep microstructures patterns. Furthermore, assessments should include the evaluation of the clinical impact of these changes in sleep structure, and the comparison of the acute effect of sleep deprivation in individuals without sleep breathing disorders.

References

1. Young T, Palta M, Dempsey J, Skatrud J, Weber S, et al. (1993) The occurrence of sleep-disordered breathing among middle-aged adults. N Engl J Med 328: 1230-1235.
2. Bixler EO, Vgontzas AN, Lin HM, Ten Have T, Rein J, et al. (2001) Prevalence of sleep-disordered breathing in women: effects of gender. Am J Respir Crit Care Med 163: 608-613.
3. Roure N, Mediano O, Durán-Cantolla J, García Río F, de la Peña M, et al. (2008) [Differences in clinical and polysomnographic variables between male and female patients with sleep apnea-hypopnea syndrome]. Arch Bronconeumol 44: 685-688.
4. Naitoh P, Antony-Baas V, Muzet A, Ehrhart J (1982) Dynamic relation of sleep spindles and K-complexes to spontaneous phasic arousal in sleeping human subjects. Sleep 5: 58-72.
5. Ehrhart J, Ehrhart M, Muzet A, Schieber JP, Naitoh P (1981) K-complexes and sleep spindles before transient activation during sleep. Sleep 4: 400-407.
6. Huupponen E, Himanen SL, Hasan J, Verri A (2003) Automatic analysis of electro-encephalogram sleep spindle frequency throughout the night. Med Biol Eng Comput 41: 727-732.
7. Berry RB, Brooks R, Gamaldo CE, Harding SM, Marcus CL, et al. (20120 American Academy of Sleep Medicine. The AASM Manual for the Scoring of Sleep and Associated Events: Rules, Terminology and Technical Specifications, Version 2.0. Darien, Illinois, American Academy of Sleep Medicine.
8. Unser M, Aldroubi A (1996) Review of Wavelets in Biomedical Applications. Proc of IEEE 84: 626-638.
9. Blanco S, D'Attellis CE, Isaacson SI, Rosso OA, Sirne RO (1996) Time-frequency analysis of electroencephalogram series. II. Gabor and wavelet transforms. Phys Rev E Stat Phys Plasmas Fluids Relat Interdiscip Topics 54: 6661-6672.
10. Blanco S, Kochen S, Rosso OA, Salgado P (1997) Applying time-frequency analysis to seizure EEG activity. IEEE Eng Med Biol Mag 16: 64-71.
11. Blanco S, Figliola A, Quiroga RQ, Rosso OA, Serrano E (1998) Time-Frequency analysis of electroencephalogram series (III): Information Transfer Function and Wavelets Packets. Physical Review E 57: 932-940.
12. Rosso OA, Blanco S, Yordanova J, Kolev V, Figliola A, et al. (2001) Wavelet entropy: a new tool for analysis of short duration brain electrical signals. J Neurosci Methods 105: 65-75.
13. Matsubayashi K, Ishiyama Y, Homma I, Ebe M (1981) Some characteristics of sleep spindles derived from automatic analysis. Sleep 4: 392-399.
14. Kumar A, Hofman W, Campbel K (1979) An Authomatic spindle analysis and detection system based on the evaluation of human ratings of the spindle quality. Walking and Sleeping 3: 325-33.

15. Kubicki S, Herrmann WM (1996) The future of computer-assisted investigation of the polysomnogram: sleep microstructure. J Clin Neurophysiol 13: 285-294.

16. Hongo T, Kubota K, Shimazu H (1963) EEG spindle and depression of gamma motor activity. J Neurophysiol 26: 568-580.

17. Gaillard JM, Aubert C (1975) Specificity of benzodiacepine action on human sleep confirmed, another contribution of authomatic analysis of polygraph recordings. Biol Spsychiatry 10: 185-197.

18. Gora J, Trinder J, Pierce R, Colrain IM (2002) Evidence of a sleep-specific blunted cortical response to inspiratory occlusions in mild obstructive sleep apnea syndrome. Am J Respir Crit Care Med 166: 1225-1234.

19. Schabus M, Dang-Vu TT, Albouy G, Balteau E, Boly M, et al. (2007) Hemodynamic cerebral correlates of sleep spindles during human non-rapid eye movement sleep. Proc Natl Acad Sci U S A 104: 13164-13169.

20. Verstraeten E (2007) Neurocognitive effects of obstructive sleep apnea syndrome. Curr Neurol Neurosci Rep 7: 161-166.

21. Cote KA, Epps TM, Campbell KB (2000) The role of the spindle in human information processing of high-intensity stimuli during sleep. J Sleep Res 9: 19-26.

22. Yang JSC, Nicholas CL, Nixon GM, Davey MJ, Anderson V, et al. (2010) Determining sleep quality in children with sleep disordered breathing: EEG spectral analysis compared with conventional polysomnography. Sleep 33: 1165-1172.

23. Vgontzas AN, Bixler EO, Tan TL, Kantner D, Martin LF, et al. (1998) Obesity without sleep apnea is associated with daytime sleepiness. Arch Intern Med 158: 1333-1337.

24. Resta O, Foschino Barbaro MP, Bonfitto P, Giliberti T, Depalo A, et al. (2003) Low sleep quality and daytime sleepiness in obese patients without obstructive sleep apnoea syndrome. J Intern Med 253: 536-543.

25. Ondze B, Espa F, Dauvilliers Y, Billiard M, Besset A (2003) Sleep architecture, slow wave activity and sleep spindles in mild sleep disordered breathing. Clin Neurophysiol 114: 867-874.

26. Himanen SL, Virkkala J, Huuponen E, Hasan J (2003) Spindle frequency remains slow in sleep apnea patients throughout the night. Sleep Med 4: 229-234.

27. Loredo JS, Ancoli-Israel S, Dimsdale JE (1999) Effect of continuous positive airway pressure vs placebo continuous positive airway pressure on sleep quality in obstructive sleep apnea. Chest 116: 1545-1549.

28. Heinzer R, Gaudreau H, Décary A, Sforza E, Petit D, et al. (2001) Slow-wave activity in sleep apnea patients before and after continuous positive airway pressure treatment: contribution to daytime sleepiness. Chest 119: 1807-1813.

29. Eskelinen V, Uibu T, Himanen SL (2007) nCPAP treatment of obstructive sleep apnea increases slow wave sleep in prefrontal EEG. Clin EEG Neurosci 38: 148-154.

30. Gleeson K, Zwillich CW, White DP (1990) The influence of increasing ventilatory effort on arousal from sleep. Am Rev Respir Dis 142: 295-300.

31. Berry RB, Bonnet MH, Light RW (1992) Effect of ethanol on the arousal response to airway occlusion during sleep in normal subjects. Am Rev Respir Dis 145: 445-452.

32. Berry RB, Asyali MA, McNellis MI, Khoo MC (1998) Within-night variation in respiratory effort preceding apnea termination and EEG delta power in sleep apnea. J Appl Physiol (1985) 85: 1434-1441.

33. Ratnavadivel R, Stadler D, Windler S, Bradley J, Paul D, et al. (2010) Upper airway function and arousability to ventilatory challenge in slow wave versus stage 2 sleep in obstructive sleep apnoea. Thorax 65: 107-112.

8

Evaluation of Sleep Quality by Actigraphy in Women with Systemic Lupus Erythematosus (SLE)

Lílian KCR[1*], Cristiane K[2], Branca DBS[3], Marco TM[4], Virgínia FMT[1]

[1]*Physiotherapist, Master´s Student. Evidence-based Healthcare Program, Federal University of São Paulo (UNIFESP), Brazil.*
[2]*Affiliate Professor. Department of Rheumatology, Federal University of São Paulo (UNIFESP), Brazil.*
[3]*Assistant Professor. Department of Rheumatology, Santa Casa de Misericórdia, São Paulo, Brazil.*
[4]*Associate Professor. Department of Sports, Federal University of Minas Gerais (UFMG), Brazil.*
[5]*Assistant Professor. Evidence-based Healthcare Program, Federal University of São Paulo (UNIFESP) and Titular Professor. Department of Rheumatology, University of Santo Amaro (UNISA), Brazil*

Abstract

Despite the small number of studies about sleep quality and its possible occurrence in SLE, it is a frequent complaint among patients. This study evaluated sleep quality using actigraphy and the Pittsburgh sleep quality index (PSQI) in 46 women with SLE and the relationship between disease activity, cumulative damage, quality of life, pain intensity, fatigue, and medication to treat the disease, as well as the influence of pain intensity (subgroups) on quality of life. The short-form 36 health survey (SF-36) assessed health related quality of life (HRQoL), the fatigue severity scale (FSS) assessed fatigue, and the visual analog scale (VAS) was used to evaluate pain intensity. The significance level was 5%. Objective and subjective measures were concordant in sleep latency. Univariate logistic regression analysis was performed using categorized VAS pain as a dependent variable, we found an association with sleep latency (actigraphy), PSQI global score, six components of the SF-36 (physical functioning, role physical or role limitations due to physical problems, bodily pain, vitality, social functioning, role emotional or role limitations due to emotional problems), and fatigue. In the final analyses, using multivariate logistic regression, the model showed that the predicting variables for HPG (high pain group) and LPG (low pain group) were sleep latency and fatigue. Perhaps we did not find associations between sleep and quality of life as other factors were more relevant, such as pain and fatigue.

Keywords: Systemic lupus erythematosus; Sleep quality actigraphy; quality of life; pain

Introduction

Systemic lupus erythematosus (SLE) is a chronic autoimmune disease, characterized by the production of several autoantibodies, where an imbalance between the action of B and T lymphocytes lead to attacks on the nucleus and cell membrane [1]. Despite the unknown origins, its etiology is multifactorial, since some factors such as genetic, hormonal, environmental, and infectious can favor its appearance [2]. SLE can reach any organs and/or systems, such as skin, joints, eyes, heart, kidneys, lungs, vascular system, and central nervous system (CNS) simultaneously or sequentially, hence it can also be classified as a multisystemic disease, marked by periods of remission and exacerbation, as well as changes in laboratory tests [3,4]. The patients are mostly young women, between 20 and 30 years of age, of fertile and productive age [5].

The presence of cytokines, responsible for the inflammatory process, disease activity, the chronic use of corticosteroids that affect the sleep-wake cycle, psychological factors, and disability in valued life activities, can impair sleep quality, increase levels of pain and fatigue, and worsen depressive mood, causing work withdrawals, help to be required to perform simple tasks (such as cleaning the house), abandonment of social activities, and isolation with a consequent negative impact on perception of quality of life [1,6-14].

Despite the small number of studies on sleep quality and its possible occurrence in SLE, it is a frequent complaint among patients, related by over 50%; the methodologies are not standardized, and, furthermore, the majority of investigations are subjective [6,7,10,15]. Only two studies, used polysomnography, a gold-standard measurement [16,17], where research revealed a longer time to fall asleep (sleep latency), frequent episodes of awakenings, restlessness, and a shorter sleep duration. In recent years, researchers have chosen to use the actigraph as an auxiliary tool to study sleep habits in special populations, such as rheumatoid arthritis (RA) [18], primary Sjögren's syndrome (pSS) [19] osteoarthritis [20], fibromyalgia [21,22], chronic back pain [23], breast cancer [24], and recently SLE [25].

Because of these findings, the primary aim of our study was to evaluate sleep quality using actigraphy in women with SLE and secondarily to determine the concordance between measurements of sleep quality and the relationship between these tools with disease activity, cumulative damage, health related quality of life, pain intensity, fatigue, and medication to treat the disease.

Methods

Participants

This cross-sectional study was approved by the local Research Ethics Committee (UNIFESP, CEP number 51425). Eighty women with SLE fulfilling the 1982 revised American College of Rheumatology (ACR) criteria [3,4], and also the SLICC new classification criteria from 2012 [26] were potentially eligible to participate in the study. The sample was aged between 18 and 69 years and those who reported sleep complaints (PSQI ≥ 5) were invited to participate in this study. The exclusion criteria

***Corresponding author:** Lílian Karla Cunha dos Reis, Evidence-Based Healthcare Program, Federal University of São Paulo (UNIFESP). 325 Carvalho de Freitas st, ap 102 bloque 1, 05728-030, São Paulo, SP Brazil;
E-mail: lilian.reis2004@gmail.com

consisted of associated rheumatic diseases, use of sleeping medication or medication that had this effect (cyclobenzaprine, antihistamines, tranquilizers, sedative hypnotics), suspected or confirmed pregnancy, and lack of interest. Thirty-four women were excluded from the study because they did not meet the inclusion criteria: nine had other associated rheumatologic conditions (06 fibromyalgia, 01 rheumatoid arthritis, 02 Sjögren's syndrome), 08 did not report sleep complaints (PSQI<5), 06 were taking sleep medication, 05 were not interested, 05 were employed and had no time to participate, and 01 patient was pregnant.

Procedure

The study began in April 2013 and ended in September 2014. All patients signed an Informed Consent Term. We collected sociodemographic and clinical data, such as age, race, education, occupation, disease duration, and medications being used at that moment. A trained researcher administered the questionnaires.

Measures

Objective sleep quality: Actigraphy [27-29] and the Pittsburgh Sleep Quality Index (PSQI) [30,31] were used to evaluate the quantitative and qualitative data about sleep quality, respectively. The actigraph is a device such a wristwatch, which evaluates the sleep-wake cycle by recording limb movements over a 15-day period. The participants were asked to push a button on the device each night when they were about to fall asleep and when they got out of bed each morning, including NAPS during the day, if they occurred (and mark these times in a sleep diary). The button needed to be pressed to mark specific times and did not start or stop recording data. The participants were requested to remove the actigraph for activities that involved water use. The information was downloaded using Motionlogger WatchWare® software, version 1.94.2.0, 2012 (Ambulatoring Monitoring Inc., Ardsley, NY, USA) and interpreted using Action-W® version 2.7, 1996-2014 Ambulatory Monitoring Inc., by the Cole-Kripke algorithm [32]. The parameters assessed included: sleep latency, the time between when the subject got into bed and fell asleep; time of wake ups after sleep onset (WASO), a measure of sleep disruption or fragmentation, defined as the total minutes of time scored as awake from the onset to the end of the sleep interval; sleep efficiency, the percentage of time that the subject is sleeping in the bed, and the total sleep time (TST) (i.e., the total time in minutes scored of the patient being asleep in their bed). The questionnaires were applied after the period that participants used the actigraph.

Subjective sleep quality: The PSQI is a self-rated questionnaire that provides an index of sleep quality for the previous month. It contains 19 different items, distributed in seven subcomponents (duration of sleep, sleep disturbance, sleep latency, daytime dysfunction, sleep efficiency, sleep quality, and use of medication). Each subcomponent is scored from 0 (better) to 3 (worse) points and results in a total range from 0 to 21, with a score ≥ 5 indicating poor sleepers and <5 good sleepers [30,31].

HR-QOL: Health-related quality of life was assessed using the Medical Outcome Study Short Form 36 Health Survey (SF-36) that consists of 36 items subdivided into eight components: physical functioning, role physical or role limitations due to physical problems, bodily pain, general health, vitality, social functioning, role-emotional or role limitations due to emotional problems, and mental health. Each component has a final score ranging from 0–100, where zero corresponds to poorer and 100 to better functional capacity and quality of life [33].

Fatigue: We used the Fatigue Severity Scale (FSS) that measures fatigue intensity over the two previous weeks, consisting of nine affirmations with scores ranging from 1-7, where 1 indicates that the subject totally disagrees with the affirmation and 7 indicates that the subject totally agrees with the affirmation. We obtained a final score through the mean of nine statements. Scores ≥ 4 indicate severe fatigue [34,35].

Pain intensity: A visual analog scale (VAS) was used to measure pain intensity, based on a straight line measured and expressed in centimeters ranging from 0-10 cm, where a higher number corresponds to a greater intensity of pain. The VAS was based on the previous week [36]. During the interview, we asked the question: "How much pain did you feel on average in the last week?"

Disease activity: The Systemic Lupus Erythematosus Disease Activity Index (SLEDAI-2K) evaluated the clinical parameters of disease activity. The scale ranges from 0-105, where 0 indicates no activity, 1-5 indicates mild activity, 6–10 indicates moderate activity, 11-19 indicates high activity, and 20+ indicates very high activity [37].

Cumulative damage: The Systemic Lupus International Collaborating Clinics/American College of Rheumatology Damage Index (SLICC/DI) assessed the cumulative damage from the disease or its sequelae in 12 organ systems (ocular, neuropsychiatric, renal, pulmonary, cardiovascular, peripheral vascular, gastrointestinal, musculoskeletal, skin, premature ovarian failure, metabolism, and neoplasm). The score of this index can range from 0-47 [38]. A rheumatologist applied both indices.

Subgroups

For the subgroup analysis, we dichotomized the SLE patients according to VAS score (0-10 cm) into a low-pain group (scores ranging from 0-4) and a high-pain group (scores ranging from 5-10) [14].

Data Analysis

Data collection was summarized using descriptive analysis, such as mean and standard deviation. For the subgroup analysis, we also used the interquartile range (IQR) value. Pearson´s correlation coefficient was used to evaluate the association between sleep quality (actigraphy and PSQI) and its predictors. It was also used to assess concordance between the sleep measurements on latency, efficiency, and total sleep time. The t-test was used to compare sleep quality and the use of medication for lupus treatment. The Mann-Whitney U test compared the subgroup variables. Regression analyses were computed to examine predictors of sleep quality and to test independent association of pain intensity with quality of life. Linear regression was performed to determine sociodemographic (age, education, occupation) and clinical variables (disease duration, pain, fatigue, use of medication) associated with each sleep quality measurement (actigraphy data and PSQI global score). This analyses is a strategy of choice, when the target is to determine the importance of a predictor variable(s) once others have already been entered into the equation [39]. The Software adopted was SPSS 2 (version 22.0) with a 5% significance level.

Results

General information: As summarized in Table 1, the sample was composed of 46 women with SLE and poor sleep quality (mean of PSQI 10.26). The age range was between 26 and 69 years with a mean of about 42.63 years, 54.35% were mixed race, 58.7% had started or completed middle school, and overall only 21.74% were employed. The mean of disease duration was 9.66 ± 7.02 years, with mild mean values of disease activity and little cumulative damage, SLEDAI-2K about 5.10 and SLICC/DI 0.80, respectively.

Overall, 65.22% of the sample had been taking prednisolone for at least 3 months, up to 10 mg/day; 60.87% antimalarial drugs (for the same period of the disease duration), the majority hydroxychloroquine (400 mg/day), and 69.56% was taking immunosuppressives, described in Table 1.

Regarding objective data about sleep, actigraphy revealed a longer mean time to fall asleep (sleep latency) of 33.86 min, compared to the general population, a mean awake duration after sleep onset of 39.01 min., a total sleep time of approximately 6.39 hours, and poor sleep quality with a mean PSQI of 10.26. Regarding health related quality of life, the lowest mean score in physical components such as role physical (or role limitations due to physical problems) was 35.33, followed by general health (mean 43.04), and bodily pain (mean 43.85). In these domains, the higher the score, the better the quality of life.

According to measurements of fatigue and pain, the results were high, with a mean and standard deviation of the fatigue severity scale of 4.11 ± 1.66 and a VAS mean above 5 cm (5.48 ± 2.63).

Table 2 exhibits data from the Pearson's correlation test relating to actigraphy data with the same PSQI domains in order to assess the consistency between both assessment methods. Two of the 46 patients did not use the actigraph correctly; therefore, data from 44 patients were included in the analysis. The WASO were not included as the PSQI did not contain this parameter separately. Of the three parameters, the only positive association was observed between sleep latency, with r=0.373 and p=0.013.

Correlations between sleep quality and its predictors: As shown in Table 3, correlations between the PSQI global score and its predictors, we did not find any association between poor sleep quality, disease activity (SLEDAI-2K), or cumulative damage (SLICC/DI). In health related quality of life, of the eight domains, we found a strong association between role emotional and higher sleep latency (r=-0.418, p=0.005), longer awakenings after sleep onset (r=-0.314, p=0.038), lower sleep efficiency (r= 0.302, p=0.046), and a strong association between PSQI global score (r=-0.398, p=0.006). In the other domains, we found positive associations only between poor sleep quality, role physical (r=-0.351, p=0.017), and mental health (r=-0.313, p=0.034).

Regarding fatigue score (FSS) and pain (VAS), the only association was between PSQI global score (p=0.048 and p=0.028, respectively). We did not find a relation between actigraphy data.

Use of medication to treat disease: We used the t-test to compare the PSQI global score and actigraphy parameters using dichotomous variables analysis (use of medication: yes or no), shown in Table 4. Patients who were not taking prednisolone presented a mean sleep duration of 408 min. (6.08 hours); on the other hand, those taking the medication exhibited a mean of 371 min (6.01 hours). This difference, which was nearly significant (p=0.056), indicated that patients using corticosteroids tend to experience shorter sleep duration. The only association that we observed was between the use of antimalarials and greater time to fall asleep (sleep latency), with a mean of 39.3 min.; patients that did not use these medications had a latency mean of 26 min. (p=0.032). We did not observe any association between immunosuppressives and sleep quality alterations. However, the patients that were taking this medication experienced more mean wake ups (WASO=43.7 min.) than those who were not. Rituximab was not included in the analysis as only one patient was using it.

Characteristics/Variables	n (%) or mean ± SD
Age, in years: mean ± SD	42.63 ± 10.1
Ethnicity: n (%)	
White	18 (39.13)
African	3 (6.52)
Mixed	25 (54.35)
Education: n (%)	
Some or completed elementary school	16 (34.8)
Some or completed middle school	27 (58.7)
Some or completed college	3 (6.5)
Occupation: n (%)	
Employed	10 (21.74)
On sick leave	6 (13.04)
Retired	8 (17.39)
Unemployed	22 (47.83)
Disease duration, in years: mean ± SD	9.66 ± 7.02
Disease activity (SLEDAI-2K)	5.10 ± 3.35
Cumulative Damage (SLICC/DI)	0.80 ± 1.27
Use of medication: n (%)	
Corticosteroids	30 (65.22)
Prednisolone (until 10 mg/day)	19
Prednisolone (until 15 mg/day)	1
Prednisolone (until 20 mg/day)	10
Antimalarials	28 (60.87)
Cloroquine diphosphate (250 mg/day)	4
Hydroxychloroquine (400 mg/day)	24
Immunossupressives	31
Azathioprine	11
Mycophenolate Mofetil	10
Methotrexate	9
Thalidomide	1
Cyclophosphamide	1
Immunobiologicals	
Rituximab	1 (2.17)
Actigraphy parameters	
Sleep latency1, 2	33.86 ± 21.17
WASO3	39.01 ± 24.26
Sleep eficciency4	91.35 ± 5.36
Total sleep time5	383.72 ± 61.48
Pittsburgh Sleep Quality Index	10.26 ± 3.24
Quality of life domains (SF-36)	
Physical Functioning	62.28 ± 24.17
Role Physical	35.33 ± 37.48
Bodily Pain	43.85 ± 22.35
General Health	43.04 ± 21.00
Vitality	53.26 ± 18.57
Social Functioning	63.08 ± 19.37
Role Emotional	55.08 ± 41.11
Mental Health	63.39 ± 18.38
Fatigue Severity Scale	4.11 ± 1.66
Fatigue (VAS) (cm)	6.08 ± 2.48
Pain (VAS) (cm)	5.48 ± 2.63

SLE: Systemic Lupus Erythematosus; SD: Standard Deviation; 1: Time to fall asleep; 2:normal value for a health adult of 15-20 min.; WASO: Wakeups After Sleep Onset; 3:normal value 5-15 min.; 4: normal value 85-90%; 5: normal value 6-8 hours; SF-36: Short-Form 36 health survey; VAS: Visual Analog Scale; SLEDAI-2K: Systemic Lupus Erythematosus Disease Activity Index; SLICC/DI: Systemic Lupus International Collaborating Clinics Damage Index.

Table 1: Descriptive analysis of demographic, clinical characteristics and scores of the 46 women with SLE.

Variables	r	p-value
Sleep latency	0.373	0.013*
Sleep efficiency	-0.134	0.385
Total sleep time	-0.172	0.573

PSQI: Pittsburgh Sleep Quality Index; r: Pearson´s correlation test; *Significant correlation (p <0.05) between actigraphy and respective PSQI domains.

Table 2: Correlation between actigraphy and respective PSQI domains.

Variables	ACT_SL	ACT_ WASO	ACT_ SE	ACT_ TST	PSQI
Disease activity (SLEDAI-2K)	–	-	-	-	-
Cumulative Damage (SLICC/DI)	-	-	-	-	-
Quality of life domains (SF-36)	-	-	-	-	-
Physical Functioning	-	-	-	-	-
Role Physical	-	-	-	-	r=0.351
	-	-	-	-	p=0.017
Bodily Pain	-	-	-	-	-
General Health	-	-	-	-	-
Vitality	-	-	-	-	-
Social Functioning	-	-	-	-	-
Role Emotional	r=0.418	r=-0.314	r=0.302	-	r=-0.398
	p=0.005	p=0.038	p=0.046	-	p=0.006
Mental Health	-	-	-	-	r=-0.313
	-	-	-	-	p=0.034
Fatigue (FSS)	-	-	-	-	r=0.294
	-	-	-	-	p=0.048
Pain (VAS)	-	-	-	-	r=0.325
	-	-	-	-	p=0.028

ACT: Actigraphy; SL: Sleep Latency, WASO: Wakeups After Sleep Onset; SE: Sleep Efficiency; TST: Total Sleep Time; PSQI: Pittsburgh Sleep Quality Index; SLEDAI-2K: Systemic Lupus Erythematosus Disease Activity Index; SLICC/DI: Systemic Lupus International Collaborating Clinics Damage Index; FSS: Fatigue Severity Scale; VAS: Visual Analog Scale; r: Pearson´s correlation test; p: significance level of correlation between sleep quality and predictors.

Table 3: Correlation between sleep quality and its predictors (n=46).

Sleep quality measurement	Class of medication	YES[1] mean ± SD	NO[2] mean ± SD	p-value[3]
Actigraphy				
Sleep duration	Prednisolone	371.0 ± 60.4	408.2 ± 57.9	0.056
Sleep latency	Antimalarials	39.3 ±22.2	26.0 ± 17.2	**0.032ł**

1: Data from the patients who was taking a certain class of medication; 2: Data from the patients who was not taking a certain class of medication; 3: Significance level after compare patients who was and who was not taking a certain class of medication (T test); ł: Significant correlation (p<0.05) between the sleep latency measured by actigraphy and use of antimalarials.

Table 4: Comparison between actigraphy variables and the use of medication (n=44).

Descriptive analysis and comparisons between subgroups: Table 5 presents the descriptive and comparative analysis data between the subgroup variables, divided according to pain intensity into a low pain group (VAS ≤ 4) and high pain group (VAS>4). In terms of disease activity and cumulative damage, there were no relations between them, without statistical significance.

In terms of actigraphy, the mean time to fall asleep (sleep latency) in the high pain group (HPG) was almost double that in the low pain group (LPG) (38.86 *vs.* 21.92 min.), with p = 0.010. Indeed, the PSQI global score was also higher in patients with high pain (mean = 11.03 *vs.* 8.30), with the same significance value (p=0.010). Of the eight health-related quality of life domains, the subgroups exhibited significant differences in six of them: physical functioning, role physical (role limitations due to physical problems), bodily pain, vitality, social functioning, and role emotional (role limitations due to emotional problems). The higher the intensity of pain, the poorer the perception of quality of life. The subgroups exhibited significant differences in the fatigue severity scale, the mean of the HPG was 41.33 *vs.* 25.92 points (p=0.003).

Regression analyses: After performing comparative analysis, we carried out linear regressions and did not find significant relations between demographic aspects (age, education, occupation, disease duration) and sleep quality. Performing univariate logistic regression analysis using categorized VAS pain as a dependent variable, we found an association with the variables shown in (Table 6): sleep latency (actigraphy), PSQI global score, six components of the SF-36 (physical functioning, role physical or role limitations due to physical problems, bodily pain, vitality, social functioning, role emotional or role limitations due to emotional problems), and fatigue (FSS). In the final analyses, described in (Table 7), using multivariate logistic regression, the model showed the predicting variables for HPG and LPG as being sleep latency (OR=1.120, p=0.030) and fatigue (FSS) (OR=4.688, p=0.005), where each unit of increase in FSS score, increased the chance of the individual belonging to the HPG 4.688 times.

Discussion

Variables	HPG (n=33)	LPG (n=13)	p-valueł
SLEDAI, mean ± SD (IQR)	5.60 ± 3.74 (3.00-6.00)	3.84 ±1.51 (2.0-5.0)	0.079
SLICC, mean ± SD (IQR)	0.84 ± 1.39 (0.00-1.00)	0.69 ± 0.94 (0.0-1.0)	0.823
Actigraphy			
Sleep latency (min.), mean ± SD (IQR)	38.86 ± 22.15 (18.7-52.7)	21.92 ±12.65 (13.0-29.1)	0.01
WASO (min.), mean ± SD (IQR)	39.75 ± 26.30 (17.6-58.4)	37.26 ± 19.38 (23.0-53.0)	0.87
Sleep eficciency (%), mean ± SD (IQR)	91.16 ± 5.70 (87.6-95.7)	91.82 ± 4.64 (87.6-95.5)	0.84
Total sleep time (min.), mean ± SD (IQR)	379.70 ± 62.40 (345.0-404.0)	393.4 ± 60.4 (341.2.-445.1)	0.45
PSQI, mean ± SD (IQR)	11.03 ± 3.00 (9.0-13.5)	8.30 ± 3.11 (5.5-11.0)	0.01
Quality of life domains(SF-36)			
Physical Functioning, mean ± SD (IQR)	55.45 ± 22.99 (42.5-75.0)	79.62 ±18.08 (75.0-92.5)	<0.001
Role Physical, mean ± SD (IQR)	23.48 ± 31.21 (0 - 50.0)	65.40 ± 36.10 (25.0-100)	<0.001
Bodily Pain, mean ± SD (IQR)	38.64 ± 19.49 (22.0-51.5)	57.08 ± 24.40 (41.0-73.0)	0.01
General Health, mean ± SD (IQR)	40.52 ± 23.15 (26.0-52.0)	49.46 ± 12.74 (38.5-59.5)	0.09
Vitality, mean ± SD (IQR)	49.85 ± 19.14 (32.5-65.0)	61.92 ± 14.22 (47.5-75.0)	0.03
Social Functioning, mean ± SD (IQR)	56.83 ± 16.57 (50.0 69.0)	78.92 ± 17.20 (75.0-94.0)	<0.001
Role Emotional, mean ± SD (IQR)	41.41 ± 39.11 (0 - 66.6)	89.77 ± 20.98 (83.5-100)	<0.001
Mental Health, mean ± SD (IQR)	59.88 ± 19.61 (40.0-76.0)	72.31 ± 11.01 (62.0-80.0)	0.06
Fatigue Severity Scale, mean ± SD (IQR)	4.59 ± 1.43 (3.27-5.89)	2.88 ± 1.61 (1.72-3.72)	0.002

HPG: High Pain Group; LPG: Low Pain Group. Ł: Mann-Whitney Test; SLEDAI-2K: Systemic Lupus Erythematosus Disease Activity Index; SLICC/DI: Systemic Lupus International Collaborating Clinics Damage Index; WASO: Wakeups After Sleep Onset; PSQI: Pittsburgh Sleep Quality Index; VAS: Visual Analog Scale.

Table 5: Descriptive analysis and comparisons between the subgroup variables.

Variables	β	S.E	p-value
Sleep latency (actigraphy)	0.055	0.025	0.027
Pittsburgh sleep quality index (PSQI)	0.313	0.130	0.016
Physical functioning (SF-36)	-0.073	0.028	0.008
Role physical (SF-36)	-0.033	0.011	0.002
Bodily pain (SF-36)	-0.045	0.019	0.020
Social Functioning (SF-36)	-0.078	0.026	0.003
Role emotional (SF-36)	-0.044	0.015	0.003
Mental health (SF-36)	-0.043	0.022	0.047
Fatigue severity scale (FSS)	0.768	0.270	0.004

SE: Standard Error. After performing the univariate analysis, we found that the patients who were in HPG had worsen results with significant values in sleep latency (actigraphy), sleep quality (PSQI), six domains of the SF-36 about quality of life and fatigue (FSS).

Table 6: Univariate logistic regression analysis predicting low pain group and high pain group.

Variables	β	S.E.	p-value
Sleep latency (actigraphy)	0.124	0.048	0.009
Fatigue severity scale (FSS)	1.545	0.546	0.005

SE: Standard Error, OR: Odds Ratio. After performed a multivariate model with all of variables that were significant in the univariate analysis, we obtained the above model, that is, in the presence of the other variables, the significant predictors for HPG and LPG are sleep latency and fatigue, according fatigue severity scale (FSS).

Table 7: Final multivariate logistic regression model with significant variables in univariate analysis.

This work presents new research in the field of SLE. The majority of studies on sleep quality in these patients have relied on subjective assessment tools. Two studies [16,17] used polysomnography (PSG), the gold-standard tool used to diagnose sleep disorders. However, in some cases, it is not feasible to use PSG due to its high cost and the necessity for specific laboratories in which patients sleep one or more nights, which disrupts the usual sleep routine [27,29]. On the other hand, actigraphy provides quantitative information and allows patients to maintain their usual sleep routine. A very recent study with SLE patients and actigraphy by Baldera-Díaz et al., [25], used actigraphy and mHealth systems for objective analyses of sleep quality. Their sample included nine SLE women who exhibited poor sleep quality, and more pain intensity, fatigue, and depression than the healthy controls, but they did not found significant differences in measures of actigraphy. We found differences between objective and subjective measures only in sleep latency, maybe because, according to Liu et al. [24], measures of actigraphy are closer to PSG than PSQI (i.e., objective data resemble other objectives, on the other hand, subjective data resembles other tools with the same characteristics). Landry et al. [40] suggested that the temporal difference between PSQI and actigraphy might explain their discrepancies, but a stronger contribution in relation to the distinction between subjective versus objective methods. Although the mean of total sleep time was <7 h, there was no significant relation between actigraphy and PSQI for this variable. Actigraphy provides indirect assessment of sleep using algorithms and automatic scoring methods to distinguish sleep from wakefulness [41]. Also, to Sadeh [42], in special populations, actigraphy tends to underestimate sleep latency and total sleep time, due to its lower specificity. Morgenthaler et al. [28], after compared PSG to actigraphy, found to be valid and reliable for detecting sleep in patients suspected of certain sleep disorders. Although our study was cross-sectional, the participants used the actigraph for 15 days, a long period of data collection regarding sleep patterns, as according to Sadeh [42], five days or longer of monitoring, reduces inherent measurement errors and increases its reliability. Besides this, according to Inoue et al. [7] fluctuations in sleep patterns can occur. Their study found an association of pain as a predictor of poor sleep quality, while in the present study, pain was related to worsening quality of life.

Data analysis showed that poor sleep presented little interference in the quality of life of patients with SLE, however we could perceive the influence of pain intensity, that is, the greater the intensity of pain in SLE patients, the longer the time spent to fall asleep, and the worse the perception of quality of life and fatigue, as when we divided the sample into subgroups (HPG and LPG), as did Waldheim et al. [14], there were indications that perhaps the increase in pain intensity caused by the disease interfered in sleep quality. The increase in sleep latency has also been observed in other studies [10,43], although only subjective evaluation tools were used for assessing sleep quality, such as PSQI, and higher scores and greater fatigue intensity worsened the perception of quality of life [12]. In the present study a cause-effect relationship of this cannot be established, due to the cross-sectional nature and small sample, but we may hypothesize that high pain intensity has a role in perception of quality of life and indirectly in sleep quality, as indicated in a recent study of [44].

In relation to disease activity and cumulative damage, probably there was no relationship because as in the study of Waldheim et al. [14], the sample showed low activity and little cumulative damage. The difference in the use of antimalarials for disease treatment was not maintained after univariate regression.

According to Menefee et al. [45], the SF-36 is a commonly used and good method to measure quality of life. In that study, higher pain intensity was also associated with poor sleep quality, longer sleep latency, and lower physical functioning to perform physical tasks such as walking. According to the authors, a sedentary lifestyle has also been associated with higher sleep disturbances. In our study, other domains related to the physical component were also negatively influenced by pain intensity (role physical, bodily pain, and vitality) [14] found an association between greater pain intensity and all SF-36 domains, fatigue, depression, anxiety, and increasing disease activity, and drew attention to the anxiety that was worse in those who knew little about the disease and its evolution. The researchers also suggested that patients with higher levels of pain and fatigue would be more likely to develop fibromyalgia. However, due to the complex nature of complaints from lupus patients such as arthralgias and myalgias, more detailed investigations on the type of pain are necessary, since it is difficult to distinguish the pain caused by lupus from other pain. As in that study, we also included women because of the elevated prevalence of the disease among females, due to genetic and hormonal origins.

In Mirbahgher et al. [9], anxiety was associated with sleep latency and sleep quality (PSQI). Indeed there was an association with pain, but not with fatigue. According to Vina et al. [43,46], the trend of performing less physical activity and taking PSL affects negatively the global sleep quality in patients with SLE; prednisolone use was reported to be associated with daytime somnolence. Although we did not analyze this variable separately, our sample with high levels of pain marked a significant value on the fatigue scale that was closely related to daytime somnolence.

Although we did not analyze anxiety and depression separately, we can see in the univariate analysis of the subgroups that the HPG obtained worse scores in the mental components, such as role emotional, social functioning, and vitality, almost achieving significance, than the LPG, although this difference was not maintained after logistic regression.

In the recent study of Inoue [7], the participants who had lower levels of pain tended also to present better sleep quality, as in the present study. Although our study was directed to self reported fatigue and we did not assess physical activity directly, Huang et al., 2007, found a positive relation with sedentary lifestyle and worse fatigue and pain; at the same time, low levels of disease activity, in other words, fatigue and pain are not always associated with the disease, but also with lifestyle and psychological factors. Even Huang et al. [47], although sleep complaints were present (72% related), they were not a predictive factor for worsening quality of life, unlike pain. Mckinley et al. [48] found higher sleep latency, although SLE patients attempted to get "enough" rest and sleep in an attempt to control fatigue and other symptoms. Therefore, fatigue is more important than quality of sleep. SLE patients tend to have problems adapting and probably require information and guidance about adaptation to enhance their ability to confront the disease, exercise safety, spiritual growth, and interpersonal relationships. In research of Mok et al. [49], achieving better control to reduce fatigue is effective in enhancing work capability, including patient perspectives for a more comprehensive assessment of SLE patients. According to Danoff-Burg et al. [50], fatigue was one of the important unmet needs in patients with SLE, due to the impact of fatigue on functional aspects, role physical, work (only 21.74% of our sample was employed, although our analyses with occupation did not reach significant values), social life, and, consequently, quality of life. In our study, it is probable fatigue is closer to higher levels of pain.

It is possible we did not find associations between sleep and quality of life because the sample in its totality already presented poor sleep quality, thus, other factors were more relevant, such as pain and fatigue. It should be recalled that one of the inclusion criteria of the study was not to have a diagnosis of fibromyalgia, as it is a disease that presents bias, with high rates of pain, fatigue and sleep alteration and could influence the objective of our study, even though the sample did not use sleep medication or muscle relaxants, despite higher levels of pain. According Iaboni´s study [16], for patients with SLE, the lack of understanding by others leads to social isolation, negatively affecting personal and professional interactions, for example; in that study 48.2% of the sample reported some level of unmet needs related to maintaining relationships.

Our study had some limitations, it is therefore very important to conduct additional investigations that include a large sample, assessments of anxiety, depression, daytime somnolence, and specific pain groups (differentiate the types of pain). It is also important to use PSG to diagnose specific sleep disorders, make comparisons with other rheumatologic diseases, and include a healthy control group, besides the continuous use of subjective measurements with objective evaluations. The most important recommendation is to continue to develop studies with non-pharmacological methods that could improve the necessities of these patients, mainly caused by the chronic disease, which has been associated with a reduction in mortality in recent years, but not necessarily with improved quality of life in patients.

Conclusion

To summarize we can perceive that until this moment, the treatment strategy in SLE, has the objective of reducing exacerbation periods and increasing remission, however aspects related to quality of life are still not a priority in health centers, since patients continue to report complaints regarding this.

Conflicts of interest

The authors declare that they have no conflict of interest and no financial relationships relevant to this article to disclose.

Acknowledgements

We would particularly like to thank the AFIP (Associação Fundo de Incentivo à Pesquisa) and CEPE (Centro de Estudos em Psicobiologia e Exercício), both from Brazil.

References

1. Yu SL, Kuan WP, Wong CK, Li EK, Tam LS (2012) Immunopathological roles of cytokines, chemokines, signaling molecules, and pattern-recognition receptors in systemic lupus erythematosus. Clin Dev Immunol.
2. Mok CC, Lau CS (2003) Pathogenesis of systemic lupus erythematosus. J Clin Pathol 56: 481-490.
3. Hochberg MC (1997) Updating the American College of Rheumatology revised criteria for the classification of systemic lupus erythematosus. Arthritis Rheum 40: 1725-1725.
4. Tan EM, Cohen AS, Fries JF, Masi AT, Mcshane DJ et al. (1982) The 1982 revised criteria for the classification of systemic lupus erythematosus. Arthritis Rheum 25: 1271-1277.
5. Hamptom T (2007) Researches probe lupus causes, treatments. JAMA 297: 141-142.
6. Furukawa M, Kiyohara C, Horiuchi T, Tsukamoto H, Mitoma H et al. (2016). Quality of life in Japanese female patients with systemic lupus erythematosus: Evaluation using the Short Form 36 Health Survey. Mod Rheumatol 26: 240-247.
7. Inoue M, Shiozawa K, Yoshihara R, Yamane T, Shima Y et al. (2017) Predictors of poor sleep quality in patients with systemic lupus erythematosus. Clin Rheumatol 36: 1053-1062.
8. Krueger JM, Rector DM, Churchill L (2007) Sleep and cytokines. Sleep Med Clin 2: 161-169.
9. Mirbagher L, Gholamrezaei A, Hosseini N, Sayed Bonakdar Z (2014). Sleep quality in women with systemic lupus erythematosus: contributing factors and effects on health-elated quality of life. Int J Rheum Dis 19: 305-311.
10. Palagini L, Tani C, Bruno RM, Gemignani A, Mauri M et al. (2014) Poor sleep quality in systemic lupus erythematosus: does it depend on depressive symptoms? Lupus 23: 1350-1357.
11. Palagini L, Mosca M, Tani C, Gemignani A, Mauri M et al. (2013) Depression and systemic lupus erythematosus: a systematic review. Lupus 22: 409-416.
12. Petri M, Bechtel B, Dennis G, Shah M, McLaughlin T et al. (2014) Burden of corticosteroid use in patients with systemic lupus erythematosus: results from a Delphi panel. Lupus 23: 1006-1013.
13. Tench CM, McCurdie I, White PD, D'Cruz DP (2000) The prevalence and associations of fatigue in systemic lupus erythematosus. Rheumatology 39: 1249-1254.
14. Waldheim E, Elkan AC, Pettersson S, Vollenhoven RV, Bergman S et al. (2013) Health-related quality of life, fatigue and mood in patients with SLE and high levels of pain compared to controls and patients with low levels of pain. Lupus 22: 1118-1127.
15. Chandrasekhara PKS, Jayachandran NV, Rajasekhar L, Thomas J Narsimulu G (2009) The prevalence and associations of sleep disturbances in patients with systemic lupus erythematosus. Mod Rheumatol 19: 407-415.
16. Iaboni A, Ibanez D, Gladman DD, Urowitz MB, Moldofsky H (2006) Fatigue in systemic lupus erythematosus: contributions of disordered sleep, sleepiness, and depression. J Rheumatol 33: 2453-2457.
17. Valencia-Flores M, Resendiz M, Castano VA, Santiago V, Campos RM et al. (1999) Objective and subjective sleep disturbances in patients with systemic lupus erythematosus. Arthritis Rheum 42: 2189-2193.

18. Clarke LL, Wilson S, Kirwan JR (2013) Using Actigraphy to Measure Sleep Patterns in Rheumatoid Arthritis: A Pilot Study in Patients Taking Night-Time Prednisone. Musculoskeletal care 11: 179-185.

19. Goodchild CE, Treharne GJ, Booth DA, Bowman SJ (2010) Daytime patterning of fatigue and its associations with the previous night's discomfort and poor sleep among women with primary Sjögren's syndrome or rheumatoid arthritis. Musculoskeletal Care 8: 107-117.

20. Campbell CM, Buenaver LF, Finan P, Bounds SC, Redding M et al. (2015). Sleep, pain catastrophizing, and central sensitization in knee osteoarthritis patients with and without insomnia. Arthritis Care Res (Hoboken) 67: 1387-1396.

21. Kop WJ, Lyden A, Berlin AA, Ambrose K, Olsen C et al. (2005) Ambulatory monitoring of physical activity and symptoms in fibromyalgia and chronic fatigue syndrome. Arthritis Rheum 52: 296-303.

22. Landis CA, Frey CA, Lentz MJ, Rothermel J, Buchwald D et al. (2003) Self-reported sleep quality and fatigue correlates with actigraphy in midlife women with fibromyalgia. Nurs Res 52: 140-147.

23. van de Water AT, Eadie J, Hurley DA (2011) Investigation of sleep disturbance in chronic low back pain: an age-and gender-matched case-control study over a 7-night period. Man Ther 16: 550-556.

24. Liu L, Fiorentino L, Rissling M, Natarajan L, Parker BA et al. (2013) Decreased health-related quality of life in women with breast cancer is associated with poor sleep. Behav Sleep Med 11: 189-206.

25. Balderas-Díaz S, Martínez MP, Guerrero-Contreras G, Miró E, Benghazi K et al. (2017) Using actigraphy and mhealth systems for an objective analysis of sleep quality on systemic lupus erythematous patients. Methods Inf Med 56: 171-179.

26. Petri M, Orbai AM, Alarcón GS, Gordon C, Merrill JT et al. (2012) Derivation and validation of the Systemic Lupus International Collaborating Clinics classification criteria for systemic lupus erythematosus. Arthritis Rheum 64: 2677-2686.

27. Ancoli-Israel S, Cole R, Alessi C, Chambers M, Moorcroft W et al. (2003) The role of actigraphy in the study of sleep and circadian rhythms. Sleep 26 (3): 342-392.

28. Morgenthaler T, Alessi C, Friedman L, Owens J, Kapur V et al. (2007) Practice parameters for the use of actigraphy in the assessment of sleep and sleep disorders: an update for 2007. Sleep 30: 519-529.

29. Zinkhan M, Berger K, Hense S, Nagel M, Obst A et al. (2014) Agreement of different methods for assessing sleep characteristics: a comparison of two actigraphs, wrist and hip placement, and self-report with polysomnography. Sleep Med 15: 1107-1114.

30. Bertolazi AN, Fagondes SC, Hoff LS, Dartora EG, da Silva Miozzo IC et al. (2011) Validation of the Brazilian Portuguese version of the Pittsburgh sleep quality index. Sleep Med 12: 70-75.

31. Buysse DJ, Reynolds CF 3rd, Monk TH, Berman SR, Kupfer DJ (1989) The Pittsburgh Sleep Quality Index: A new instrument for psychiatric practice and research. Psychiatry Res 28: 193-213.

32. Monitoring A (2002) Action-W User's Guide Version 2.4. Ardsley, NY: Ambulatory Monitoring.

33. Ciconelli RM, Ferraz MB, Santos W, Meinão I, Quaresma MR (1999) Brazilian-Portuguese version of the SF-36. A reliable and valid quality of life outcome measure. Rev Bras Reumatol 39: 143-50.

34. Krupp LB, LaRocca NG, Muir-Nash J, Steinberg AD (1989) The fatigue severity scale: application to patients with multiple sclerosis and systemic lupus erythematosus. Arch Neurol 46: 1121-1123.

35. Mendes MF, Pavan K, Marangoni BE, Schmidt KB (2008) Cross-cultural adaptation of the fatigue severity scale for the Portuguese language/Cross-cultural of the fatigue severity scale. Med reabil 69-71.

36. Carlsson AM (1983) Assessment of chronic pain. I. Aspects of the reliability and validity of the visual analogue scale. Pain 16: 87-101.

37. Gladman DD, Ibanez D, Urowitz MB (2002) Systemic lupus erythematosus disease activity index 2000. J Rheumatol 29: 288-291.

38. Gladman D, Ginzler E, Goldsmith C, Fortin P, Liang M et al. (1996) The development and initial validation of the Systemic Lupus International Collaborating Clinics/American College of Rheumatology damage index for systemic lupus erythematosus. Arthritis Rheum 39: 363-369.

39. Kutner MH, Nachtsheim C, Neter J (2004) Applied linear regression models (4th edtn), Boston: McGraw-Hill/Irwin.

40. Landry GJ, Best JR, Liu-Ambrose T (2015) Measuring sleep quality in older adults: a comparison using subjective and objective methods. Front Aging Neurosci 7:166.

41. De Souza L, Benedito-Silva AA, Pires MLN, Poyares D, Tufik S et al. (2003) Further validation of actigraphy for sleep studies. Sleep 26: 81-85.

42. Sadeh A (2011) The role and validity of actigraphy in sleep medicine: an update. Sleep Med Rev. 15: 259-267.

43. Vina ER, Green SL, Trivedi T, Kwoh CK, Utset TO (2013) Correlates of sleep abnormalities in systemic lupus: A cross-sectional survey in an urban, academic center. J Clin Rheumatol 19: 7-13.

44. Palagini L, Mauri M, Faraguna U, Carli L, Tani C et al. (2016) Insomnia symptoms, perceived stress and coping strategies in patients with systemic lupus erythematosus. Lupus 25: 988-996.

45. Menefee LA, Frank ED, Doghramji K, Picarello K, Park JJ et al. (2000) Self-reported sleep quality and quality of life for individuals with chronic pain conditions. Clin J Pain 16: 290-297.

46. Da Costa D, Bernatsky S, Dritsa M, Clarke AE, Dasgupta K et al. (2005) Determinants of sleep quality in women with systemic lupus erythematosus. Arthritis Rheum 53: 272-278.

47. Huang HC, Chou CT, Lin KC, Chao YF (2007) The relationships between disability level, health-promoting lifestyle, and quality of life in outpatients with systemic lupus erythematosus. J Nurs Res 15: 21-32.

48. Mckinley PS, Ouellette SC, Winkel GH (1995) The contributions of disease activity sleep patterns, and depression to fatigue in systemic lupus erythematosus. Arthritis Rheum 38: 826-834.

49. Mok CC, Cheung MY, Ho LY, Yu KL, To CH (2008) Risk and predictors of work disability in Chinese patients with systemic lupus erythematosus. Lupus 17: 1103-1107.

50. Danoff-Burg S, Friedberg F (2009) Unmet needs of patients with systemic lupus erythematosus. Behav Med 35: 5-13.

How Much Does Depressive Mood Affect Sleep for High School Students?

Seoyoun Kim*, Hyojae Kim, Min Jeong Kim, Jaehong Park, Joohee Kim, Yesol Min, Tae Kyung Kim, Younggyun Lee, Jinhee IM and Sohee Kim

Korea International High School in Jeju, Daejeong-eup, Seogwipo-si, Jeju-do, Korea

***Corresponding author:** Seoyoun kim, Korea International High School in Jeju, Daejeong-eup, Seogwipo-si, Jeju-do, Korea, E-mail: syounkim16@kis.ac

Abstract

Background: This research examined gender variations in depressive mood for high school students affected by emotional upset and how such depressive mood affect their sleep quality.

Methods: This research was conducted for 2 months from September 2015 to October 2015. Both males and females were divided into normal group and depressive group by Zung Self-rating Depression Scale (ZSDS). Each group adopted the Pittsburgh Sleep Quality Index (PSQI) to measure sleep quality. Chi-Square test and AVOVA analysis through SPSS-21 were used as statistics methods.

Results: Analysis was made on a total of 155 students (83 male, 72 female students) that submitted clear answers to the questionnaire. There were 86 students in the normal group and 69 students on the depressive group according to the ZSDS. More female students had depressive mood than male students with 52.8% and 37.3% respectively but without particular statistical meaning. The average ZSDS for all high school students was 43.38 and the average PSQI was 5.39.

The number of male students in the normal and depressive group who were diagnosed with sleep disorder were 2 (3.8%) and 9 (29.0%) respectively. But the number of female students in the normal and depressive group who were diagnosed with sleep disorder were 11 (32.4%) and 33 (86.8%) respectively, which was quite meaningful result. Both males and females shared a meaningful result over sleep latency, sleep disturbance, use of sleep medication, and daytime functional disturbance among 7 items of PSQI for sleep quality, and female students had a significantly meaningful result over sleep duration, habitual sleep effects.

Conclusions: This research showed that sleep quality of all high school students was not too bad but it can be problematic for those with depressive mood. Especially, female students with hormone changes and emotional instability were diagnosed with sleep disorder more than male students.

Keywords: Depression; Sleep; Zung self-rating depression scale (ZSDS); Pittsburgh sleep quality index (PSQI); High school students

Introduction

Sleep is one of important physiological processes, accounting for one third of biorhythm of entire life. According to studies conducted in the western countries, 25-40% of adolescents experience sleep disturbance [1,2]. Similar reports on Asian countries, a report on China states 16.9% of adolescents experience sleep disturbance [3].

Although a slight difference in prevalence appears to exist based on these numbers only, it is difficult to accurately determine the difference due to lack of comparative studies of Asian and western countries on the topic. However, it is clear that a significant number of adolescents experience sleep disturbance.

Adolescents' normal sufficient sleep duration is defined as eight or more hours of sleep on an average school night [4]. Normal sleep is essential for student heath; however, they take sleep insufficient for their required amount of sleep due to various factors.

According to international studies, sleep duration decreases in students in higher grades [5,6]. According to National Sleep Foundation Sleep in American Poll, proportion of students who take 8 or less hours of sleep was 16% for 6th graders, whereas 75% for 12th graders [7]. In particular, there was a report that in Korea, among Asian countries with high level of academic stress, students' average sleep hours is 4.9 hours [5]. Such insufficient sleep in the adolescent period results in negative impacts on mood, attention, and school performance.

Judith Owens stated that contributing factors of insufficient sleep include biologic processes such as hormonal change, electro-media, school start times, caffeine, medical illness, and mental health issues such as depressive mood [8]. The mood disorders among the factors have a bidirectional relationship with sleep disturbance where the former can worsen the latter and can result from the latter [9].

Depressive disorder in adolescence has become a serious issue as its prevalence is reportedly 12.3% in the U.S., and 41.3% in Korea [10,11]. In particular, the primary causes of high prevalence of adolescent depression include schools that exclude developmental features, overall societal pressure on academic performance, uncertainty of future, and anxiety about college entrance [12,13]. In particular, adolescence is a transitional period to adulthood, with instability due to emotional, cognitive and physical change.

Depressive symptoms shown in this period can lead to persistent sadness, failure in school performance, and reduced motivation, resulting in various problem behaviors. In addition, various physical problems such as loss of appetite, depressed mood, anxiety disorder, altered sleeping, and psychosomatic symptoms may be exhibited [14,15].

In particular, as untreated depression may continue to adulthood and develop into major depressive disorder, it is important to investigate the association between early depressive mood and sleep disturbance in adolescence.

Association between depressive state and sleep disturbance in adolescence has been demonstrated by several studies. Pigeon, et al. [16] reported that women experiencing sleep disturbance have low expectation of their own health and physical and mental health symptoms more frequently. In addition, adolescents with sleep disturbance develop depressive symptoms more often than adolescents without sleep disturbance, and the symptoms maintained [17,18].

Research on the relationship between sleep disturbance and depressive symptoms have been conducted continuously because various factors affect the relationship. For example, demographics, family, school, intersexual relationships, and social factors may affect it [19]. In addition, gender difference may exist. While most studies reported prevalence of sleep disturbance was higher among female students than male students, the opposite results have also been reported [20,21].

The conflicting results may suggest that a variety of factors contribute to results in addition to sample size and location of studies. In the end, it was found that although sleep disturbance in adolescence occurs due to a variety of factors, studies show inconsistent results. However, these studies shared in common that their results were similar to the studies on sleep disturbance due to mental status.

In Korea, fact-finding surveys on high school students' sleep disturbance are lacking, and research on gender difference in effect of depressive mood status on sleep disturbance are also yet to be done.

This study was conducted with KIS students to investigate the effect of depressive mood on sleep disturbance, despite small sample size, under the assumption that, as excellent students from around Korea selected by rigorous testing, their variation in academic history can be minimized, and that, due to expensive tuition fees, parents' economic level and biography based on peer review status can be minimized.

Methods

This study adopted a cross-sectional study design in which high school students' depressive mental status was surveyed and its relationship with sleep disturbance was examined. Study participants consisted of 9th-12th male and female students from KIS, Jeju, Korea. Study period was two months from September to October, 2015. All students were included in the study, but the students who did not participate in the survey and who provided inadequate responses were excluded form analysis.

All survey participants participate in the survey after being informed on the purpose of the study and giving written informed consent. The survey was conducted using two types of questionnaires. First, the depressive mood was surveyed with Zung Self-rating Depression Scale (ZSDS), and sleep quality and disturbances was surveyed with the Korean version Pittsburgh Sleep Quality Index (PSQI).

Participants were classified into normal and depressive groups based on the results of ZSDS; then, each group's association with PSQI was investigated. The ZSDS consists of 20 items with 4-point scale on self-reported symptoms, with a total score of 80 points. Depression items were scored as follows; 1=a little of the time, 2=some of the time, 3=a good part of the time, 4=most of the time [22,23].

The worst possible psychological status scores 80 points, and the best possible psychological status scores 20 points. Total ZSDS score may be associated with clinical relevance.

The ZSDS were interpreted as follows: normal range (20-44), mildly depressed (45-59), moderately depressed (60-69), and severely depressed (70 and above). In this study, ZSDS scores of 44 or less were classified into the normal group, and ZSDS scores of 45 or more were classified into the depressive group.

The PSQI is a self-administered questionnaire on overall status of sleep in the past 1 month, consisting of 19 items. It represents overall status of sleep using seven components: Subjective sleep quality, sleep latency, sleep duration, habitual sleep efficiency, sleep disturbances, use of sleep medication, and daytime function [23].

Each component is scored on 0-3 point scale with a total of 21 points. The total scores of 6 points or more indicates poor sleep quality, and is defined as having sleep disturbance [24]. That is, high the PSQI scores indicate poor sleep quality.

Statistical analysis

In terms of statistical analyses, Chi-Square test and analysis of variance (ANOVA) were conducted using the Statistical Package for Social Sciences Software (SPSS-version 21). Descriptive analyses were performed to describe prevalence of depressive symptoms in male and female students as well as all participating students.

To investigate the effect of depressive mental status on sleep quality by gender, two-way ANOVA was performed. To investigate if the depressive mental status varied in gender, Chi-Square test was performed.

More specifically, for symmetric measures, Pearson's product moment correlation coefficient was used for interval scale, and Spearman rank-order correlation coefficient was used for ordinal scale. Means and standard deviations were calculated for sub-scale scores of each group. The p-value of <0.05 were considered the level of statistical significance difference.

Results

Students who provided adequate responses on the survey were 83 male and 72 female students, and 155 students in total. The proportions of male and female participants were 53.6% and 46.4%, respectively. Students' grades were well-distributed between 9th-12th grades.

The mean age of all participants was 17.08 years; the mean age of male participants was 17.08 years; and the mean age of female participants was 17.07 years. The mean ZSDS score of all participants was 43.39, and the mean PSQI score was 5.38.

Does depressive mood state vary between genders?

Distribution in the ZSDS to investigate mood state of each group is shown in Figure 1. In the total student population, the normal group included 86 students (55.5%), and the depressive group included 69 students (44.5%).

In terms of gender, the normal and the depressive groups included 52 (62.7%), 31 (37.3%) male students, and 34 (47.2%), 38 (52.8%) female students, respectively, showing higher proportion of depressive mood in female students. The mean ZSDS score also was also found to be higher in female students, with 41.92 for male and 45.08 for female students ($P<0.05$) (Figure 1).

It was investigated if the mean ZSDS score varied among the total student group, male student group, and female student group. First, the mean ages of the normal and the depressive group in the total student group were 17.12/17.03 years, and the mean ZSDS score were 37.58/50.62. The mean ages of the normal and the depressive group in the male student group were 17.0/17.23 years, and the mean ZSDS score were 37.27/49.71. The mean ages of the normal and the depressive group in the female student group were 17.30/16.86 years, and the mean ZSDS score were 38.06/51.37, respectively.

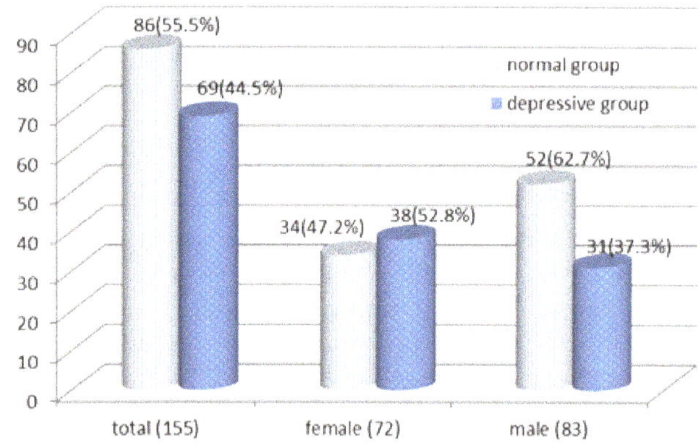

Figure 1: Distribution of normal and depressive group with sexual differences.

Does depressive mood state including gender influence poor sleep?

Distribution of normal sleep and sleep disturbance based on the PSQI of each group is shown in Figure 2. It was found that in the total student group, the numbers of students with normal sleep and sleep disturbance were 87 (56.1%)/68 (43.9%) respectively, with the mean PSQI score of 5.38.

In the normal mood state based on the ZSDS, the numbers of students with normal sleep and sleep disturbance were 73 (84.9%)/13(15.1%) respectively, with the mean PSQI score of 3.84, and in the depressive group, the numbers were 14 (20.3%)/55 (79.7%) respectively, with the mean PSQI score of 7.32, suggesting depressive mood state have greater impact on poor sleep ($p<0.05$).

However, in the comparison of the normal and depressive group by gender showed slight different results. First, among male students, in the normal group, the numbers of students with normal sleep and sleep disturbance were 50(96.2%)/2(2%) respectively, with the mean PSQI score of 3.40, and also in the depressive group, the numbers were 22(71.0%)/9(29.0%) respectively, with the mean PSQI score of 6.92.

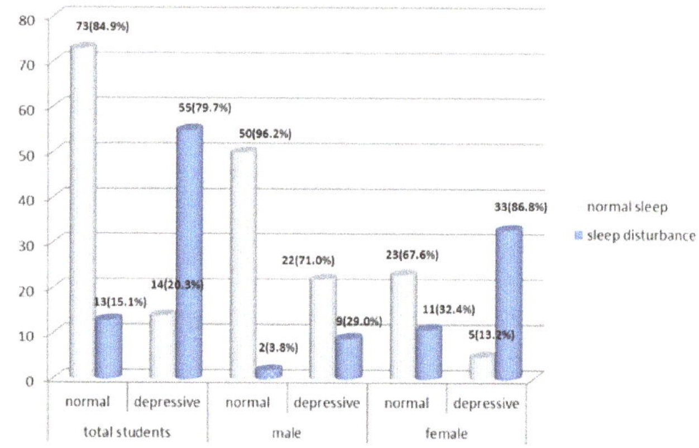

Figure 2: Distribution of sleep disturbance with Mood state changes.

The standard deviation of the PSQI scores was large at 6.92 ± 3.22, while mean scores were high. This suggests that sleep disturbance did not vary significantly among male students ($p>0.05$).

However, among female students, in the normal group, the number of students with normal sleep and sleep disturbance were 23 (67.6%)/11(32.4%) respectivey, with the mean PSQI score of 4.50, and in the depressive group, the numbers were 5(13.2%)/33(86.8%) respectively, with the mean PSQI score of 7.47, suggesting significant impact of mood on poor sleep ($p<0.05$) (Table 1).

		Normal group	Depressive group
Total	Age (years)	17.12	17.03
High school students	ZSDS	37.58	50.62
	PSQI	3.84	7.32
Male students	Age (years)	17.3	16.86
	ZSDS	38.06	51.37
	PSQI	4.5	7.47
Female students	Age (years)	17	17.23
	ZSDS	37.27	49.71
	PSQI	3.4	6.92

Table 1: Mean values of age, ZSDS, PSQI in normal and depressive groups.

What is the effect of depressive mood state on sleep quality subscales?

Although it was found that sleep disturbance vary between males and females in their mood states, it is also important to examine which sleep quality is affected. In each group, the effect on seven subscales of PSQI was examined.

First, the total student group showed a significant difference in five subscales among normal and depressive group PSQI subscales: Sleep latency (0.47 ± 0.077/1.13 ± 0.107), sleep duration (1.09 ± 0.090, 1.62 ± 0.113), sleep disturbance (0.77 ± 0.049, 1.29 ± 0.066), use of sleep medication (0.27 ± 0.061/0.90 ± 0.134), and daytime dysfunction (1.07 ± 0.075/1.77 ± 0.088) ($p<0.05$) (Table 2).

	Normal (52)	Depressive (31)	p-value
Subjective sleep quality	0.06 ± 0.025	0.10 ± 0.055	0.478
Sleep latency	0.47 ± 0.077	1.13 ± 0.107	0
Sleep duration	1.09 ± 0.090	1.62 ± 0.113	0
Habitual Sleep efficiency	0.12 ± 0.035	0.33 ± 0.092	0.029
Sleep disturbance	0.77 ± 0.049	1.29 ± 0.066	0
Use of sleep medication	0.27 ± 0.061	0.90 ± 0.134	0
Daytime dysfunction	1.07 ± 0.075	1.77 ± 0.088	0

Table 2: PSQI difference between total normal and depressive students.

Male students showed a significant difference in four subscales among normal and depressive group the PSQI subscales: Sleep latency (0.50 ± 0.097/1.19 ± 0.170), sleep disturbance (0.71 ± 0.069, 1.39 ± 0.110), use of sleep medication (0.21 ± 0.074/1.03 ± 0.205), and daytime dysfunction (0.94 ± 0.084/1.61 ± 0.152) ($p<0.05$) (Table 3).

	Normal	Depressive	p-value
Subjective sleep quality	0.04 ± 0.027	0.23 ± 0.120	0.138
Sleep latency	0.50 ± 0.097	1.19 ± 0.170	0.001
Sleep duration	0.87 ± 0.110	1.23 ± 0.178	0.091
Habitual Sleep efficiency	0.13 ± 0.048	0.45 ± 0.166	0.075
Sleep disturbance	0.71 ± 0.069	1.39 ± 0.110	0
Use of sleep medication	0.21 ± 0.074	1.03 ± 0.205	0.001
Daytime dysfunction	0.94 ± 0.084	1.61 ± 0.152	0

Table 3: PSQI difference between normal and depressive male students.

Female students showed a significant difference in five subscales among normal and depressive group PSQI subscales: Sleep latency (0.41 ± 0.127/1.08 ± 0.138), sleep duration (1.44 ± 0.135/1.95 ± 0.125), sleep disturbance (0.85 ± 0.062/1.21 ± 0.077), use of sleep medication (0.35 ± 0.102/0.79 ± 0.178), and daytime dysfunction (1.26 ± 0.136/1.89 ± 0.098) ($p<0.05$) (Table 4).

These results suggest that both male and female students in the depressive state have difficulty with sleep induction. This insomnia pattern results in daytime dysfunction due to insufficient hours of sleep when the focus on study is required, making it difficult for students to engage in school life.

In addition, as frequency of taking drugs to solve this pattern increases, students may develop drug dependency, and vicious cycle of poor sleep and quality of school life may occur.

	Normal	Depressive	p-value
Subjective sleep quality	0.09 ± 0.049	0.00 ± 0.00	0.083
Sleep latency	0.41 ± 0.127	1.08 ± 0.138	0.001
Sleep duration	1.44 ± 0.135	1.95 ± 0.125	0.007
Habitual Sleep efficiency	0.09 ± 0.049	0.24 ± 0.096	0.173
Sleep disturbance	0.85 ± 0.062	1.21 ± 0.077	0.001
Use of sleep medication	0.35 ± 0.102	0.79 ± 0.178	0.037
Daytime dysfunction	1.26 ± 0.136	1.89 ± 0.098	0

Table 4: PSQI difference between normal and depressive female group.

Discussion

High school students are in the adolescence transitioning from childhood to adulthood with rapidly occurring major changes in physical, emotional, and social aspects. The students develop self-identity by overcoming this period [25]. Many students experience difficulty in adjusting to these changes, and a variety of stresses including academic performance and relationship building. If they are exposed to chronic stress, depression is likely to develop through interaction with various factors such as genetic diathesis [26]. When the depression is not properly addressed and continues into adulthood, drug overuse, sexually reckless behavior, sense of alienation, and suicidal thoughts and behaviors may occur frequently or worsen [27]. Therefore, it is imperative to facilitate normal school life and pee relations through proper assessment of depression and reducing maladjustment in the early adolescence. First, epidemiology of adolescent depression needs to be understood. In the total population, the depressive mood rate is fairly high at 44.5%. This result may result from a lack of emotional support as the KIS is a private dormitory school and located in a rural area, and therefore, they are cut off from family. As a related study result, Liu et al. reported that results vary according to student age and grade, and students from incomplete families with little peer review experience sleep disturbance [28]. Regarding reports on separate results for male and female, there is a report that depression prevalence rate is higher for women than men [29], and there is a report of opposite result [30]. In our study, female students' depression prevalence rate was 52.8%, higher than male students' 37.3%. For such higher prevalence of depression in women, both biological cause of hormonal change such as menstruation and social cause such as psychological conflict experienced as they realize male-dominant society have been presented as explanations [15].

The sleep deprivation, the most important aspect of life, is the most important aspect of adolescence in the developmental process because it interferes with daily life due to unpleasant mood, reduced concentration, and excessive daytime sleepiness, and results in memory loss and dissatisfaction with interpersonal relationships [8]. Therefore, research efforts on role of sleep are needed as part of efforts to improve quality of life and enhance sense of happiness in adolescence. As a result, many reports have been produced on correlation between depressive mood and sleep in adolescence, a mentally immature stage. In terms of physiological aspect, although sleep appears to be a passive state due to reduced cognition and response to what is happening around, active state due to high level of interaction in central nervous system (CNS) is maintained during sleep. Because of the CNS stimulation, people are affected by many hormones during sleep. Sleep propensity and sleep architecture are in turn controlled by the interaction of two time-keeping mechanisms in the central nervous system, circadian rhythm and sleep-wake homeostasis [31]. In particular, thyroid hormone secreted during sleep modulates loss of appetite and weight loss; luteinizing hormone modulates nervousness; and corticosteroid hormone modulates stress. Unstable sleep in adolescence cause disturbance in the hormones. In addition, when women begin to have menstruation, sleep disturbance is more frequently observed in female students who are affected by follicular hormone and luteinizing hormone imbalance [31,32]. In our study, the proportion of the students who experience sleep disturbance was found to be 43.9%, and in the depressive mood state, the proportion of sleep disturbance was 15.1% for male, and 79.7% for female, showing higher sleep disturbance rate in female students.

In our study, both male and female students showed the problem of sleep induction of sleep latency and sleep disturbance among seven sleep quality subscales of PSQI. In proportion to this result, in the next day, both male and female students complained of daytime dysfunction. In contrast, Seblewngel Lemma, et al. [33] with universal students as study participants reported that those who complained low sleep latency also showed low daytime dysfunction rate. This results demonstrate that poor sleep quality indicate worsening poor daytime dysfunction. In particular, KIS students in our study are under severe pressure on academic performance as the school is a prestigious private school. These students have strong perfectionism. Perfectionism shows the personality of having a high and rigid standard with regard to performance, fear of failure and excessive self-criticism [34]. The perfectionism has been reported to have a direct negative impact on sleep and psychological functioning [34]. Most students with high academic achievement seek perfectionism. Lan Guo, et al. [29] reported that the students with below-average academic pressure complains sleep disturbance less. This suggests that academic pressure serves as a stressor that influences sleep disturbance. Due to this aspect, prevalence of depression and sleep disturbance was found to be higher in our study than in other studies on relationship between sleep and mood.

Conclusion

In conclusion, this study demonstrated that depressive mood is closely associated with sleep disturbance in adolescence. Also, our research showed that sleep quality of all high school students was not too bad but it can be problematic for those with depressive mood. Especially, female students with hormone changes and emotional instability were diagnosed with sleep disorder more than male students. Such results imply that mental state of high school students can disturb their healthy sleep and can affect general well-being state negatively. Adolescence is when the conflict between needs for sleep and social life occurs. There is no way to prevent sleep deprivation due to academic aspect of preparation for future. However, it would be possible to provide careful attention and sufficient care to the students in an early stage of depressive state, since sleep and depression are in a mutually dependent relationship as discussed earlier. This is expected to contribute to good sleep by minimizing at least the effect on mood change among various factors of poor sleep.

References

1. Lazaratou H, Dikeos DG, Anagnostopoulos DC, Sbokou O, Soldatos CR (2005) Sleep problems in adolescence. A study of senior high school students in Greece. Eur Child Adolesc Psychiatry 14: 237-243.
2. García-Jiménez MA, Salcedo-Aguilar F, Rodríguez-Almonacid FM, Redondo-Martínez MP, Monterde-Aznar ML, et al. (2004) [The prevalence of sleep disorders among adolescents in Cuenca, Spain]. Rev Neurol 39: 18-24.
3. Liu X, Uchiyama M, Okawa M, Kurita H (2000) Prevalence and correlates of self-reported sleep problems among Chinese adolescents. Sleep 23: 27-34.
4. Wheaton AG, Ferro GA, Croft JB (2015) School Start Times for Middle School and High School Students - United States, 2011-12 School Year. MMWR Morb Mortal Wkly Rep 64: 809-813.
5. Yang CK, Kim JK, Patel SR, Lee JH (2005) Age-related changes in sleep/wake patterns among Korean teenagers. Pediatrics 115: 250-256.
6. Loessl B, Valerius G, Kopasz M, Hornyak M, Riemann D, et al. (2008) Are adolescents chronically sleep-deprived? An investigation of sleep habits of adolescents in the Southwest of Germany. Child Care Health Dev 34: 549-556.
7. https://sleepfoundation.org/sleep-polls-data/sleep-in-america-poll/2006-teens-and-sleep.
8. Owens J (2014) Adolescent Sleep Working Group; Committee on Adolescence. Insufficient sleep in adolescents and young adults: an update on causes and consequences. Pediatrics 134(3): e921-932.
9. Chen MC, Burley HW, Gotlib IH (2012) Reduced sleep quality in healthy girls at risk for depression. J Sleep Res 21: 68-72.
10. National Survey on Drug Use and Health (NSDUH) (2005) Depression among adolescent. The NSDUH Report. December 30.
11. Ministry of Health and Welfare (2009) Support for depression screening and treatment for children & adolescents with ADHD.
12. Hong YS (2004) The effects of life stress and self-esteem for adolescent suicidal behaviors. Studies on Korean Youth 15(2): 153-182.
13. Hong SO, Eum KS, Bae OH (2003) A study on social support and stress of adolescent. Korea Association of Family Relations 8(1): 139-155.
14. Tylee A, Gandhi P (2005) The importance of somatic symptoms in depression in primary care. Prim Care Companion J Clin Psychiatry 7: 167-176.
15. Petersen AC, Sarigiani PA, Kennedy RE (1991) Adolescent depression: Why more girls? J Youth Adolesc 20: 247-271.
16. Pigeon WR, Cerulli C, Richards H, He H, Perlis M, et al. (2011) Sleep disturbances and their association with mental health among women exposed to intimate partner violence. J Womens Health (Larchmt) 20: 1923-1929.
17. Roane BM, Taylor DJ (2008) Adolescent insomnia as a risk factor for early adult depression and substance abuse. Sleep 31: 1351-1356.
18. Xu Z, Su H, Zou Y, Chen J, Wu J, et al. (2012) Sleep quality of Chinese adolescents: distribution and its associated factors. J Paediatr Child Health 48: 138-145.
19. Stores G (1999) Children's sleep disorders: modern approaches, developmental effects, and children at special risk. Dev Med Child Neurol 41: 568-573.
20. Ohida T, Osaki Y, Doi Y, Tanihata T, Minowa M, et al. (2004) An epidemiologic study of self-reported sleep problems among Japanese adolescents. Sleep 27: 978-985.
21. Chung KF, Cheung MM (2008) Sleep-wake patterns and sleep disturbance among Hong Kong Chinese adolescents. Sleep 31: 185-194.
22. Zung WW (1971) A rating instrument for anxiety disorders. Psychosomatics 12: 371-379.
23. ZUNG WW (1965) A SELF-RATING DEPRESSION SCALE. Arch Gen Psychiatry 12: 63-70.
24. Buysse DJ, Reynolds CF 3rd, Monk TH, Berman SR, Kupfer DJ (1989) The Pittsburgh Sleep Quality Index: a new instrument for psychiatric practice and research. Psychiatry Res 28: 193-213.
25. Wallerstein RS (1998) Erikson's concept of ego identity reconsidered. J Am Psychoanal Assoc 46: 229-247.
26. Bemporad JR, Lee KW (1996) Affective disorders. In Kestenbaum CJ and Williams DT (Eds). Handbook of clinical assessment of children and adolescent. New York University Press 629-649.

27. Fleming JE, Offord DR (1990) Epidemiology of childhood depressive disorders: a critical review. J Am Acad Child Adolesc Psychiatry 29: 571-580.

28. Kovacs M (1996) Presentation and course of major depressive disorder during childhood and later years of the life span. J Am Acad Child Adolesc Psychiatry 35: 705-715.

29. Lan Guo, Jianxiong Deng, Yuan He, Xueqing Deng, Jinghui Huang, et al. (2014) Prevalence and correlates of sleep disturbance and depressive symtoms among Chinese adolescents: a cross-sectional survey study. BMJ Open 4(7): e005517.

30. Liu X, Zhao Z, Jia C, Buysse. DJ (2008) Sleep patterns and problems among chinese adolescents. Pediatrics 121: 1165-1173.

31. Leproult R, Van Cauter E (2010) Role of sleep and sleep loss in hormonal release and metabolism. Endocr Dev 17: 11-21.

32. Yan L, Silver R (2015) Neuroendocrine underpinnings of sex differences in circadian timing systems. J Steroid Biochem Mol Biol. Oct 22. pii: S0960-0760(15)30111-4. doi: 10.1016/j.jsbmb.2015.10.007.

33. Lemma S, Gelaye B, Berhane Y, Worku A, Williams MA (2012) Sleep quality and its psychological correlates among university students in Ethiopia: a cross-sectional study. BMC Psychiatry 12: 237.

34. Brand S, Kirov R, Kalak N, Gerber M, Pühse U, et al. (2015) Perfectionism related to self-reported insomnia severity, but not when controlled for stress and emotion regulation. Neuropsychiatr Dis Treat 11: 263-271.

10

Obstructive Sleep Apnea among Players in the National Football League

April J Rogers[1-2], Kevin Xia[3], Kyaw Soe[3], Azizi Seixas[1], Felix Sogade[4], Barbara Hutchinson[5], Dorice Vieira[1], Samy I McFarlane[6*] and Girardin Jean-Louis[1]

[1]*Center for Healthful Behavior Change (CHBC), Division of Health and Behavior, Department of Population Health, New York University Medical Center, New York, NY 10016, USA*

[2]*Department of Health Service Administration, St. John's University, Queens, NY 11439, USA*

[3]*Department of Medicine, Jersey Shore University Medical Center, Neptune, NJ 07753, USA*

[4]*Department of Cardiology, Health Service of Central Georgia, Macon, Georgia 31201, USA*

[5]*President of Chesapeake Cardiac Care, Annapolis, Maryland, 21401, USA*

[6]*Department of Medicine, Division of Endocrinology, State University of New York, Downstate Medical Center, Brooklyn, NY 11203, USA*

***Corresponding author:** Samy I. McFarlane, Department of Medicine, Division of Endocrinology, State University of New York, Downstate Medical Center, Brooklyn, NY 11203, USA, E-mail: smcfarlane@downstate.edu

Abstract

Objective: Obstructive sleep apnea (OSA) is a common sleep-disordered breathing condition that has emerged as a significant public health problem given its increased prevalence over the past decade. The high prevalence of obesity and large waist circumference among NFL players are two risk factors that might contribute to the high susceptibility of football players to develop OSA. National Football League linemen might be particularly vulnerable since they tend to have a higher body mass index. In this scoping review, we aim to bring attention to the limited research regarding OSA among National Football League players and highlight the negative consequences of OSA in an attempt to increase awareness of the urgent need for further research in this area.

Methods: Search terms associated with obstructive sleep apnea and football were used to examine Google Scholar, EMBASE, CINAHL, PubMed, ProQuest, and Web of Science Plus for relevant studies. All relevant studies were included and documented.

Results: Findings included (n=4) studies of interest. All 4 studies revealed a near or slightly above 50% prevalence of OSA in the investigated cohorts (mostly retired NFL linemen). Most participants in the study (active NFL players) showed symptoms associated with a sleep-disorder breathing condition (snoring).

Conclusion: OSA requires more attention from the research and medical community. As suggested by results in the 4 studies included in this paper, OSA and associated symptoms are prevalent in the NFL population. Further research is required to investigate the extent of OSA and OSA risk in this population. There is an urgent need to conduct OSA risk surveillance in the athletic community.

Keywords: Obstructive sleep apnea; Sleep Apnea; Hypertension; Insufficient sleep

Introduction

Sleep is vital for human survival and adequate bodily functioning [1,2]. When adequate sleep quality is experienced, the body responds in an efficacious manner as observed in optimal body metabolism and heightened cognitive awareness, which can promote better decision-making [3]. In the sports world, in order to be competitive and perform at optimal levels, it is paramount to receive efficient sleep [4]. In recent years, sleep-disordered breathing such as obstructive sleep apnea (OSA) has gained notoriety in the athletic community. OSA has been implicated as a medical condition that affects millions of Americans [5]. In the National Football League (NFL) community, the prevalence of OSA is estimated to range from 14% to 19%, and the prevalence in the general USA population is estimated at 2-5% [4,5]. During an apnea episode, which is characteristic among persons with OSA, the individual stops breathing for a short period of time resulting in forced awakening, disrupting the individual's sleep and reduces total sleep time and compromises their overall sleep health [6]. The restriction of airflow leads to impairment of baroreceptor modulation of sympathetic nerve activity; such dysregulation can exacerbate arteriosclerosis, hypertension and other cardio-metabolic disorders [7].

OSA has been proposed as an important risk factor in the cause of death among NFL players such as Reggie White, who played professionally for the Philadelphia Eagles and the Green Bay Packers. Other notable NFL players diagnosed with OSA include Tony Dorsett, Warren Sapp, Aaron Taylor, Percy Harvin and Ja Marcus Russell [7]. Research has revealed that football players have a higher prevalence of obesity, de ined as body mass index (BMI) > 30 kg/m^2 [8,9]. Obesity is among the many predictors of OSA risk [10]. Currently, there is limited information regarding the association of obstructive sleep apnea among American professional football players. Thus, the purpose of this scoping review is to evaluate the current literature on the impact of OSA among NFL players.

Methods

Research objectives were addressed using a scoping review methodology. The aim of a scoping review is to: 1) map relevant concepts and identify gaps in research [11] and 2) provide a comprehensive overview of the literature without engaging in the appraisal of multiple study outcomes [11]. The procedures of a scoping review consists of (1) identifying the research questions (2) identifying relevant studies, (3) study selection (4) charting the data (5) collating, summarizing and reporting the results and (6) an expert advisory consultation exercise [11]. Search terms were identified and agreed upon by authors and a medical librarian from New York University School of Medicine. Our literature search included a study of six databases; Google Scholar, EMBASE, CINAHL, PubMed, ProQuest, and Web of Science Plus. The following combination of terms was used to conduct a search in each database: (National football players or national football player OR professional football players or professional football player or national football league or NFL) and (Cardiovascular disease or cardiovascular diseases or heart disease or heart failure or vascular disease) and (Sleep disordered breathing OR apnea or apneas or sleep hypopneas) and (hypertension OR high blood pressure). A diagram illustrating the inclusion and exclusion of studies included is shown in Figure 1.

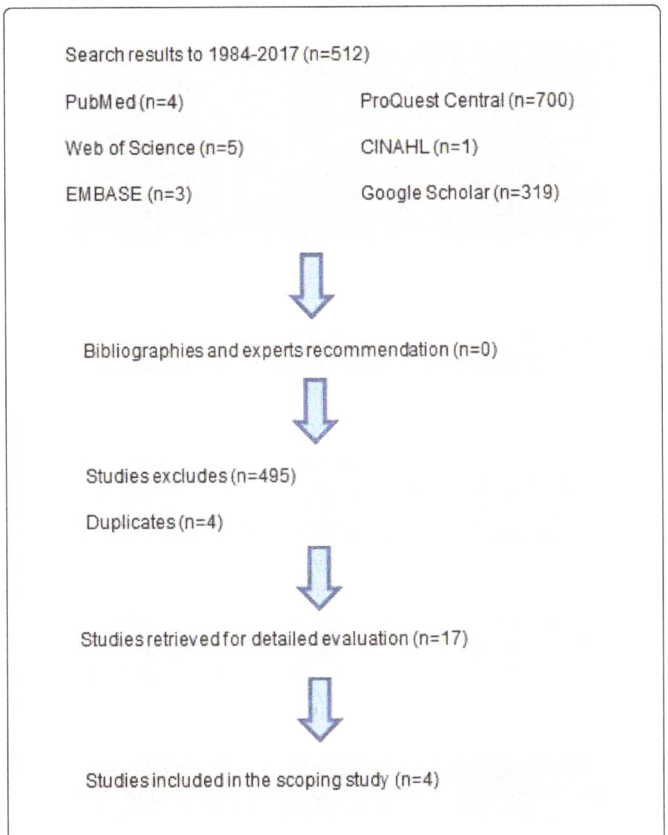

Figure 1: A flow chart using databases.

All articles were manually reviewed to identify any relevant studies. Grey literature was excluded; literature study was exclusive to peer-reviewed articles between 1984-2017. Citations were managed using bibliographic software manager endnote [11]. Eligibility criteria placed emphasis on whether studies provided a direct or broad description of the associations of obstructive sleep apnea among national league football players with cardiovascular disease and related sleep breathing disorders. The titles and abstracts of each citation were screened by the lead author; all relevant peer-reviewed articles were procured for full-text version.

Results

Searches were carried out during the month of June 2017. All databases were searched independently, and all articles returned were compiled and saved in Endnote. All duplicates were removed, and after final screening and data extraction (n=4). Of the 512 references recorded, 495 were excluded during the initial screening process. The remaining 17 articles were reviewed in-depth and 4 articles were included in this scoping review. A flow chart of this process can be found (Figure 1).

Relevant information was extracted from each paper and charted to highlight the following: author, year of publication, study title, method, theme, outcome and limitations.

Authors	Year	Method	Themes	Outcome
Hyman et al.	2012	Logistic regression	Sensitivity and specificity of use of BMI for obesity	Of 129 NFL players, nearly half played linemen. After 1-32 years out from retirement most prevalent conditions were OSA and HTN; 42% reporting both
Albuquerque et al.	2010	Case control	Prevalence of SDB in retired NFL players	Of 257 retired NFL players; SDB was present in 52.3%. Defensive linemen were more likely to have SDB (61%vs. 46%; p= 0.02) than non-linemen
Rice et al.	2010	Cross sectional cohort study	Prevalence of SDB in active NFL players	Of 137 active NFL players recruited from 12 different teams 100% reported snoring; observed apneas in 23.9%; Moderate SDB in 4.4%; no significant differences between linemen and non-linemen
Luyster et al.	2017	Retrospective analysis	Compared OSA risk in retired NFL players to CARDIA sleep study participants	Retired NFL players have greater prevalence of OSA

Table 1: Collating, summarizing and reporting the result.

Discussion

The purpose of this scoping study was to organize and evaluate the limited literature regarding obstructive sleep apnea among NFL players and to increase awareness of the adverse effects of untreated OSA. As noted from NFL recruitment surveys, average NFL linemen weigh over 300 lbs; and this is now the norm compared with 3 decades ago (300 players in 2017 over 300 lbs., 10 players in 1986) [12]. This trend starts at the college level and has continued on this trajectory. There is an unprecedented need for further studies on the health of NFL linemen, fueled by the unmeasured dangers of NFL athletes increasing in size, weight, and BMI. The widow of Reggie White has called for increased awareness of OSA through an education campaign launched by a foundation under his name as well as health initiatives promoted by different organizations in the league [13]. For clinicians, there is a paucity of peer-reviewed information on OSA among NFL players. Failure to treat OSA can increase the risk of stroke and cardiovascular disease [8]. The effects of OSA are rampant, not only regarding the quality of sleep and daytime performance, but there is also a tremendous influence on the circulatory system [8,14]. Repeated and recurrent nightly episodes of dyspnea from airflow collapse leads to retention of carbon dioxide and low oxygenation [15]. This can result in increased heart rate and respiratory drive provoked after many apneic cycles per hour per night of raised stress hormones and catecholamine that leads to elevated blood pressures [16]. Over time, the incremental effect would exacerbate comorbid factors such as preexisting hypertension, metabolic syndrome, dyslipidemia, coronary artery disease and the chances of mortality from a stroke, heart attack or both [16].

Limitations

The data from the studies included in this scoping study were largely in support of the presence of OSA among linemen in the NFL. This is consistent with the hypothesis of the scoping study: NFL players are more predisposed to OSA than are non-NFL players. However, there are multiple confounding factors and limitations from the studies that should be further explored.

The power of the studies included is an important limitation. The study conducted by Rice et al. shows a negligible incidence of OSA among linemen and non-linemen. The study further revealed that investigators fell short on their recruitment goals. Drop out or inability to complete study for any number of reasons reduced the sample size even smaller.

Volunteer bias was an issue in several studies and was mentioned by Albuquerque et al. as a limitation in their study. Their study, which favored the hypothesis that NFL linemen suffered from a higher prevalence of OSA, could have been affected by the concerns of the participants that led them to volunteer for the study. The volunteers could have been concerned with having some or all of the symptoms of OSA or its associated comorbidities such as high blood pressure. The study, therefore, could have excluded those individuals that were not aware of their symptoms and or chose not to participate. Again, volunteer drop-out or inability to complete the study reduced the sample size.

Generalization of the collected data from the studies presently is difficult in part due to the limitations mentioned above, but may also be due to lack of specific factors such as ethnicity. Ethnicity of the participants was collected, but the percentage of each ethnic group regarding the presence of OSA was not reported. This may be because ethnicity was not seen as a risk factor in the development of OSA. There are even fewer studies done on whether certain races/ethnicities have a higher prevalence of developing OSA among NFL players. However, it is widely well documented that certain chronic comorbidities such as diabetes and hypertension do affect certain races/ethnicities greater, such as Blacks [8]. Other studies have found that minorities tend to experience less sleep quantity and quality than do whites [16]. Furthermore, since NFL participants were all male between the ages of 23-28 years, application of the findings to the general population must be done cautiously.

The accuracy and validity of using BMI as a predictor of obesity is questioned because it does not take into account muscle mass, bone density and body composition [15]. In addition to obesity, other attributes that put a linemen or non-linemen at risk for OSA could be dependent on other variables such as other comorbidities (diabetes and cardiovascular disease) [16]. Many studies used measurements such as neck circumference and hip-to-waist ratio in addition to BMI. Other researchers propose the use of DEXA scan for better estimation of body fat composition for determination of true obesity [15].

The accuracy and validity of home sleep apnea testing (HSAT) were called into question and this modality for OSA detection was commonly used across the studies in the scoping study. The gold standard for which HSAT is compared against is polysomnography in inpatient sleep study. In general practice, physicians would refer individuals suspected of OSA from the initial screening questionnaire to undergo overnight polysomnographic sleep study. This has been the gold standard to assess sleep apnea. In-patient sleep studies may not involve the physician directly over the course of the night but involves implementing multiple monitoring modalities. Some of the data recorded include rapid eye movement (REM) occurrence and brain wave activity via electroencephalogram (EEG), possible cardiac arrhythmias via electrocardiogram (ECG), carbon dioxide levels, muscle tone and whether substances have been utilized to induce sleep such as alcohol and medications. Compared with lab-based sleep studies, HSAT may be preferred because of convenience, accessibility, and lower costs (no overnight staff). Rice et al. state there was data loss (22 of 159) in their study from the single channel portable unattended home study reporting apnea/hypopnea episodes. The HSAT results in Rice et al. study were compared to results of the general population with OSA that was produced by polysomnography. Two different machines could have an unreported amount of variation. Furthermore, there are multiple types of HSAT and some studies reported which type was used while others did not.

Conclusion

Lifestyle changes such as weight reduction to reduce OSA severity is widely known as a method to mitigate the symptoms of OSA. However, for most NFL linemen weight reduction may not be feasible for their active careers. For this population, greater emphasis needs to be placed on adherences to OSA treatment such as Continuous Positive Airway Pressure (CPAP). Noncompliance to CPAP should be closely followed by clinicians to investigate the root reasons if noncompliance occurs. If non-adherence to CPAP is in the form of discomfort or perceived stigma of wearing a mask, increased educational awareness and successful treatment testimonials can open opportunities to increase adherence. Further studies are required to improve the rate of screening NFL players for OSA risk. The potential impact of treating OSA may have a positive influence in athletic agility and increase players performance in addition to decreasing risk for cardiovascular disease and sudden cardiac death.

Acknowledgments

Gaganjot Parmar, who provided support with the literature review.

Funding

This research is supported by the National Heart, Lung, and Blood Institute (NHLBI) (R25HL116378)

References

1. Ellenbogen JM (2005) Cognitive benefits of sleep and their loss due to sleep deprivation. Neurology 64: E25-27.
2. Valentino IIIDJ, O'Donnell AE (2006) Reasons and referrals for sleep medicine consultation in obstructive sleep apnea. Chest 130: 264S-b-264S.
3. Williams NJ, Jean LG, Ravenell J, Seixas A, Islam N, et al. (2016) A community-oriented framework to increase screening and treatment of obstructive sleep apnea among blacks. Sleep Med 18: 82-87.
4. Ravenell J, Seixas A, Rosenthal DM, Williams O, Ogedegbe C, et al. (2016) Effect of birthplace on cardiometabolic risk among blacks in the Metabolic Syndrome Outcome Study (MetSO). Diabetol Metab Syndr 8:14.
5. Diaz AM, Chatila W, Lammi MR, Swift I, D'Alonzo GE, et al. (2014) Determinants of CPAP Adherence in Hispanics with Obstructive Sleep Apnea. Sleep Disord 878213.
6. George CF, Kab V, Levy AM (2003) Increased prevalence of sleep-disordered breathing among professional football players. In: Solutions ss. Sleep apnea and NFL players. N Engl J Med. pp: 367-368.
7. Luyster FS, Dunn RE, Lauderdale DS, Carnethon MR, Tucker AM, et al. (2017) Sleep-apnea risk and subclinical atherosclerosis in early-middle-aged retired National Football League players. Nat Sci Sleep 9: 31-38.
8. Buell JL, Calland D, Hanks F, Johnston B, Pester B, et al. (2008) Presence of metabolic syndrome in football linemen. J Athl Train 43: 608-616.
9. Rogers A, Ravenell J, Donat M, Sexias A, Ogedegbe C, et al. (2015) Predictors of obstructive sleep apnea risk among Blacks with metabolic syndrome. J Obes Overweight 1: 1104
10. Reuters T. Web of Science. 2012.
11. Pokharel Y, Basra S, Lincoln AE, Tucker AM, Nambi V, et al. (2014) Association of body mass index and waist circumference with subclinical atherosclerosis in retired NFL players. South Med J 107: 633-639.
12. Abernethy WB, Choo JK, Hutter AM (2003) Echocardiographic characteristics of professional football players. J Am Coll Cardiol 41:280-284.
13. George CF, Kab V, Kab P, Villa JJ, Levy AM (2003) Sleep and breathing in professional football players. Sleep Med 4:317-325.
14. Ripka WL, Modesto JD, Ulbricht L, Gewehr PM (2016) Obesity impact evaluated from fat percentage in bone mineral density of male adolescents. PLoS One 11: e0163470.
15. Halson SL. (2014) Sleep in elite athletes and nutritional interventions to enhance sleep. Sports Med 44: 13-23.
16. Batool AS, Goodwin JL, Kushida CA, Walsh JA, Simon RD, et al. (2016) Impact of continuous positive airway pressure (CPAP) on quality of life in patients with obstructive sleep apnea (OSA). J Sleep Res 25: 731-738.

On the Comparison of the Effectiveness of Acupuncture and Medication Therapy on Improving Sleep Disorders in Women Suffering from Generalized Anxiety Disorder

Sajedeh Behtaj*

Alborz Science and Research Branch, Islamic Azad University, Iran.

***Corresponding author:** Sajedeh Behtaj, Alborz Science and Research Branch, Islamic Azad University, Iran, E-mail: sajedeh.behtaj@yahoo.com

Abstract

This study aims to compare the effectiveness of acupuncture and medication therapy on improving sleep disorders in women suffering from Generalized Anxiety Disorder. This study is a quasi-experimental with pretest-posttest, control group, and follow-up period. The study population included all women suffering from generalized anxiety disorder and sleep disorder. Purposive sampling was used to select the sample. Using this method, 45 participants were selected and randomly assigned to three groups: acupuncture, medication therapy, and control groups. Acupuncture group received 12 to 15 treatment sessions (2-3 times a week) in DU20, HT7, PC6, Kid6, Ren12, UB62, Sp6, Anmian and Ear-shen men. Medication therapy group were taken drugs under the supervision of a psychiatric while the control group received no intervention over this period. In order to analyze the data, repeated measures were used in the statistical SPSS software version 21. The results showed that both acupuncture and medication therapy programs improve sleep disorder in women with generalized anxiety disorder; however, the acupuncture was more effective than medication therapy.

Keywords: Generalized anxiety disorder; Acupuncture effectiveness; Sleep disorder

Introduction

Sleep disorders, i.e. dissatisfaction with the quality or quantity of sleep, are along with complaints about the difficulty in falling asleep and in keeping sleeping [1]. Sleep quality has a key role in one's health and well being. Any sleep disorder, in addition to causing mental health problems, physically reduces the person's ability. Those suffering from sleep disorders are easily aroused and get angry. Furthermore, one's cognitive function and concentration level to deal with daily activities are reduced [2]. The results have shown that the mean frequency of hospitalization per month for people suffering from insomnia, compared with those with no history of sleep disorders, has almost doubled [3]. Sleep deprivation also leads to a decrease in function of the immune system and in function of hypothalamus, pituitary and adrenal during subsequent days, glucose tolerance, hypertension and increased risk of cardiovascular events, decreased maximum ability in anaerobic power and level [4].

Generalized anxiety disorder is a pervasive disorder in which a person is constantly worried about future events and is afraid of them. This subject leads to chronic and morbid concern about future events [5]. This disorder is characterized by intrusive and pervasive fears and daily dysfunction. People suffering from the generalized anxiety disorder are obsessed with non-controllable concerns (Pending concerns). Diagnosis of generalized anxiety disorder depends on the existence of two key symptoms: concern (e.g. negative preoccupation of future events) and physiological overstimulation (e.g. muscle tension, sleep disturbance, feelings of tuning). Concern is regarded as the most prominent symptom of generalized anxiety disorder. Concern is a cognitive activity which is determined by the perception of a potential risk in the future (for instance, If I fail licensing exam next week, I won't be able to find a job). Concerns are often to gain control and to prevent the occurrence of negative events in the future (What can I do to avoid failing the exam) [6-8].

People suffering from generalized anxiety disorder first seek medical treatment because of some problems including physical difficulties, sleep disorders, muscle tension, indigestion, restlessness, boredom susceptibility, irritability as well as those problems occurring during individuals' leisure activities. In this disorder, there is distortion in the management of facts and risks, particularly in people who are concerned about their own and their family members' health, safety, welfare. They face cognitive distortions in perceiving the coming events [9]. In addition, studies have shown that there is a positive relationship between concerns in generalized anxiety disorder and other maladaptive emotion regulation strategies and psychopathology such as suppression rumination [10].

Previous studies examining the relationship between anxiety disorders and sleep problems show that one of the areas being severely affected by anxiety disorders is sleep quality and quantity. For example, Short in his study claimed that insomnia symptoms are directly associated with anxiety [11]. He also showed that anxiety treatment reduces symptoms of insomnia. In this regard, Wang also indicated that sleep disorder is closely related to problems such as hypertension, diabetes, hyperlipidemia, depression, and anxiety. He also showed that 54% of individuals suffering from sleep disorder have an anxiety disorder too [12].

For the treatment of sleep disorders, the effectiveness of various treatment methods including Cognitive Behavioral Therapy (CBT), medication therapy, herbal therapy, yoga, acupuncture, meditation and the like is separately studied. The research on the side effects of medication therapy indicates that long-term use of these medications may have undesirable consequences. For example, the results of the study conducted by Feiz Abadi, et al. showed that the use of Benzodiazepines causes negative side effects including forgetfulness, drowsiness, fatigue, headache, weakness, exhaustion, irritability, and confusion. Benzodiazepines also affect the motor system, causing slowness of movement and impaired motor skills. Furthermore, the research has shown that taking these medications affect the liver enzymes and cause increased alkaline phosphatase.

Although the most common method to treat sleep problems is taking drugs, scientific evidence suggests that the effectiveness of non-pharmaceutical approaches, due to their long-term durability and lack of side effects, are recommended by physicians. For example, CBT which consists of a specific set of techniques that strengthen the bed-sleep connection, realign the homeostatic mechanisms and the circadian rhythm and decrease anxiety and rumination about sleep [13].

One of the methods of alternative medicine is acupuncture which has been of concern over recent years in the world as well as in Iran. Clinical advances in the acupuncture research, along with side effects of conventional medication treatment of chronic pains, have significantly increased the use of acupuncture over the past decades. It is estimated that over half a million therapist outside China have used acupuncture to treat diseases [14]. According to clinical evidence, acupuncture is a safe non-medication approach to treat insomnia. The first official organization reporting the effect of acupuncture on many diseases, including sleep disorder was the World Health Organization. In 1996, this organization, based on clinical trials, announced a list of diseases which can be treated by acupuncture. Spence et al. as a result of their research on a five-week clinical trial on 18 young patients suffering from anxiety and insomnia showed that acupuncture not also reduces anxiety but also decreases the number of waking-up times [15].

The results of the research regard the mechanism of acupuncture effect on sleep quality as follows:

- Adjusting the chemical transmitters (neurotransmitters) such as serotonin, noradrenaline, dopamine, and neuropeptide Y Gapa in the nervous system, which lead to positive psychological effects including enhanced good-temperedness, reduced anxiety and depression as well as stress management.
- Stimulating the secretion of Beta-endorphin and increasing the activity of opioid receptors in the central nervous system.
- Decreasing the sympathetic activity of nervous system and creating a relaxing effect.
- Improving blood flow by regulating the activity of the Nitricoxide synthase enzyme.

According to what was mentioned above, the researcher in this study is to compare the effectiveness of two methods of medication therapy and acupuncture therapy on improving sleep disorders in women suffering from generalized anxiety disorder. The results will be of great implications for researchers, physicians, and patients.

Methodology

This study is a pilot study with pre and posttest and control group design. The sample of the study consisted of forty five 18-70 year-old women referring to the clinic. Fifteen participants were randomly assigned to the acupuncture therapy group. Fifteen subjects were also randomly placed in the medication therapy (Zolpidem, diazepam, clonazepam, alprazolam) group and the remaining 15 patients were in the control group. Inclusion criteria were as follows: lack of therapeutic intervention at the same time, getting a score of 6 and higher in Pittsburgh's test, confirmed anxiety by questionnaire, complaints of insomnia for at least a month. The exclusion criteria included: developing medical insomnia, pregnancy, inflammation or infection in the acupuncture points. To collect data in the pretest and posttest phases, Structured Clinical Interview for DSMIV (SCID DSM-IV) Clinical Version (SCID-CV), Pittsburgh Sleep Quality Index (PSQI), Beck Anxiety Inventory, and Ketel Anxiety Questionnaire were used. In order to analyze the data, repeated measures were used in the statistical SPSS software version 21.

Findings

To compare the effectiveness of acupuncture and medication therapy on sleep disorders in women suffering from generalized anxiety disorder, the scores of participants with acupuncture and medication therapy in total score of Pittsburgh sleep quality questionnaire before and after the intervention and well as during follow-up period were statistically analyzed using repeated measures analysis are shown in Table 1.

One of the assumptions of repeated measures test is Mauchly test. It should be noted that Green Haos-Gasser index will be used if the Mauchly test is significant. On the other hand, sphericity index will be employed. The results for all aspects of the questionnaire and its total score in the acupuncture and medication therapy groups are shown in Table 2.

Dimension	Time periods	Acupuncture		Medication therapy		Control group	
		Mean	Standard deviation	Mean	Standard deviation	Mean	Standard deviation
Sleep mental quality	Pre- intervention	46/2	63/0	80/2	56/0	33/2	72/0
	Post-intervention	73/0	45/0	66/1	72/0	86/1	63/0
	follow-up	73/0	45/0	66/1	72/0	40/2	50/0
Delays in falling asleep	Pre- intervention	33/2	89/0	80/2	41/0	33/2	72/0
	Post-intervention	13-Jan	63/0	73/1	96/0	2	65/0
	follow-up	06-Jan	45/0	60/1	05-Jan	40/2	63/0

Sleep duration	Pre- intervention	60/2	63/0	66/2	48/0	66/1	72/0
	Post-intervention	40/0	50/0	06-Jan	22-Jan	33/2	48/0
	follow-up	60/0	63/0	1	13-Jan	2	06-Jan
Beneficial sleep	Pre- intervention	66/2	48/0	53/2	99/0	93/1	03-Jan
	Post-intervention	26/0	45/0	26/0	70/0	20-Feb	77/0
	follow-up	26/0	45/0	26/0	70/0	13-Feb	63/0
Sleep disorders	Pre- intervention	33/2	48/0	66/2	48/0	53/2	63/0
	Post-intervention	1	34/0	66/1	48/0	33/2	48/0
	follow-up	1	34/0	66/1	48/0	20-Feb	67/0
Daily dysfunction disorder	Pre- intervention	2	92/0	20-Feb	77/0	46/2	51/0
	Post-intervention	80/0	56/0	93/1	96/0	46/2	63/0
	follow-up	80/0	56/0	2	84/0	46/2	51/0
Total score of sleep quality questionnaire	Pre- intervention	40/14	88/1	66/15	63/1	13	92/1
	Post-intervention	33/4	11-Jan	10	3	80/15	65/1
	follow-up	46/4	18-Jan	26-Sep	84/2	60/16	19-Feb

Table 1: Descriptive indices of scores over three periods in sleep quality indices.

Mauchly sphericity test	**Indices**			
	W Mauchly	**Chi-square**	**df**	**Sig.**
sleep mental quality	75/0	66/14	2	25/0
Delays in falling asleep	329/0	30/3	2	001/0
Sleep duration	293/0	33/11	2	001/0
Beneficial sleep	265/0	19/18	2	01/0
Sleep disorders	76/0	30/7	2	028/0
Daily dysfunction disorder	115/0	38/58	2	001/0
Total score of sleep quality questionnaire	490/	27/19	2	001/0

Table 2: Mauchly Sphericity Test results to examine the assumptions of repeated measures.

As it can be observed in Table 3, the results show that the within-subjects index is significantly different in treatment and control group with regard to at least one of the pre- intervention, post-intervention, and follow-up tests since Green Haos-Gasser and sphericity tests are significant. The between-subjects results also showed that there is no significant difference between acupuncture and medication therapy groups in terms of delay in falling asleep, sleep duration, and beneficial sleep; however, there is a significant difference between these two groups regarding other domains and total score of the sleep quality questionnaire.

Dimensions	**Index**	**Test**	**Sum of squares**	**df**	**Mean of squares**	**F**	**Sig.**	**Eta**
Sleep mental quality	Within-subjects	Sphericity test	41/08	2	54/20	54/103	001/0	78/0
		Time * Group	80/1	2	90/0	53/4	001/0	13/0
		Error	43415	56	198/0	-	-	-

	Between subjects	Group	43444	1	43444	32/17	001/0	38/0
		Error	55/19	28	69/0	-	-	-
Delays in falling asleep	Within-subjects	Green Haos-Gasser	18/28	43119	52/23	57/54	001/0	66/0
		Time * Group	067/0	43119	056/0	129/0	767/0	005/0
		Error	44/14	50/33	431/0	-	-	-
	Between subjects	Group	40/6	1	40/6	91/4	36586	14/0
		Error	48/36	28	43130	-	-	-
Sleep duration	Within-subjects	Green Haos-Gasser	75/69	43117	52/59	50/93	001/0	77/0
		Time * Group	35/1	43117	43115	81/1	187/0	36678
		Error	88/20	81/23	637/0	-	-	-
	Between subjects	Group	43180	1	43180	48/2	126/0	36739
		Error	17/36	28	43129	-	-	-
Beneficial sleep	Within-subjects	Green Haos-Gasser	88/108	1	88/108	78/149	001/0	84/0
		Time * Group	089/0	1	089/0	122/0	729/0	004/0
		Error	35/20	28	72/0	-	-	-
	Between subjects	Group	044/0	1	044/0	076/0	78/0	003/0
		Error	44/16	28	587/0	-	-	-
Sleep disorders	Within-subjects	Green Haos-Gasser	22/27	1	22/27	90/155	001/0	840
		Time * Group	556/0	1	556/0	43177	36739	102/0
		Error	88/4	56	087/0	-	-	-
	Between subjects	Group	94/6	1	94/6	43154	001/0	45/0
		Error	44/8	28	30/0	-	-	-
Daily dysfunction disorder	Within-subjects	Green Haos-Gasser	43401	43106	69/9	36/18	001/0	39/0
		Time * Group	68/4	43106	41/4	36/8	006/0	23/0
		Error	68/15	70/29	528/0	-	-	-
	Between subjects	Group	43206	1	43206	32/12	002/0	30/0
		error	44/36	28	43130	-	-	-
Total score of sleep quality questionnaire	Within-subjects	Green Haos-Gasser	68/1286	32/1	66/971	05/330	001/0	92/0
		Time * Group	48/81	32/1	53/61	90/20	001/0	42/0
		Error	15/109	13697	94/2	-	-	-
	Between subjects	Group	17/344	1	17/344	79/37	001/0	57/0
		Error	77/253	28	33025	-	-	-

Table 3: Results of within-subjects and between-subjects for acupuncture and medication therapy groups.

In Table 4, the results of Trace Pillai's multivariate analysis of variance to compare sleep quality dimensions and its total score based on variable Control Group is shown. Considering this information, it can be said that groups differ regarding their total score and sleep disorders dimensions. It means that there is a difference in the sleep disorder at least between one of the tests (pre-intervention and post-intervention, follow-up) in acupuncture and medication therapy groups. Bonferroni post hoc test was used to evaluate the differences and the results are presented below.

Source of variation	Value	DF Hypothesis	DF error	F	Sig.
Sleep mental quality	78/0	2	27	54/3	001/0
Delays in falling asleep	686/0	2	27	43341	001/0
Sleep duration	785/0	2	27	19/49	001/0
Beneficial sleep	84/0	2	27	78/149	001/0
Sleep disorders	848/0	2	27	90/155	001/0
Daily dysfunction disorder	410/0	2	27	38/9	001/0
Total score of sleep quality questionnaire	934/0	2	27	62/189	001/0

Table 4: The results of Trace Pillai's multivariate analysis of variance to compare sleep quality dimensions and its total score based on variable Group.

Results presented in Table 5 show that there are significant differences between acupuncture and medication therapy groups with regard to sleep quality, delays in falling asleep, sleep disorders, daily dysfunction disorder and total score of sleep quality questionnaire. Based on descriptive statistics, mean, and standard deviation of sleep quality dimensions and their total score and due to the significant differences between medication therapy and acupuncture groups regarding the aforementioned indices, it can be concluded that acupuncture therapy is more effective in improving sleep order in women suffering from generalized anxiety disorder.

Dimension	Group i	Group j	Mean difference (i-j)	Standard error	Sig.
Sleep mental quality	acupuncture	medication therapy	733/0	176/0	001/0
Delays in falling asleep	acupuncture	medication therapy	53/0	241/0	36586
Sleep duration	acupuncture	medication therapy	378/0	240/	36861
Beneficial sleep	acupuncture	medication therapy	044/0	162/0	78/0
Sleep disorders	acupuncture	medication therapy	556/0	116/0	001/0
Daily dysfunction disorder	acupuncture	medication therapy	844/0	241/0	002/0
Total score of sleep quality questionnaire	acupuncture	medication therapy	91/3	635/0	001/0

Table 5: Bonferroni test results for sleep quality total scores and dimensions over time periods in acupuncture and medication therapy groups.

Results and Discussion

The results showed that both acupuncture and medication therapy programs improve sleep disorder in women with generalized anxiety disorder; however, the acupuncture was more effective than medication therapy.

With regard to the effect of acupuncture on improving and enhancing sleep quality, the results of the current study are in line with the results of research conducted by Zhao [16]. Considering the emphasis on the role of acupuncture in improving sleep disorder, the results of this study are consistent with the results of Yuxin's study. Yuxin reported that the number of participants' nightmare attacks was halved after one week of acupuncture and there were no such attacks after two weeks. Using PET scan, MRI and EEG, he showed that acupuncture had a significant impact on cortical structure, frontal cortex, medial temporal lobe, and limbic areas (Amygdala, Hypothalamus, and Hippocampus). Hence, it has been effective in reducing anxiety.

The results of this study and the research findings by Spence, et al. are in a same vein. In a five-week clinical trial on 18 young patients suffering from anxiety and insomnia, they show that acupuncture, in addition to reducing anxiety, significantly increases the brain endogenous melatonin secretion. According to the measurements of polysomnography (sleepography), it improved all sleep-related factors such as increased total sleep time and decreased frequency of waking-up times [15].

Considering the literature in explaining the effect mechanism of acupuncture in improving sleep quality and mood disorders, researchers have emphasized on the following cases: Adjusting the chemical transmitters (neurotransmitters) such as serotonin, noradrenaline, dopamine, and neuropeptide Y Gapa in the nervous system, which lead to positive psychological effects including enhanced good-temperedness, reduced anxiety and depression as well as stress management. Stimulating the secretion of Beta-endorphin and increasing the activity of opioid receptors in the central nervous system. Decreasing the sympathetic activity of nervous system and creating a relaxing effect. Improving blood flow by regulating the activity of the Nitricoxide synthase enzyme [16,17].

Accordingly, it can be argued that acupuncture can be effective in the treatment of sleep disorders in individuals suffering from anxiety disorders. However, there are a few research studies on long-term effects of acupuncture. Today, acupuncture has many advocators in different Asian, European, and American countries. Many people around the world, besides pain cure and relieve, use it to prevent the diseases. Even a group of men and women referring to clinics strive to improve their life quality, relaxation, increased calmness, and health by using acupuncture. This group, in addition to providing equal nutrition and blood supply to various parts of the body cells, transfer proper energy to different parts of the body cells through the regulation of the body's energy in energy channels and chakras. In this regard, it strengthens individuals' central and peripheral nervous system, power, and physical strength [18-22].

It also encourages further study on a large scale and fundamental research on the mechanism on another region of brain action. Furthermore, there is the possibility of using another methods namely laser acupuncture, auricular acupuncture, etc. The above mentioned research is only practical on women. It is also advised to do furthered examinations on men as well [22-26].

References

1. Tehran, Ravan N (2013) Diagnostic and Statistical Manual of Mental Disorders. (Translated by Yahya Sayyed Mohammadi, 2014) (Fifth edn), American Psychiatric Association pp: 215-218.
2. Khushab, Hadi (2013) Comparing the views of physicians, nurses, and patients on risk factors associated with patients' sleep problems. J Health Promot Manag 2: 17-18.
3. Thase ME (2005) Correlates and consequences of chronic insomnia. Gen Hosp Psychiatry 27: 100-112.
4. Ayas NT, White DP, Manson JE, Stampfer MJ, Speizer FE, et al. (2003) A prospective study of sleep duration and coronary heart disease in women. Arch Intern Med 163: 205-209.
5. Ganji, Mahdi (2014) Psychopathology, DSM-5, Savalan Publication Center Tehran.
6. Diagnostic and statistical manual of mental disorders (2000) (4th edn, Text Revision). American Psychiatric Association , Washington DC
7. Stapinski LA, Abbott MJ, Rapee RM (2010) Evaluating the cognitive avoidance model of generalised anxiety disorder: Impactof worry on threat appraisal, perceived control and anxious arousal. Behav Res Ther 48: 1032-1042.
8. Hupper JD, Sanderson WC (2007) Psychotherapy for Generalized Anxiety Disorder. Textbook of anxiety disorders.
9. Allgulande C (2012) Generalized Anxiety Disorder: A Review of Recent Findings. J Exp Clin Med 4: 88-91.
10. Aldao A, Mennin DS (2012) Paradoxical cardiovascular effects of implementing adaptive emotion regulation strategies in generalized anxiety disorder. Behav Res Ther 50: 122-130.
11. Short NA, Allan NP, Raines AM, Schmidt NB (2015) The effects of an anxiety sensitivity intervention on insomnia symptoms. Sleep Med 16: 152-159.
12. Wang L, Song Y, Li F, Liu Y, Ma J, et al. (2014) Effect of wen Dan Tang on insomnia-related anxiety and levels. Neural Regen Res 9: 205-212.
13. Anderson KN (2018) Insomnia and cognitive behavioural therapy-How to assess your patient and why it should be a standard part of care. J Thorac Dis 10: 94-102.
14. Navidi, Asghar A (2002) Basic and Clinical Principles of Acupuncture. Tabib Publication Center 70-74.
15. Spence DW, Kayumov L, Chen A, Lowe A, Jain U, et al. (2004) Acupuncture increases nocturnal melatonin secretion and reduces insomnia and anxiety: A preliminary report. J Neuropsychiatry Clin Neurosci 16: 19-28.
16. Zhao K (2013) Acupuncture for the treatment of insomnia. Int Rev Neurobial 111:217-34.
17. Gao X, Xu C, Wang P, Ren SH, Zhou Y, et al. (2013) Curative effect of acupuncture and moxibustion on insomnia: A randomized clinical trial. J Tradit Chin Med 33(4): 428-432
18. Feyzabadi Z, Jafari F, Kamali SH, Ashayeri H, Badiee Aval S, et al. (2014) Efficacy of Viola odorata in Treatment of Chronic Insomnia. Iran Red Crescent Med J 16: e17511.
19. Gao L, Zhang M, Gong H, Bai L, Dai XJ, et al. (2014) Differential activation patterns of FMRI in sleep-deprived brain: Restoring effects of acupuncture. Evid Based Complement Alternat Med (465760).
20. Haljin, Depi R, Vitborn, Susan Kras (2007) Psychopathology: Clinical views on mental disorders, Volume II, Translated by Yahya Sayyed Mohammadi, 2005. Tehran: Nashre Ravan.
21. Han KH, Kim SY, Chung SY (2014) Effect of acupuncture on patients with insomnia: Study protocol for a randomized controlled trial. Trials 15: 403.
22. He Y, Chen J, Pan Z, Ying Z (2014) Scalp acupuncture treatment protocol for Anxiety disorders: A case report. Glob Adv Health Med 3(4): 35–39.
23. Lu C, Yang XJ, Hu J (2014) Efficiency comparison between acupuncture smoothing Liver and regulating Spleen method for menopausal insomnia. Zhongguo Zhen Jiu 34: 759-762.
24. Tawfiq RA, Nassar NN, El-Eraky WI, El-Denshary ES (2014) Enhanced efficacy and reduced side effects of diazepam by Kava combination. J Adv Res 5: 587-594.
25. Mehran R (2011) Acupuncture from the perspective of the West. J Anesth Pain Med 1: 2-3.
26. Yao HF, Zhang HF, Chen XL (2012) Observation on therapeutic effect of scalp-acupoint catgut embedding for 33 cases of insomnia patients. Zhen Ci Yan Jiu 37: 394-397.

12

Parasomnias and Childhood Adversity in an Adult Psychiatric Population

Giovanni Mansueto, Sara Palmieri and Carlo Faravelli*

Department of Health Sciences, Psychology and Psychiatry Unit, University of Florence, Florence, Italy

***Corresponding author:** Carlo Faravelli, Department of Health Sciences, Psychology and Psychiatry Unit, University of Florence, via di San Salvi 12, 50135, Florence, Italy, E-mail: carlo.faravelli@unifi.it

Abstract

Background: A wide evidence suggest that sleep disorders and psychopathology could be related each other, as well as, that childhood adversities (CAs) may be associated with both. However, the relationship between CA and sleep disorders in psychiatric patients is still unclear. This study aims to explore the hypothesis that CA could be associated with sleep impairments in a sample of psychiatric patients.

Method: 351 psychiatric patients and 177 controls draw from the general population were recruited. Sleep symptoms were assessed by FPI. CAs were evaluated by FPI and CECA-Q. Chi-square, Fisher's test, Odds Ratios, Binary Logistic Regression were performed.

Results: Patients with childhood sexual abuse (CSA) showed higher rate of nightmares, bruxism, somnambulism and pavor nocturns than those without CSA. Cases with negligence of father or mother reported higher rate of terminal insomnia and nightmares than patients without neglect. Controls with childhood physical abuse (CPA) showed higher rate of pavor nocturns.

Conclusion: CA could be related with sleep impairments in adulthood, moreover, seems to be a specific relationship between childhood sexual abuse and parasomnia. The association CAs-parasomnia seems to be more relevant among psychiatric cases than in the general population.

Keywords: Childhood adversity; Insomnia; Parasomnia; Psychopathology

Introduction

Descriptive and cross-sectional studies provide a robust evidence of a possible connection between sleep disturbances and psychopathology, showing an excess of sleep impairments in a wide array of psychiatric disorders as well as a psychiatric comorbidity among patients with insomnia and parasomnia [1-9].

Current evidence suggests that childhood adversities (CAs) might be linked with both psychopathology and sleep disorders [10-12]. CAs are commonly defined as life events that may occur during childhood and/or adolescence, such as childhood abuse (emotional, physical, or sexual), neglect, and loss event (parental loss and/or divorce) [10].

Substantial evidence from both cross-sectional and prospective studies indicates that childhood abuse and neglect are strongly associated with the development, persistence, and severity of adult psychopathology such as anxiety, PTSD [10,11], depression [13], psychosis [14], eating disorder, and personality disorder [10]. On the other hand, controversial findings have been reported about the role of early loss events [10,13,14].

Although a recent review by Kajeepeta et al. [12] suggested that sleep problems could be related with exposure to adversity during childhood, the relationship between CAs and sleep disorders in psychiatric patients remains still unclear. Indeed, we do not own a very robust amount of data confirming the role of early stress on sleep problems in psychiatric patients, as only two studies [15,16] have extensively evaluated this possible association. In this regard, Schafer and Bade [15] showed that high stress load in childhood was associated with prolonged sleep onset latency, decreased sleep efficiency and increased number of body movements during sleep. Faravelli et al. [16] showed that childhood abuse (physical and/or sexual) seems to increase by nearly 3 times the risk of recurrent nightmares.

Moreover, the research has largely focused on the relationship between CAs and insomnia [12], in part neglecting the role of parasomnia. Parasomnia is defined as an arousal disorder, characterized by unusual behaviours during sleep, such as nightmares, bruxism, sleep terrors, and somnambulism [2]. CAs seem to be associated with both nightmare and bruxism [16-20], while on the basis of our knowledge, any study has evaluated the relationship between CAs and experience of pavor and somnambulism in adulthood yet. In order to provide additional evidences to previous studies [12,15-20] the current research aims: (a) to evaluate the relationship between CA and sleep impairments in a representative sample of psychiatric patients, exploring the hypothesis that CAs could be associated with a cluster of sleep impairments; (b) to explore the association between CA and sleep disorders also in a control group of subjects drawn from a general population, in order to evaluate if the relationship CA-sleep disorders is present only in the psychiatric patients.

Methods

This research is part of the PSI-FIELDS (Factors in Early Life, Diagnoses, and Symptoms) project, an observational, multidisciplinary, and trans-nosological study. During a two-month period it was possible to contact and interview 351 consecutive patients admitted, within one week of the interview, to all the psychiatric in-and outpatient facilities of Tuscany.

Exclusion criteria were: age >75 years, neurological and/or neurocognitive impairment, disorders that might compromise the ability to give informed consent, pregnant or breast-feeding, substance abuse and/or addiction. A group of 177 people randomly drawn from the general population living in the same catchment area and matched with the psychiatric cases for age, gender and education made up the controls. The study protocol was approved by the local ethics committee and participants provided written informed consent.

Measure

DSM-IV diagnoses were made using the Structured Clinical Interview for DSM-IV Axis I Disorders [21]. Sleep impairments, insomnia and parasomnia symptoms were assessed by the Florence Psychiatric Interview (FPI) [22]. Each symptom is scored on a 5-point severity scale (0=absent, 1=dubious, 2=mild, 3=moderate and 4=severe). A score of at least 2 was considered for a symptom to be present. Sleep disorders were assessed referring to the last month. The FPI [22], a semi structured interview for evaluating the psychopathology in the community, is basically made up of the items from several well established rating scale combined in a single instrument. 121 symptoms are systematically explored, independent of the subject's diagnosis. As the interview uses a typically bottom up method, diagnoses may be obtained by specific algorithms: the correspondence with the Structured Clinical Interview for DSM-IV Axis I Disorders [21] is almost complete [22]. Moreover, sociodemographic information, life events, treatments received are also recorded. The FPI has shown good reliability [22].

The presence of childhood adversity was investigated by means of the Childhood Experience of Care and Abuse Questionnaire (CECA-Q) [23] and through a structured interview for early trauma included in the FPI [22]. CA was evaluated as follows: (a) presence of loss events whenever a death or separation (for 1 year or more) from parents was reported; (b) presence of sexual or physical abuse events when the CECA-Q or the interview revealed the presence of physical and/or sexual abuse; (c) presence of neglect was based on the CECA-Q scores in the scales "Mother's Neglect" and "Father's Neglect" using the proposed cut-off [23]. Insofar as the CECA-Q responses were concerned, we did not consider events that occurred after the age of 15. Life events were evaluated by experts who were not involved in the interview and who were blind to the patient or control status of the subjects.

According to previous studies [16,24], we have avoided using operational diagnoses due their high rate of comorbidity and lack of specificity. The lack of diagnostic specificity seems to be common in psychiatry, indeed, having one single diagnosis is unusual in psychiatry with the comorbidity being the rule, rather than the exception [25]. Furthermore, it has been shown that early adversities seem to influence differentially specific symptom profiles rather than specific diagnoses [16].

It is conceivable that CAs might produce sleep symptom patterns that range transdiagnostically. Thus, we have assessed the relationship between CAs and sleep impairments in a representative sample of psychiatric patients according to a transnosographic perspective.

Statistics

Chi-square (Fisher's test when needed) and Odds Ratios were performed. Moreover, as childhood adversities were not independent of each other, we adopted the stepwise forward conditional method of binary logistic regression for controlling the multicollinearity.

Thus, binary logistic regression analyses, with each sleep symptoms (absence vs presence), as dependent variable, and CAs (sexual abuse, physical abuse, loss of mother, loss of father, mother neglect, father neglect) as independent variables were performed. Separate binary logistic regression analyses were performed for each sleep symptoms.

The statistical analyses were performed using SPSS for Windows 20.0 [26].

Results

Patients and controls resulted comparable for gender (females: 64.1% vs 61%, χ^2=0.48, df=1, p=0.48) age (44.03 ± 13.22 vs 42.48 ± 12.82, t (df)=-1.28 (526), p=0.19) and educational level (mean education years: 11.23 ± 4.02 vs 11.53 ± 3.57 t (df)=0.83 (526), p=0.40).

Patients were more frequently single than those in the control group (54.4% vs 19.2%, χ^2=59.64, df=1, p<0.001).

As regards the clinical sample the most represented diagnostic category was the major depression (n=139; female: 74.1%), followed by panic disorder (n=113; female: 69.9%), psychosis (n=87; female: 52.9%), bipolar disorder (n=71; female: 56.3%), obsessive-compulsive disorder (n=71; female: 62%), eating disorder (n=57; female: 73.7%) and social phobia (n=53; female: 64.2%). No significant associations were found between drug use-treatments received and sleep impairments.

CA and sleep impairments in adult psychiatric population

Cases with childhood sexual abuse (CSA) compared with those without CSA were characterized by an excess of nightmare (20.1% vs 12.2%, χ^2=4.13, df=1, p=0.04), somnambulism (42.9% vs 14.5%, χ^2=8.15, df=1, fisher exact test p=0.01) bruxism (23.4% vs 13.5%, χ^2=4.43, df=1, p=0.03) and pavor nocturns (23.6% vs 13.6%, χ^2=4.32, df=1, p=0.03).

Moreover, compared with cases without neglect, patients with early experience of father neglect showed a higher prevalence of nightmares (12.3% vs 6.1%, χ^2=4.18, df=1, p=0.04), while cases with mother neglect shower a higher rate of terminal insomnia (13.3% vs 22.6%, χ^2=5.01, df=1, p=0.02).

Binary logistic regression analyses, adjusted for CAs co-occurrence, confirmed that: sexual abuse was associated with somnambulism (β=1.48, p=0.008, OR=4.41, 95% CI=1.46-13.25), bruxism (β=0.67, p=0.03, OR=1.95, 95% CI=1.03-3.67), and pavor nocturnus (β=0.67, p=0.04, OR=1.96; 95% CI=1.03-3.72); father neglect was associated with nightmares (β=0.77; p=0.04, OR=2.17, 95% CI=1.01-4.62); mother neglect was associated with terminal insomnia (β=0.64, p=0.02, OR=1.89, 95% CI=1.07-3.33).

Dividing patients according to their DSM-IV diagnoses, similar patterns of results were found across different diagnostic categories: the association between CA and sleep impairments is not diagnosis-specific (Table 1).

		Initial insomnia	Middle insomnia	Terminal Insomnia	Somnambulism	Nightmares	Bruxism	Pavor nocturnus	Altered sleep–wake cycles
	% Cases with CA	ORa [95% CI]	ORa [95% CI]	ORa [95% CI]	ORa [95% CI]	ORa [95% CI]	ORa [95% CI]	ORa [95% CI]	ORa [95% CI]
At least one CA	53.80%	0.91 [0.58-1.41]	1.22 [0.79-1.88]	1.43 [0.94-2.18]	2.20 [0.67-7.17]	1.26 [0.82-1.93]	1.10 [0.66-1.84]	1.56 [0.91-2.65]	1.42 [0.89-2.27]
Physical abuse	23.40%	1.17 [0.69-1.99]	1.30 [0.77-2.19]	1.52 [0.92-2.52]	0.89 [0.24-3.72]	1.56[0.95-2.57]	1.20 [0.67-2.14]	1.34 [0.74-2.42]	1.11 [0.65-1.90]
Sexual abuse	15.70%	1.34 [0.71-2.51]	1.17 [0.64-2.13]	1.28 [0.71-2.29]	**4.40 [1.46-13.25]**	**1.81 [1.01-3.24]**	**1.95 [1.03-3.67]**	**1.96 [1.03-3.72]**	1.16 [0.63-2.16]
Loss of mother	13.40%	1.14 [0.59-2.20]	1.35 [0.69-2.57]	1.23 [0.66-2.29]	1.08 [0.23-4.99]	0.76 [0.40-1.44]	0.82 [0.37-1.78]	1.05 [0.49-2.23]	1.11 [0.57-2.15]
Loss of father	18.20%	0.92 [0.52-1.62]	1.06 [0.57-1.76]	1.08 [0.63-1.87]	1.84 [0.56-6.08]	0.91 [0.53-1.59]	1.11 [0.58-2.11]	1.37 [0.72-2.59]	1.65 [0.94-2.91]
Mother Neglect	18.20%	1.73 [0.93-3.20]	1.68 [0.93-3.05]	**1.89 [1.07-3.33]**	1.84 [0.56-6.06]	1.16 [0.67-1.98]	1.23 [0.65-2.32]	1.10 [0.57-2.13]	1.28 [0.72-2.28]
Father Neglect	8.80%	1.31 [0.58-2.95]	1.52 [0.68-3.42]	1.25 [0.59-2.62]	0.78 [0.10-6.22]	**2.17 [1.01-4.62]**	1.79 [0.80-4.01]	1.14 [0.47-2.77]	0.95 [0.42-2.14]

Table 1: Association of childhood adversity and sleep impairments in adult psychiatric cases (n=351). CA=childhood adversity; a=adjusted for age and gender; Significant findings are marked in bold.

CA and sleep impairments in adult controls draw from the general population

Subjects with childhood physical abuse (CPA) showed higher rate of pavor nocturns (40% vs 11.4%, χ^2=6.83, df=1, p value Fisher's exact test=0.02, OR=5.2, 95% CI=1.34-20.07) than those without CPA. None other significant associations were found between CAs and sleep impairments in control group.

Discussion

The current study highlighted that among adult psychiatric patients CSA was associated with nightmares, bruxism, pavor and somnambulism, as well as, that father and mother neglect were related with nightmares and terminal insomnia respectively. On the other hand, no significant association was found between childhood loss events and sleep impairments. Moreover, among subjects draw form the general population, except for the association CPA-pavor, none significant relationships were found between CAs and sleep impairments.

Our findings are consistent with previous studies showing that nightmares are significantly associated with both child abuse and neglect [16-18]. Dreaming is considered as being a relevant process for emotional adaptation to emotionally salient and traumatic events [17,18,27]. It might be that disturbed dreaming may arise and persist when dreaming fails to accomplish its putative function of emotional regulation during sleep [18]. Furthermore, as suggested by Duval et al. [18], the exposure to stressful events in traumatized individuals, implies an increased risk of activation of memories and schemas related to CA, with nightmares possibly resulting from this mental activity.

Our study may support previous evidence [19,20] about the association between CSA and bruxism. Furthermore, the experience of CSA seems to increase the risk of pavor and somnambulism in adulthood. Unfortunately, no data from the literature evaluated the role of CA on pavor and/or sleep walking in adulthood, thus comparisons on this issue are not possible.

Moreover, we found that insomnia might be related with mother neglect, but we could not prove its association with child abuse as reported by previous studies [12]. This result is only apparently inconsistent with the literature [12], since previous studies were conducted on patients with primary insomnia [28] and alcohol-dependent patients [29], while we focused on a sample of merely psychiatric patients. It is therefore conceivable that the clinical nature of our sample contributed to this contradictory finding. Finally, in agreement with Agargun et al. [17], our results highlight that childhood loss events seem not to be associated with sleep impairments in adulthood.

Summing up, our findings suggest that could be a specific relationship between CSA and parasomnia, since no other form of CA appears to be strongly related with it, and no other sleep problems seem to be related with CSA. Thus, the relationship between CA and sleep impairments in adult psychiatric patients seems to be specific according to the type of CA and pattern of sleep symptoms. The underlying mechanism linking CA to sleep disorders in adulthood is still unclear. On the one hand the increased corticotropin-releasing hormone (CRH) and the hypothalamic-pituitary-adrenal (HPA) axis hyperactivity, induced by CA, may act as a pathway to sleep disorders in adulthood [12]. Furthermore, from a social perspective it could be argued that children exposed to CA, grow up in disorganized families and thus never learn good sleeping habits: this has a negative impact on sleep pattern that can persist into adulthood [12].

Moreover it should be considered that the relationship between CA and sleep disorders could be biased by current psychopathology, since CA may induce psychiatric diseases that in turn could be related to sleep disorders. Indeed, our findings showed that the relationship CA-sleep disorders seems more relevant in psychiatric patients rather than in a control group of subjects draw form the general population. Further investigation of the underlying pathways linking CA to sleep diseases will be an important issue for subsequent research.

Some methodological issues should be considered when interpreting the results of this study: (a) CAs were assessed by subjective retrospective reports, thus recall bias (memory distortions, search for meanings) may have influenced these results, although research suggests good reliability of retrospective assessment of CA [30]; (b) CA and sleep symptoms are based on subjective data therefore they should be overestimated; (c) the cross-sectional data precludes conclusions regarding causal relationships; (d) since that our research did not primary planned to assess sleep disorders, the sleep symptoms were evaluated only by the FPI rather than by specific instruments focused on sleep parameters. Strengths of the study were: (a) a large sample size; (b) a wide range of CA were evaluated.

Conclusion

CA may be related with sleep problems in adulthood, but probably it exist a specific relationship between CSA and parasomnia. Moreover the effect of CAs on sleep impairments in adulthood seems more specific in the psychiatric population rather than in the general population. However, the cross-sectional design of this study does not allow us to make further speculation on this issue, thus longitudinal studies will be necessary to confirm the findings of the present study, as well as to clarify the underlying pathways on the relationship between CA, psychopathology, and sleep impairments in adulthood.

On the clinical ground, in order to facilitate meaningful formulations and treatment plans, the assessment of CA should not be overlooked in anamnesis and treatment of sleep impairments.

Conflict of Interest

Authors declared no conflict of interest.

References

1. Lam SP, Fong SY, Ho CK, Mandy WM, Wing YK (2008) Parasomnia among psychiatric outpatients: a clinical, epidemiologic, cross-sectional study. J Clin Psychiatry 69: 1-478.
2. Morin CM, Ware JC (1996) Sleep and psychopathology. Appl Prev Psychol 5: 211-224.
3. Harvey AG, Jones C, Schmidt DA (2003) Sleep and posttraumatic stress disorder: A review. Clin Psychol Rev 23: 377-407.
4. Swart ML, van Schagen AM, Lancee J, van Den Bout J (2013) Prevalence of nightmare disorder in psychiatric outpatients. Psychother Psychosoma 82: 267-268.
5. Szelenberger W, Niemcewicz S, Dabrowska AJ (2005) Sleepwalking and night terrors: psychopathological and psychophysiological correlates. Int Rev Psychiatry 17: 263-270.
6. Alves AC, Alchieri JC, Barbosa GA (2013) Bruxism: Masticatory implications and anxiety. Acta Odontol Latinoam 26: 15-22.
7. Carra MC, Huynh N, Lavigne G (2012) Sleep bruxism: a comprehensive overview for the dental clinician interested in sleep medicine. Dent Clin North Am 56: 387-413.
8. Manfredini D, Landi N, Romagnoli M, Bosco M (2004) Psychic and occlusal factors in bruxers. Aust Dent J 49: 84-89.
9. Manfredini D, Ciapparelli A, Dell'Osso L, Bosco M (2005) Mood disorders in subjects with bruxing behavior. J Dent 33: 485-490.
10. Carr CP, Martins CMS, Stingel AM, Lemgruber VB, Juruena MF (2013) The role of early life stress in adult psychiatric disorders: a systematic review according to childhood trauma subtypes. J Nerv Ment Dis 201: 1007-1020.
11. Verdolini N, Attademo L, Agius M, Ferranti L, Moretti P, et al. (2015) Traumatic events in childhood and their association with psychiatric illness in the adult. Psychiatr Danub 27: 60-70.
12. Kajeepeta S, Gelaye B, Jackson CL, Williams MA (2015) Adverse childhood experiences are associated with adult sleep disorders: a systematic review. Sleep Med 16: 320-330.
13. Infurna MR, Reichl C, Parzer P, Schimmenti A, Bifulco A, et al. (2016) Associations between depression and specific childhood experiences of abuse and neglect: a meta-analysis. J Affect Disord 190: 47-55.
14. Varese F, Smeets F, Drukker M, Lieverse R, Lataster T, et al. (2012) Childhood adversities increase the risk of psychosis: a meta-analysis of patient-control, prospective-and cross-sectional cohort studies. Schizophr Bull 38: 661-671.
15. Schafer V, Bade K (2013) Relationship Between Early-life Stress Load and Sleep in Psychiatric Outpatients: A Sleep Diary and Actigraphy Study. Stress Health 29: 177-189.
16. Faravelli C, Castellini G, Fioravanti G, Lo Sauro C, Pietrini F, et al. (2014) Different Childhood Adversities Are Associated with Different Symptom Patterns in Adulthood. Psychother Psychosoma 83: 320-321.
17. Agargun MY, Kara H, Ozer OA, Selvi Y, Kiran U, et al. (2003) Nightmares and dissociative experiences: The key role of childhood traumatic events. Psychiatry Clin Neurosci 57: 139-145.
18. Duval M, McDuff P, Zadra A (2013) Nightmare frequency, nightmare distress, and psychopathology in female victims of childhood maltreatment. J Nerv Ment Dis 201: 767-772.
19. Messer AA (1992) Bruxism, neck pain, and a history of child sexual abuse. J Med Assoc Ga 81: 637-640.
20. Molina OF, dos Santos CR, Marquezan RF, Cano ML, da Silva FF, et al. (2015) Changes of Several Psychological Measures in the Patients with Craniomandibular Disorders, Bruxing Behavior and Sexual Abuse History. J Adv Neurosci Res 2: 9-15.
21. First MB, Spitzer RL, Gibbon M, Williams JBW (1995) Structured Clinical Interview for DSM-IV Axis I Disorders-Patient Edition (SCID-I/P, Version 2.0). Biometrics Research Department, New York State Psychiatric Institute, New York, USA.
22. Faravelli C, Bartolozzi D, Cimminiello L, Cecchi C, Cosci F, et al. (2001) The Florence Psychiatric Interview. Int J Methods Psychiatr Res 10: 157-171.
23. Bifulco A, Bernazzani O, Moran PM, Jacobs C (2005) The childhood experience of care and abuse questionnaire (CECA-Q). Br J Clin Psychol 44: 563-581.
24. Faravelli C, Amedei SG, Rotella F, Faravelli L, Palla A, et al. (2010) Childhood traumata, Dexamethasone Suppression Test and psychiatric symptoms: a trans-diagnostic approach. Psychol Med 40: 2037-2048.
25. Kessler RC, Chiu WT, Demler O, Merikangas KR, Walters EE (2005) Prevalence, severity, and comorbidity of 12-month DSM-IV disorders in the National Comorbidity Survey Replication. Arch Gener Psychiatry 62: 617-627.
26. (2011) IBM SPSS Statistics.
27. Stickgold R (2008) Sleep-dependent memory processing and EMDR action. J EMDR Pract Res 2: 289-299.
28. Bader K, Schafer V, Schenkel M, Nissen L, Schwander J (2007) Adverse childhood experiences associated with sleep in primary insomnia. J Sleep Res 16: 285-296.
29. Zhabenko N, Wojnar M, Brower KJ (2012) Prevalence and correlates of insomnia in a Polish sample of alcohol-dependent patients. Alcohol Clin Exp Res 36: 1600-1607.
30. Fisher HL, Craig TK, Fearon P, Morgan K, Dazzan P, et al. (2009) Reliability and comparability of psychosis patients' retrospective reports of childhood abuse. Schizophr Bull 37: 546-553.

Physical and Psychological Stress and Sleep Efficiency before and after Introducing a New Sleep Surface

Bert H Jacobson* **and Taylor P Monaghan**

School of Applied Health and Educational Psychology, Health and Human Performance, Oklahoma State University, USA

***Corresponding author:** Bert H Jacobson, School of Educational Studies, 204 Willard Hall, Stillwater, Oklahoma, USA, E-mail: bert.jacobson@okstate.edu

Abstract

Background: It has been long assumed that stress interferes with sleep, but less has been attributed to the converse of poor sleep contributing to stress.

Study question: Can an older sleep surface contribute to poor sleep and thus, stress and will a new sleep surface provide better sleep, thus less stress.

Methods: Forty-six participants rated physical and psychological signs of stress and sleep efficiency for three weeks while sleeping in their own beds. Following baseline measures participants' beds were replaced by new, unmarked beds and they again rated their stress and sleep efficiency.

Results: Average age of participants' bed was 11.27 yrs. Physical and psychological signs of stress were reduced significantly ($p<0.01$) from pre- to post-assessments. Similarly, sleep efficiency improved significantly ($p<0.01$) between pre- and post-assessments.

Conclusions: Replacing an older mattress that may have lost adequate support and comfort may result in a better night's sleep thereby reducing stress brought on by a lack of sleep. It was suggested that a simple principal step in acquiring better sleep is to consider a new sleep surface rather than to opt for pharmaceuticals to achieve better sleep.

Keywords: Sleep; Bed; Mattress; Quality; Stress

Introduction

The National Sleep Foundation suggest that the amount of sleep varies with age, lifestyles, and health status and indicate that as we grow from infancy to adult hood we require less and less sleep [1]. Additionally, the NSF suggests that the average adult needs between seven and nine hours of sleep per night. However, in 2013 it was estimated that Americans average 6.8 hours per night and that 40% of Americans average six or less hours per night [2]. Sleep deprived individuals exhibit impairment in several areas such as operating machinery, [3] lack of focus, [4] sustained attention, reaction time, and cognitive processing speed [5]. These impairments contribute to a high degree in loss of work productivity and workplace injury [1,6-11]. Recently, researchers have suggested a strong and complex link between lack of sufficient sleep and cardiovascular health [12] as well as mood instability [13].

Idiopathic musculoskeletal pain has been associated with both stress and sleep interference [14]. Indeed, pain severity is associated with lack of sleep quality and stress is thought to be related to pain severity, thus contributing to poor sleep along with additional health problems [15]. Also, the quality of sleep is often compromised by pressure pain which relates to the comfort and support of the sleep surface [16]. Many individuals continue to sleep in their beds even after the mattress has lost its support and structure integrity. Anecdotally, it is suggested that a mattress 5 to 7 years old may not provide the adequate support or comfort, however; this varies with original quality, use, and inherent anthropometric changes in the user [17]. In one of our previous studies, we found the average age of the participants' beds was 9.7 years, [18] which contributed in part, to back stiffness and pain upon waking. Presently no universal prescription exists for recommending mattress qualities meeting specific sleep needs of the general population [19].

Neurologically, the regulation of sleep, behavior, and emotion is closely related [20], thus physiologically stress may result in poor sleep quality or duration. Gregory and Sadeh [21] suggest that short sleep escalates stress hormone production which hinders sleep. Additionally, significant increased risk of depression and anxiety is associated with sleeping difficulties [22]. Furthermore, self-reported short sleep duration may be an indicator of emotional stress and sleep disturbances [23].

It has been proposed that the relationship between stress and sleep is bidirectional, in that stress can interfere with sleep and that lack of sleep can increase stress levels [24]. Further, Doane [24] concluded that prior day stress is related to shorter sleep duration and that sleep efficiency is associated with greater stress that next day. One study reported that sleep deprived participants reported significantly greater subjective stress, anger, and anxiety in response to a low-stressor condition [21]. Conversely, mental stress, worry, and anxiety contribute to sleep loss and is related to sleep stage fragmentation [25]. Research has demonstrated that stress has a strong association to impaired sleep [25] and that life stress may be both a predisposing and a precipitating basis of poor sleep [26,27] which can be linked to anxiety, depression, and mood disorders [28-30]. Furthermore, disturbed sleep has been indicted as a factor in both morbidity and mortality [31].

The purpose of this study was to determine subjective, physical, and emotional stress along with sleep disturbances before and after the introduction of new bedding systems in a population sleeping on beds greater than five years old.

Methods

Participants

A total of 46 participants (women=23 and men=23) who owned and slept on commercially made spring mattresses older than 5 years volunteered for the study. After reading a written description of the conditions of the study, all participants signed an informed consent document approved by the University Institutional Review Board. The participants were solicited based on a pre-stress screening and bed age survey. Survey responses indicated that participants were moderately active and without diagnosed mental health conditions or using medication for sleep disorders. Additionally, participants were asked to complete a demographic survey containing items such as age, height, weight, and age of their bed (Table 1).

Variable	Males (n=23)	Females (n=23)	Total (N=46)
	Means, +SD	Means, +SD	Means, +SD
Age (yrs)	48.24, +11.35	44.13, +12.29	46.11, +11.38
Ht. (cm)	178.63, +8.64	165.24, +5.92	171.91, +9.63
Wt. (kg)	74.63, +12.46	56.55, +11.68	77.43, +16.87
Bed age			11.27, +4.27

Table 1: Demographic variable means by gender.

Procedures

Prior to the onset of the study, participants were asked to complete a 14 item survey concerning sleep habits and stress related to behaviors manifested by anxiety, stress, and sleep. The items of the stress survey were taken from previously developed and validated stress surveys [17,32-39] and were organized to fit a five-point Likert-like scale with 1=never, 2=about once this week, 3=about twice this week, 4=about every other day, and 5=nearly every day.

The directions given the participants were: "Have you had any of the following things happen to you during the past week? If so, simply circle one of the numbers preceding each of those items". Stress related items on the survey included psychological and physiological stress items and sleep related stress items. Among examples of psychological stress markers were anxiety, worrying, nervousness, among examples of physiological stress markers were digestive problems, chest pain, and tight neck muscles, and examples of sleep related stress were difficulty falling asleep, insomnia, waking tired, and disturbing dreams.

Physiological stress items, psychological and physiological stress items, and sleep stress items were randomly distributed throughout the questionnaire but grouped for analysis. A 10 subject test-retest analysis found the survey to be moderately high in reliability (r=0.78).

Following previously published protocol, the pre-test period required participants to sleep in their own beds or older beds and rate their stress each week for a three-week period [Jacobson, Bader] in order to establish a baseline. Participants rated their stress at the end of each week and were advised to avoid rating their stress following an unusually bad day, heavy alcohol consumption, or any extraordinary emotional or physical event that would not be considered the norm.

In addition to the multiple pre- and post-stress surveys, participants were asked simultaneously to subjectively rate efficiency as their total amount of sleep to total time in bed by using a 100 mm visual analogue scale in which a 50 reflects that the participant slept on only half of the time he/she was in bed. All participants were given instructions on how to calculate sleep efficiency based on the suggestion posited by Breus [32].

At the completion of the pre-test, the experimental phase began with the delivery and setup of the new bed. The beds were medium-priced, unlabeled box-spring mattresses with a medium-firm sleep surface. Each mattress contained foam encased bonnell springs, dense fiber pads with foam, and a damask cover. The new beds were the same size as those that the participants' had slept on originally and participants continued to use their own linen, blankets and pillows. After the delivery of the bedding system, participants rated stress symptoms and sleep to bed ratio at the end of each week for four weeks.

Statistical analysis

A factor analysis was used to cluster the survey items into similar categories. This resulted in the 14 items to be categorized into three types of stress experiences (physical stress symptoms=8 items, psychological stress symptoms=4 items, and sleep stress symptoms=2 items). Among examples of physical stress items were: muscle tension, headache, irritable. Examples of psychological stress items were: worrying, tenseness, keyed-up, and examples of sleep items were: insomnia, difficulty wakening, and disturbing dreams.

To prevent an atypical week of stress from skewing the data the three weekly pre-test stress ratings were aggregated into one pre-test data set. Similarly, the four-week post-test stress ratings were combined to form two post-test data sets; one after the first two weeks and one after weeks 3 and 4 in order to obtain a mid-test and a post-test. Pre- and post-tests scores for each stress category (physical, psychological, and sleep) were analyzed using ANOVAs with repeated measure and Newman-Keuls post-hoc test. An alpha level of $p<0.01$ was considered to reflect significant differences between pre- and post-test means.

Results

The survey taken by the participants indicated that the average age of their beds was 11.27 years (SD+4.27 years) with a range between 6 and 18 years, well over the recommended usage (Table 1). All analyses were conducted by controlling for bed age, participants' age, and bed cost. A repeated measures ANOVA analysis of pre-, mid-, and post-test physical stress yielded a significant ($p<0.001$) difference among means ($F=43.67$) and the post-hoc tests indicated that significant differences existed between pre- and post-test, between mid- and post-test, but not between pre-and mid-tests (Tables 2 and 3).

Variable	N	Mean ± SD	-95% CI	+95% CI
Physical Pre	46	2.57 ± 1.33	-2.74	2.31
Physical Mid	46	2.40 ± 1.00	-2.56	2.24
Physical Post	46	1.73 ± 0.94	-1.82	1.82

Table 2: Pre-mid, and post-physical stress means, standard deviations, confidence intervals and probability: F=43.67, p<0.001

	Physical Pre	**Physical Mid**	**Physical Post**
Physical Pre		0.23	<0.001*
Physical Mid	0.23		<0.001*
Physical Post	<0.001*	<0.001*	

Table 3: Newman-Keuls post hoc test of physical stress (*Significant at p<0.01).

For psychological stress similar results were found in that a significant (p<0.001) difference existed among means (F=11.86) with the post-hoc tests reflecting significant differences between pre- and post-test, between mid- and post-test, but not between pre-and mid-tests (Tables 4 and 5).

Variable	**N**	**Mean ± SD**	**-95% CI**	**+95% CI**
Psych Pre	46	1.70±		1.85
Psych Mid	46	1.44±		1.54
Psych Post	46	1.37±		1.48

Table 4: Pre-mid, and post-psychological stress means, standard deviations, confidence intervals and probability: F=11.85, p<0.001.

	Psych Pre	Psych Mid	Psych Post
Psych Pre		<0.001*	<0.001*
Psych Mid	<0.001*		0.35
Psych Post	<0.001*	0.35	

Table 5: Newman-Keuls post hoc test of psychological stress (*Significant at p<0.01).

Similarly, for the sleep/stress category, mean differences were significant (p<0.001) among means (F=14.56) and the post-hoc analysis found significant differences between pre- and post-test, between mid- and post-test, but not between pre-and mid- tests (Tables 6 and 7). A follow-up of the participants resulted in a 97% agreement that the change in beds resulted in greater comfort and sleep quality. Participant's sleep ratio was measured and defined as the amount of time spent in bed compared to the amount of time the participant felt he/she slept. Participant's sleep efficiency improved significantly (p<0.01) between pre- and post-measurements.

Variable	N	Mean ± SD	-95% CI	+95% CI
Physical Pre	46	1.93 ± 1.13	-2.12	1.74
Physical Mid	46	1.84 ± 1.02	-2	1.65
Physical Post	46	1.47 ± 0.78	-1.61	1.34

Table 6: Pre-, mid, and post-sleep stress means, standard deviations, confidence intervals and probability: F=1.58, p<0.001.

	Sleep Pre	**Sleep Mid**	**Sleep Post**
Sleep Pre		0.22	<0.001*
Sleep Mid	0.22		<0.001*
Sleep Post	<0.001*	<0.001*	

Table 7: Newman-Keuls post hoc test of psychological stress (*Significant at p<0.01).

Discussion

Among common psychological signs of stress are depression, worry, moodiness, and irritability, common physical signs include aches, digestive disorders, muscle tension, and headache, and signs of sleep interference include difficulty falling asleep and insomnia. These factors were included in the 14 item stress survey in which the participants subjectively rated their stress from never to nearly every day at the end of each week, before and after changing from their old beds to new beds. Of the three stress categories, the pre-physical stress indicators were more prominent with sleep disturbance showing a 32% reduction with the introduction of a new sleep surface. The sleep stress association and the psychological stress improved 22.2% and 22.0% respectively from pre- to post-evaluations.

Several previously conducted studies have found that that stress correlates with sleep [30,34]. Conversely, the lack of sleep whether from work-related duties or other demands can result in stress-like symptoms both physical and psychological in nature. Others studies [29,33] have indicated that reduced sleep is related to anxiety, irritability, anger, and depression.

The current study demonstrated that the participants' beds averaged over a decade in use (Mean=11.27 years). These results of better sleep efficiency resemble those of Enck and associates [19] who determined that new mattresses provided statistically better sleep quality than "old" mattresses (8-yr). It is reasonable to assume that a bed used over ten years may not fulfill the users sleep needs adequately.

The participants' beds may have been compromised due to age and use thereby having lost both structure integrity and support qualities. Such beds may not afford the comfort of a sound sleeping surface and may result in physical discomfort which can interfere with sleep [36,37] thus adding to daytime stress. Additionally, many experience body changes over 10 years due to work-related conditions, physical changes, and aging which may warrant looking into a new sleep surface rather than to depend on pharmaceuticals to achieve better sleep.

The results of the present study reflect a significant improvement in the three stress-related categories after the removal of the old beds and delivery of the new beds. Furthermore, participants indicated they slept more while in the new bed than when sleeping in their old bed.

A limitation to this study is that the subjects acted as their own control without a true control group. As has been noted previously [36] a control group is not practical in a study such as this since a control or sham bed would constitute the introduction of yet another new sleep surface. The question becomes, what should be the makeup of a sham bed? The current research was based on previous protocols in which no sham beds were used [19,38,39], but rather compared firmness of separate beds or adjustable beds. One study [40] did compare new beds to beds 8-yrs old and found significantly greater sleep quality in the newer beds.

Similar to the current study, a placebo effect may have resulted in the initial positive responses to stress by the mere fact that a "new" mattress was available. Others have addressed the possibility of a placebo effect [37]. While a placebo effect may have been present in the initial stages of the study. We suggest that if a placebo effect had compromised the post-observations it must have been present at the first data collection point (mid-test), however, the significant improvement in each stress category continued to the end of the study. Placebo sustainability varies by the variables observed, but eventually the placebo effect begins to diminish. It is likely that once the "new" wears off, the efficacy of the intervention diminishes. Additionally, the sample size may be considered small, however; similar studies [39,40] involved fewer participants.

Mimicking previous studies, the current study employed a medium-firm [37,41,42] innerspring mattress as the experimental bedding system. However, no universal standards presently define the firmness of mattresses. Such definitions are the construct of the mattress companies. Continued research in the area should focus on sleeping surface comparisons and assessment of the longevity and sustainability of the support and comfort of the bedding system.

References

1. National Sleep Foundation. Sleep in America Poll. Summary of the Sleep in America Poll [cited 2014; Available from: http://sleepfoundation.org/sites/default/files/2005_summary_of_findings.pdf.
2. Jones JM, In U.S., 40% Get Less Than Recommended Amount of Sleep. Available from: http://www.gallup.com/poll/166553/less-recommended-amount -sleep.aspx. Accessed 1/29/2015.
3. Howard ME, Jackson ML, Berlowitz D, O'Donoghue F, Swann P, et al. (2014) Specific sleepiness symptoms are indicators of performance impairment during sleep deprivation. Accid Anal Prev 62: 1-8.
4. Chua EC, Yeo SC, Lee IT (2014) Sustained attention performance during sleep deprivation associates with instability in behavior and physiologic measures at baseline. Sleep, 37: 27-39.
5. Louca M, Short MA (2014) The effect of one night's sleep deprivation on adolescent neurobehavioral performance. Sleep 37: 1799-1807.
6. Nakata A (2011) Effects of long work hours and poor sleep characteristics on workplace injury among full-time male employees of small- and medium-scale businesses. J Sleep Res 20: 576-584.
7. Chilcott LA, Shapiro CM (1996) The socioeconomic impact of insomnia. An overview. Pharmacoeconomics 10 Suppl 1: 1-14.
8. Drake C, Richardson G, Roehrs T, Scofield H, Roth T (2004) Vulnerability to stress-related sleep disturbance and hyperarousal. Sleep 27: 285-291.
9. Godet-Cayré V, Pelletier-Fleury N, Le Vaillant M, Dinet J, Massuel MA, et al. (2006) Insomnia and absenteeism at work. Who pays the cost? Sleep 29: 179-184.
10. Hillman DR, Murphy AS, Pezzullo L (2006) The economic cost of sleep disorders. Sleep 29: 299-305.
11. Ohayon MM, Lemoine P (2004) [Sleep and insomnia markers in the general population]. Encephale 30: 135-140.
12. Miller MA, Cappuccio FP (2013) Biomarkers of cardiovascular risk in sleep-deprived people. J Hum Hypertens 27: 583-588.
13. Bowen R, Balbuena L, Baetz M, Schwartz L (2013) Maintaining sleep and physical activity alleviate mood instability. Prev Med 57: 461-465.
14. Molina J, Dos Santos FH, Terreri MT, Fraga MM, Silva SG, et al. (2012) Sleep, stress, neurocognitive profile and health-related quality of life in adolescents with idiopathic musculoskeletal pain. Clinics (Sao Paulo) 67: 1139-1144.
15. Graham JE, Streitel KL (2010) Sleep quality and acute pain severity among young adults with and without chronic pain: the role of biobehavioral factors. J Behav Med 33: 335-345.
16. Addison RG, Thorpy MJ, Roth TA (1986) survey of the United States public concerning the quality of sleep. Sleep Research 16: 244.
17. The Better Sleep Council. Replacing a Mattress. Available from: http://bettersleep.org/mattresses-and-more/caring-for-a-mattress/replacing-a-mattress. Accessed 4/29/2015.
18. Jacobson BH, Wallace T, Gemmell H (2007) Subjective rating of perceived back pain, stiffness and sleep quality following introduction of medium-firm bedding systems. Journal of Chiropractic Medicine 5: 28-134.
19. Enck P, Walten T, Traue HC (1999) [Associations between back pain, quality of sleep and quality of mattresses. Double-blind pilot study with hotel guests]. Schmerz 13: 205-207.
20. Vgontzas AN, Chrousos GP (2002) Sleep, the hypothalamic–pituitary–adrenal axis, and cytokines: multiple interactions and disturbances in sleep disorders. Endocrinology and Metabolism Clinics of North America 31: 15-36.
21. Minkel JD, Banks S, Htaik O, Moreta MC, Jones CW, et al. (2012) Sleep deprivation and stressors: evidence for elevated negative affect in response to mild stressors when sleep deprived. Emotion 12: 1015-1020.
22. Jackson ML, Sztendur EM, Diamond NT, Byles JE, Bruck D (2014) Sleep difficulties and the development of depression and anxiety: a longitudinal study of young Australian women. Arch Womens Ment Health 17: 189-198.
23. Vgontzas AN, Lin HM, Papaliaga M, Calhoun S, Vela-Bueno A, et al. (2008) Short sleep duration and obesity: the role of emotional stress and sleep disturbances. Int J Obes (Lond) 32: 801-809.
24. Doane LD, Thurston EC (2014) Associations among sleep, daily experiences, and loneliness in adolescence: evidence of moderating and bidirectional pathways. J Adolesc 37: 145-154.
25. Akerstedt T (2006) Psychosocial stress and impaired sleep. Scand J Work Environ Health 32: 493-501.
26. Bernert RA, Merrill KA, Braithwaite SR, Van Orden KA, Joiner TE Jr (2007) Family life stress and insomnia symptoms in a prospective evaluation of young adults. J Fam Psychol 21: 58-66.
27. The Better Sleep Council. How Stressed are We? ; Available from: http://bettersleep.org/better-sleep/healthy-sleep/stress-sleep. Accessed 5/1/2015.
28. Insel PM, Roth WT Core Concepts in Health. (10thedn.) 2006, Mountain View (CA): Mayfield Publishing Company.
29. Roberts RE, Roberts CR, Chen IG (2001) Functioning of adolescents with symptoms of disturbed sleep. Journal of Youth and Adolescence 30: 1-18.
30. Szelenberger W, Soldatos C (2005) Sleep disorders in psychiatric practice. World Psychiatry 4: 186-190.
31. Åkerstedt T, Sleep and stress, in Sleep Related Disorders and Internal Diseases. 1987, New York, NY, Springer Publishing Company 183-191.
32. Breus MJ Calculating your perfect bedtime sleep efficiency. http://blog.doctoroz.com/oz-experts/calculating-your-perfect-bedtime-and-sleep-efficiency. Accessed 4/29/2015.
33. Fuligni AJ, Hardway C (2006) Daily Variation in Adolescents' Sleep, Activities, and Psychological Well-Being. Journal of Research on Adolescence 16: 353-378.
34. Härmä M (2006) Workhours in relation to work stress, recovery and health. Scand J Work Environ Health 32: 502-514.

35. Feng GS, Chen JW, Yang XZ (2005) Study on the status and quality of sleep-related influencing factors in medical college students. 26: 328-331.

36. Jacobson BH, Gemmell HA, Hayes BM, Altena TS (2002) Effectiveness of a selected bedding system on quality of sleep, low back pain, shoulder pain, and spine stiffness. J Manipulative Physiol Ther 25: 88-92.

37. Jacobson BH, Wallace TJ, Smith DB, Kolb T (2008) Grouped comparisons of sleep quality for new and personal bedding systems. Appl Ergon 39: 247-254.

38. Garfin SR, Pye SA (1981) Bed design and its effect on chronic low back pain--a limited controlled trial. Pain 10: 87-91.

39. Scharf MB, Stover R, McDannold M, Kaye H, Berkowitz DV (1997) Comparative effects of sleep on a standard mattress to an experimental foam surface on sleep architecture and CAP rates. Sleep 20: 1197-1200.

40. Bader GG, Engdal S (2000) The influence of bed firmness on sleep quality. Appl Ergon 31: 487-497.

41. Kovacs FM, Abraira V, Peña A, Martín-Rodríguez JG, Sánchez-Vera M, et al. (2003) Effect of firmness of mattress on chronic non-specific low-back pain: randomised, double-blind, controlled, multicentre trial. Lancet 362: 1599-1604.

42. Hadler NM, Evans AT (2004) Medium-firm mattresses reduced pain-related disability more than firm mattresses in chronic, nonspecific low-back pain. ACP J Club 141: 12.

14

Physiological Basis of Alternative Therapies to Alleviate Sleep Disturbances

Palaniappan K[1*] and Thenappan A[2]

[1]*University of Newcastle, Singapore*

[2]*White Memorial Medical Center, Los Angeles, USA*

[*]**Corresponding author:** Palaniappan K, University of Newcastle Singapore 355, Jalan Bukit Ho Swee, Block B, Room B-407, Singapore 169567, E-mail: Kavitha.Palaniappan@newcastle.edu.au

Abstract

Prevalence of various types of sleep disturbances have been increasing at an alarming rate in the past few decades and have also been associated with several physiological as well as psychological problems. Pharmaceutical hypnotics have been the first-line of pharmacotherapy to be used for the treatment of such sleep disturbances. However, in the past two decades, complementary and alternative therapies have gained grounds in this field and reviews have been done on some of these therapies. Some of the notable therapies that have been reviewed extensively include homeopathic remedies, ayurvedic preparations, acupuncture and cognitive behavioral therapy. However, the literature lacks an extensive comparative study of the physiological explanations behind these alternative approaches to enhance sleep and this study aims to fill in that gap. Various studies pertaining to alternative approaches to enhance sleep such as nutritional interventions, herbal medicines, essential oils, acupuncture, bright light therapy, music therapy, massage and touch therapies, yoga and tai-chi are reviewed here, thereby providing a potent source of information for both clinicians and patients on these specific alternative therapies to alleviate sleep disturbances. The physiological basics of homeopathy and Ayurveda are beyond the scope of this review. Apart from reviewing the physiological elucidations behind the simpler alternative therapies suggested, their effectiveness over a wide range of people is also reviewed in this study.

Keywords: Sleep disturbances; Alternative therapies; Homeopathic remedies; Ayurvedic preparations; Acupuncture; Cognitive behavioral therapy

Introduction

In common man's terms, sleep is a state of rest for the body. It is a time when our body is at rest; only basic functions are happening involuntarily and our mind is at rest. The Oxford Dictionary defines sleep as "a condition of body and mind such as that which typically recurs for several hours every night, in which the nervous system is relatively inactive, the eyes closed, the postural muscles relaxed and consciousness practically suspended" [1]. From a behavioral standpoint, sleep is a reversible behavioral state of perceptual disengagement from, and unresponsiveness to, the environment [2]. Invention of EEG in 1929 has shed some light on brain functions during these dark hours of sleep. A typical sleep starts with NREM (Non Rapid Eye Movement) sleep and that includes slow wave sleep stages N1, N2 and N3 [3]. This is followed by REM sleep, often called "active sleep" and is identified by its characteristic low-amplitude (small), high-frequency (fast) waves and alpha rhythm, as well as the eye movements for which it is named [4]. Though the definition of sleep may vary from person to person, each and every one of us need a good night's sleep to feel one's self next day. Good sleep is that which happens spontaneously and regularly by itself. We don't need any external aids for it to happen. After a good sleep, one should wake up energized for the rest of the day ahead.

In prehistoric times, sleep was simply thought of as a coping mechanism for primitive organisms to seek shelter during the dangerous period of darkness. This adaptive behavior would have also helped them conserve energy that would have been expended otherwise. However, in the present day scenario, sleep is closely tied with the bio physiology of our body functions. Several studies have confirmed the importance of adequate, sound sleep as an essential ingredient for physical, psychological and social well-being [5]. Hence, sleep is a basic key to good health along with proper nutrition and exercise.

The public health domain has been increasingly recognizing difficulties with initiating and maintaining sleep among all age groups of people. This lack of good sleep is associated with several complications, ranging from physiological to psychological issues, workplace and road accidents, human errors and impaired performance. Basically, sleep disturbances are characterized by difficulty to fall asleep at night, frequent waking up during night and problems of waking up earlier than expected or required in the morning. So, how much sleep do we actually need? For everything in life, we need balance: inside and outside of us, balance in diet and digestion, balance in thought and action, and balance in day and night. Similarly, we need balance in time being awake and time being asleep in the rate of 2:1. We need about 8 hours of restful sleep every day in order to prevent neurobehavioral deficits [6] and to enable us to function in a balanced way throughout our day to day life. However, sleep architecture changes continuously and considerably with age and varies among people. Newborns generally sleep for about 16-18 hours a day and that reduces to about 10 hours for 3-12 year olds and teenagers. Typical adult needs 7-8 hours of restful sleep a day. As we age, we get less of sleep due to other physiological issues like wear and tear of the body like arthritis, body aches, frequent need to use the restroom, etc. Scientific studies have also proved that less than [6] hours of sleep for 4 or more consecutive nights together can impair glucose metabolism [7], immune functions [8], can cause changes in appetite regulation [9] and can also impair cognitive performance and mood [10].

Severe sleep disturbances are usually treated with prescribed medications that are actually intended for short term use. These medications may have other adverse side effects when used for a longer term, which happens to be the case in most situations [11]. On the other hand, sleep disturbances if detected at an earlier and milder stage, can be treated with several types of alternative therapies which possibly do not have any other adverse side effects. Certain authorities as well recommend the use of conventional non-pharmacological interventions to overcome sleep disturbances [12]. A study by Pearson et al. indicated that about 72% of the study participants who used complementary alternative medicine to improve their sleep agreed that their sleep did improve to some extent after treatment. In the same study, it was also found that the complementary and alternative medicine for treating insomnia was more preferred by young and the more educated population [13].

Some of the alternative approaches to enhance sleep include certain kinds of sleep promoting foods (nutritional medicine), herbal medicines and essential oils (aromatherapy), acupuncture or acupressure, bright-light therapy, massage and touch therapy, music therapy, tai chi and yoga. These specific approaches have been chosen for this study as these approaches have generally been considered as old-folks remedies and very little stress is laid on their physiological significance in the literature.

Nutritional Interventions for Enhancement of Sleep

Melatonin is a major hormone of the circadian system as it plays an important role in the regulation of human sleep by controlling both the circadian rhythm and the homeostatic mechanisms [14]. The amino acid L-tryptophan is converted to melatonin through a series of enzymatic reactions in the pineal gland [14]. Under general circumstances, retinal light exposure suppresses the production of melatonin, thereby stimulating wakefulness [15]. As increase in melatonin can eventually promote sleep, several nutritional interventions have been studied to increase the melatonin production by manipulating tryptophan through diet. Such strategies include a high protein diet that contains more tryptophan, a carbohydrate rich diet in order to increase the ratio of free tryptophan to branched-chain amino acids, and a high-fat meal to increase free tryptophan. Silber and Schmitt have indicated that tryptophan doses as low as 1g can improve sleep latency and subjective sleep quality [16]. For example, this can be achieved by consuming approximately 300 g of turkey or approximately 200g of pumpkin seeds [17].

Lindseth et al. conducted a study wherein the diets of 44 adults were manipulated either to be high protein (56% protein, 22% carbohydrate, 22% fat) or high carbohydrate (22% protein, 56% carbohydrate, 22% fat) or high fat (22% protein, 22% carbohydrate, 56% fat) for four days. It was found that a high protein diet reduced wake episodes and a high carbohydrate diet reduced the sleep-onset latencies [18]. In another study, it was found that a high fat diet affected adversely the total sleep time [19]. Lunchtime food intake, even if it is just a liquid meal, be it of a high caloric or low caloric content is said to increase the sleep duration [20]. Afaghi et al. have indicated that a high glycemic index diet given 4 hours before sleep is capable of improving the sleep-onset latency compared to low glycemic index diet [21]. Likewise, another study also indicated that a high-carbohydrate meal given 45 minutes before bedtime led to increased REM sleep, decreased light sleep and wakefulness [22]. Additionally, L-Theanine which is present in tea is said to promote feelings of calmness, decrease alertness and thereby increase sleep onset [23].

Herbal medicines and essential oils

Certain herbs are said to release tension and stress and mainly help people who fall asleep, but wake up and cannot go back to sleep again. Some of the examples of herbs that can help to enhance the quality of sleep include lemon balm (Melissa officinalis), valerian (Valeriana officinalis), Passion flower (Passiflora incarnata), Chamomile (Matricaria recutita), Linden flower (Tilia americana), Hops (Humulus lupulus) and adrenal tonic herbs such as Ginseng (Eleutherococcus senticosus).

Lemon balm (Melissa officinalis) is from the mint family and has been used for reducing stress, anxiety, pain, indigestion problems and for improving sleep and appetite since the Middle Ages [24]. Scientific studies have indicated that lemon balm has the capacity to inhibit the breakdown of the sedative neurotransmitter gamma amino butyric acid (GABA) [25].

Valerian (Valeriana officinalis) is also another herb that has been used as a sleeping aid for a long time [26]. Valerian is said to induce a calming effect by binding to GABA type A receptors and thereby regulating the excitability of the nervous system [27]. A meta-analysis study revealed that valerian is capable of improving the sleep quality [28]. Further, as the metabolites of valerian are rapidly detoxified in the liver, they probably do not cause any adverse side effects [29].

Passionflower (Passiflora incarnata) is a traditional herb that has been used for anxiety [30], insomnia [31], seizures [32] and hysteria [33]. It acts by increasing the levels of GABA in the brain, which in turn leads to relaxation due to reduced activity of brain cells [31].

Chamomile (Matricaria recutita) is a gentle herb that is most often used in the form of tea and is considered safe for both adults and children. The active ingredients in chamomile are said to bind to benzodiazepine receptors and demonstrate central nervous system (CNS) depressant activity, anxiolytic activity and anticonvulsant activity [34].

Linden flowers have also been used as anxiolytics for several years. One study has indicated that Tilia americana var. mexicana has both anxiolytic and sedative effects due to the presence of beta-sitosterol in them [35]. Another study also highlights the depressant activity of Tilia americana var. mexicana on the CNS [36].

It was found that hop pickers got tired very easily due to their hand-mouth activity and thereby transfer of hop resins [37]. On further studies, the relaxing effect of hops (Humulus lupulus) was attributed to the specific chemical component dimethylvinyl carbinol and traditionally it has been used as CNS depressant, to treat headache, insomnia, anxiety, stress and restlessness [38]. In some countries, hop baths are being used to decrease hot flashes in menopausal women [39]. Several studies have also highlighted that a combination of hops and valerian extracts have been used for inducing sleep [40].

It was discussed earlier that sleep deprivation caused behavioral changes and certain herbs have also been used to mitigate these changes. One such example is Eleutheroside E, which is a principal component of Eleutherococcus senticosus, an adrenal tonic herb which was found to alleviate the behavioral alterations induced by sleep deprivation [41].

Sleep disturbances can be resolved to some extent by inhaling essential oils. The mechanism of action of such oils is mainly due to their biochemical, psychological and energetic properties [42]. The biochemical constituents of these essential oils such as esters, coumarins and monoterpenols are known to act on nerve cell function by antagonizing specified neuronal receptors or binding to other receptors [43]. Not only animal studies have demonstrated the sedative effects of certain essential oils such as lavender [44], sweet orange [45], rose [46], cedar [47], bergamot [48], valerian and lemon [49]; but human studies have also shown similar results.

The oil that has been studied predominantly was lavender oil (Lavandula angustifolia), either alone or blended with other oils. Lavender oil was found to increase sleepiness in a group of healthy students [50] and also improve the quality of sleep up to one week in midlife women with insomnia after treatment [51]. Sleep quality after treatment with lavender oil was also found to increase among CCU patients with ischemic heart disease [52]. The quality of daytime wakefulness and continuous sleep at night were both improved among elderly patients when exposed to lavender oil [53].

Using aroma sticks made by blending lavender and valerian oil was found to be effective in cancer patients who had sleep issues [54]. In a study, during the analysis of perception of sleep, 97% of the study population composed of psychogeriatric patients indicated that they had a refreshing night's sleep after treatment with a blend of lavender, basil (Ocimum basilicum), juniper (Juniperus communis) and sweet marjoram (Origanum majorana) [55].

Peppermint oil was also found to increase total sleep time and decrease fatigue and depression among healthy adults [56]. Jasmine oil was reported to increase sleep efficiency and also to reduce sleep movement [57]. More studies need to be done in humans as far as other essential oils that have proved to be useful to enhance sleep in animals.

Acupuncture/Acupressure

Acupuncture is an important aspect of Traditional Chinese Medicine (TCM) that dates back to 4000 years ago [58]. Studies on randomized controlled trials of acupuncture used for insomnia treatment revealed that acupuncture did improve sleep efficiency and quality as well as daytime functioning [59]. A few other prominent reviews on acupuncture include the studies by Chen et al. [60], Cheuk et al. [61], Huang et al. [62] and Yeung et al. [63].

Auricular acupressure has been shown to be effective in improving the sleep quality of cancer patients [64], patients with obstructive sleep apnea syndrome [65] and also in nurses working three shifts [66]. A meta-analyses report stated that the acupuncture on Sanyinjiao acupoint, also known as Spleen 6 (SP6) proved to be a good remedy for sleep disturbances [67]. Another study highlighted 96% effectiveness of acupuncture on Shenmen (HT7) and Fuliu (KI7) acupuncture sites in 288 cases of insomnia [68]. 96.5% effectiveness was reported in a study which concentrated on the acupuncture sites Ezhongxian (MS1), EpangxianI (MS2), Pishu (BL20) and Xinshu (BL15) [69]. Yet another study indicated 96% efficiency through the sites Baihui (Du20) and Sishenchong (Extra6) for the treatment of insomnia [70].

Acupuncture and acupressure are said to play an active role in the neuro-chemical modulatory activity that involves dopamine, serotonin and endogenous opioids and this characteristic enables them to serve as an effective enhancer of sleep [71]. The brain-derived neurotrophic factor (BDNF) has been well-established as a sleep regulator [72]. In a study, decreased serum BDNF levels were seen in insomnia patients compared to sleep-healthy controls [73]. Acupuncture basically acts to enhance sleep by modulating BDNF and this principle was applied in a study which found that acupuncture was highly effective in improving sleep quality in the elderly population [74].

Bright light therapy

Circadian rhythm is a biological clock within the human body that follows a 24-hour cycle responding primarily to light and darkness in one's environment. This clock works harmoniously with the homeostatic mechanisms and controls neurological and endocrine functions, temperature regulations and sleep wake periods [75]. Releasing of certain hormones and neurotransmitters and in turn their function in regulating multiple organ functions are happening constantly inside our body in an auto pilot mode based on these circadian rhythms. However, the invention of light bulbs followed by the easy flip of switch to keep the light going indefinitely had made us to go to bed according to our physical clocks instead of our own biological clocks. Inventions of electricity, socialization, advancement in technologies, globalization and outsourcing have disturbed our bodies' natural rhythm in innumerable ways.

When these rhythms are disturbed some disorders begin to surface. Insomnia, characterized by difficulty in initiating sleep at conventional bedtime and earlier than normal morning awakening is one of the major disorders associated with the abnormalities in the timing of circadian rhythms [76]. Two kinds of bright light therapy are generally used to treat such insomnia. Morning bright light therapy is used for sleep-onset insomnia and evening bright light therapy is used for early morning awakening insomnia. That is, a delayed circadian rhythm can be advanced or shifted to an earlier time by exposure to bright light in the morning and an early circadian rhythm can be delayed or retimed to later by exposure to bright light in the evening.

Individuals exposed to bright light in the range of 2500 lux were able to advance their sleep-onset times when compared to individuals exposed to dim light of 300 lux [77]. Likewise, in another study, sleep-onset times and wake-up times were all significantly advanced after exposure to bright light in the morning [78]. Bright light masks in the morning also showed similar results [79]. Positive changes in the sleep latency and daytime dysfunction were noticed when healthy elders were exposed to bright light of 10,000 lux in the morning for about half-hour [80]. In one study, where the participants wore short-wavelength blue light glasses that had blue light-emitting diodes for two hours soon after waking up in the morning were able to advance their sleep-onset by 2.5 hours [81].

Likewise, the wake-up time of study participants was significantly delayed by exposing them to bright white light of 2500 lux in the evenings [82]. In another study, along with delaying the wake-up time, an increase in total sleep time was also noticed on exposure to bright light of 2500 lux in the evenings [83].

Massage and touch therapies

Massage and touch therapies are said to increase blood circulation, relieve pain and lower body stiffness by balancing the nervous system and boost the morale, thereby improving the quality of sleep [84]. Back massage for about 6 minutes was found to be useful in promoting sleep in critically ill older men [85]. Touch therapy along with preferred music (chosen from a selection of 4 pieces: in Hüseyni, Saba, Rast and Uşşak maqams) and preferred aroma (chosen from a selection of 9 varieties: lavender, mint, orange, rose, chamomile, Asiatic dayflower, rosemary, common sage and linden) was found to have positive effects on sleep [84]. Another study has also reported that therapeutic touch has a relaxation response of vasodilation which can in turn induce sleep [86].

Music therapy

Considering all the alternative approaches, music is identified as the relatively inexpensive and a readily available therapy that can be easily self-administered [87]. Music is said to act on the limbic system of the brain and affect the modulation of endogenous opiods and oxytocin, thereby enhancing sleep [88]. Beccaloni [89] and Pittman and Kridli [90] have shown that music helps to resolve pre-operative anxiety and Engwall and Dupplis indicated that music also helps to overcome post-operative pain [91].

Several studies conducted among a wide range of populations ranging from university students, elders in the community, patients in hospitals and rehabilitation centers, etc. have reported that music improves the quality of sleep. Some of the notable studies include the ones done by Jespersen and Vuust [92] on traumatized refugees; Ryu et al. [93] in a South Korean hospital on patients who have gone through coronary angiography; Bloch et al. [94] where it was found that music improved sleep latency and sleep efficiency in schizophrenia patients; Deshmukh et al. [95] in India on depressed patients; Harmat et al. [96] among students from a Hungarian university; Lai and Good [97] among the elders in the Taiwan community; Hernandez-Ruiz [98] in abused women in a shelter at USA; Johnson [99] on older women; Kullich et al. [100] in an Austrian rehabilitation center; Renzi et al. [101] in a hospital on patients who have gone through anorectal operation in Italy; Richards [85] and Zimmerman [102] among in-patients in hospitals of USA.

Even though all the above mentioned studies brought to light the fact that music can enhance sleep, there isn't enough evidence in the literature to identify a protocol for the intervention strategy. Hence, more studies need to be done to categorize the specific pieces of music that would enhance sleep, an appropriate time frame and duration to play the music and methods to create a suitable ambience so that the study participants put in their full attention to the music that is being played to them. This protocol becomes necessary as it has been indicated that the efficiency of the music played depends on the listener's enjoyment [103] and most of the time the listener's preferred music has more beneficial effects rather any random music [104].

Yoga and tai chi

Mind-body therapies such as yoga and tai chi have been more popular among the older population and are nowadays slowly gaining grounds among the younger generations too. Having originated in the eastern part of the world and slowly loosing grounds there, these practices are forging ahead and are being embraced more widely in the western part of the world. The biological mechanisms by which these mind-body therapies exert their holistic effects are yet to be deciphered.

Manjunath et al.'s study indicated that yoga improved sleep latency and total sleep better than herbal medicines [105]. In one study, decreased nocturnal awakenings and faster return to sleep after nocturnal awakenings were noticed in young adults who were performing Bikram Yoga [106]. Significant improvement in the total sleep quality was noticed in a group of elderly participants living in old age homes after yoga intervention [107]. Jonathan et al. reported that older adults who went in for yoga intervention showed significant improvements in overall sleep quality, sleep efficiency, sleep latency and duration [108].

One study on tai chi indicated that it improved sleep quality and sleep duration outcomes in older adults [109]. Another study reported that tai chi was significantly more effective than low-impact exercise on improving sleep latency, sleep quality and efficiency and also in increasing sleep duration [110]. An ECG-based sleep spectrogram revealed improved sleep stability among participants who practiced tai-chi for about 12 weeks [111]. A recent study that used DNA methylation as an epigenetic biomarker has indicated that regular practice of tai-chi could be associated with significant and beneficial epigenetic changes [112].

Conclusion

This review gives a broad idea of the various types of complementary and alternative methods and their physiological mode of action to alleviate sleep disturbances. Researchers are now concentrating on such methods as the widely used pharmacological therapies have the limitation of their inability to be used as a long-term intervention due to their potential side effects. Reviews of research activities in terms of other alternative methods such as Homeopathy and Ayurveda to treat sleep disorders are beyond the scope of this article. Further research on exercises, massage, touch and music therapy for the treatment of sleep disorders with more clinically relevant evidences is encouraged as current research in these fields is still in their infancy. It was also noticed that several studies, especially pertaining to tai chi are in Mandarin and translation of these would enable the scientific community to benefit from them as well.

References

1. Sleep - definition of sleep in English from the Oxford dictionary.
2. Carskadon, MA, Dement WC (2000). Normal human sleep: an overview. Princ. Pract. Sleep Med 2: 16-25.
3. Neu D, Mairesse O, Verbanck P, Linkowski P, Le Bon O (2014) Non-REM sleep EEG power distribution in fatigue and sleepiness. J Psychosom Res 76: 286-291.
4. Natural Patterns of Sleep | Healthy Sleep. at
5. Nakata A (2011) Effects of long work hours and poor sleep characteristics on workplace injury among full-time male employees of small- and medium-scale businesses. J Sleep Res 20: 576-584.
6. Van Dongen HPA, Maislin G, Mullington JM, Dinges DF (2003) The cumulative cost of additional wakefulness: dose-response effects on neurobehavioral functions and sleep physiology from chronic sleep restriction and total sleep deprivation. Sleep 26: 117-126.
7. Spiegel K, Leproult R, Van Cauter E (1999) Impact of sleep debt on metabolic and endocrine function. Lancet 354: 1435-1439.
8. Krueger JM, Majde JA, Rector DM (2011) Cytokines in immune function and sleep regulation. Handb Clin Neurol 98: 229-240.
9. Spiegel K, Tasali E, Penev P, Van Cauter E (2004) Brief communication: Sleep curtailment in healthy young men is associated with decreased leptin levels, elevated ghrelin levels, and increased hunger and appetite. Annals of Internal Medicine 846.
10. Belenky G, Wesensten NJ, Thorne DR, Thomas ML, Sing HC, et al. (2003) Patterns of performance degradation and restoration during sleep restriction and subsequent recovery: a sleep dose-response study. J Sleep Res 12: 1-12.
11. Hardy M, Kirk-Smith MD, Stretch DD (1995) Replacement of drug treatment for insomnia by ambient odour. Lancet 346: 701.

12. Wang MY, Wang SY, Tsai PS (2005) Cognitive behavioural therapy for primary insomnia: a systematic review. J Adv Nurs 50: 553-564.
13. Pearson NJ, Johnson LL, Nahin RL (2006) Insomnia, trouble sleeping, and complementary and alternative medicine: Analysis of the 2002 national health interview survey data. Arch Intern Med 166: 1775-1782.
14. Sleep and sleep disorders: a neuropsychopharmacological approach. Springer Science+Business Media (2006).
15. Principles and practice of sleep medicine. Elsevier Saunders (2011).
16. Silber BY, Schmitt JA (2010) Effects of tryptophan loading on human cognition, mood, and sleep. Neurosci Biobehav Rev 34: 387-407.
17. Halson SL (2014) Sleep in elite athletes and nutritional interventions to enhance sleep. Sports Med 44 Suppl 1: S13-23.
18. Lindseth G, Lindseth P, Thompson M (2013) Nutritional effects on sleep. West J Nurs Res 35: 497-513.
19. Grandner MA, Kripke DF, Naidoo N, Langer RD (2010) Relationships among dietary nutrients and subjective sleep, objective sleep, and napping in women. Sleep Med 11: 180-184.
20. Zammit GK, Kolevzon A, Fauci M, Shindledecker R, Ackerman S (1995) Postprandial sleep in healthy men. Sleep 18: 229-231.
21. Afaghi A, O'Connor H, Chow CM (2007) High-glycemic-index carbohydrate meals shorten sleep onset. Am J Clin Nutr 85: 426-430.
22. Porter JM, Horne JA (1981) Bed-time food supplements and sleep: effects of different carbohydrate levels. Electroencephalogr Clin Neurophysiol 51: 426-433.
23. Jang HS, Jung JY, Jang IS, Jang KH, Kim SH, et al. (2012) L-theanine partially counteracts caffeine-induced sleep disturbances in rats. Pharmacol Biochem Behav 101: 217-221.
24. Kopparapu N (2012) Natural sleep Aids; Boon or Bane. J. Pharm. Res 5: 4950-4956.
25. Awad R, Levac D, Cybulska P, Merali Z, Trudeau VL, et al. (2007) Effects of traditionally used anxiolytic botanicals on enzymes of the gamma-aminobutyric acid (GABA) system. Can J Physiol Pharmacol 85: 933-942.
26. Bent S, Padula A, Moore D, Patterson M, Mehling W (2006) Valerian for sleep: a systematic review and meta-analysis. Am J Med 119: 1005-1012.
27. Wheatley D (2005) Medicinal plants for insomnia: a review of their pharmacology, efficacy and tolerability. J Psychopharmacol 19: 414-421.
28. Fernández-San-Martín MI, Masa-Font R, Palacios-Soler L, Sancho-Gómez P, Calbó-Caldentey C, et al. (2010) Effectiveness of Valerian on insomnia: a meta-analysis of randomized placebo-controlled trials. Sleep Med 11: 505-511.
29. von der Hude W, Scheutwinkel-Reich M, Braun R (1986) Bacterial mutagenicity of the tranquilizing constituents of Valerianaceae roots. Mutat Res 169: 23-27.
30. Dhawan K, Kumar S, Sharma A (2001) Anti-anxiety studies on extracts of Passiflora incarnata Linneaus. J Ethnopharmacol 78: 165-170.
31. Elsas SM, Rossi DJ, Raber J, White G, Seeley CA, et al. (2010) Passiflora incarnata L. (Passionflower) extracts elicit GABA currents in hippocampal neurons in vitro, and show anxiogenic and anticonvulsant effects in vivo, varying with extraction method. Phytomedicine 17: 940-949.
32. Sarris J (2007) Herbal medicines in the treatment of psychiatric disorders: a systematic review. Phytother Res 21: 703-716.
33. The desktop guide to complementary and alternative medicine: an evidence-based approach (2001).
34. Medina JH, Viola H, Wolfman C, Marder M, Wasowski C, et al. (1998) Neuroactive flavonoids: new ligands for the Benzodiazepine receptors. Phytomedicine 5: 235-243.
35. Aguirre-Hernández E, Rosas-Acevedo H, Soto-Hernández M, Martínez AL, Moreno J, et al. (2007) Bioactivity-guided isolation of beta-sitosterol and some fatty acids as active compounds in the anxiolytic and sedative effects of Tilia americana var. mexicana. Planta Med 73: 1148-1155.
36. Aguirre-Hernández E, Martínez AL, González-Trujano ME, Moreno J, Vibrans H, et al. (2007) Pharmacological evaluation of the anxiolytic and sedative effects of Tilia americana L. var. mexicana in mice. J Ethnopharmacol 109: 140-145.
37. Tyler VE, Tyler VE (1987) The new honest herbal: a sensible guide to the use of herbs and related remedies. G.F. Stickley Co.
38. Newall CA, Anderson LA, Phillipson JD (1996) Herbal medicines: a guide for health-care professionals. Pharmaceutical Press.
39. Zanoli P, Rivasi M, Zavatti M, Brusiani F, Baraldi M (2005) New insight in the neuropharmacological activity of Humulus lupulus L. J Ethnopharmacol 102: 102-106.
40. Vonderheid-Guth B, Todorova A, Brattström A, Dimpfel W (2000) Pharmacodynamic effects of valerian and hops extract combination (Ze 91019) on the quantitative-topographical EEG in healthy volunteers. Eur J Med Res 5: 139-144.
41. Huang LZ, Wei L, Zhao HF, Huang BK, Rahman K, et al. (2011) The effect of Eleutheroside E on behavioral alterations in murine sleep deprivation stress model. Eur J Pharmacol 658: 150-155.
42. Battaglia S (2003) The complete guide to aromatherapy. International Centre of Holistic Aromatherapy.
43. Bowles EJ (2003)The chemistry of aromatherapeutic oils. Allen & Unwin.
44. Guillemain J, Rousseau A, Delaveau P (1989) Neurodepressive effects of the essential oil of Lavandula angustifolia Mill. Ann Pharm Fr 47: 337-343.
45. Faturi CB, Leite JR, Alves PB, Canton AC, Teixeira-Silva F (2010) Anxiolytic-like effect of sweet orange aroma in Wistar rats. Prog Neuropsychopharmacol Biol Psychiatry 34: 605-609.
46. de Almeida RN, Motta SC, de Brito Faturi C, Catallani B, Leite JR (2004) Anxiolytic-like effects of rose oil inhalation on the elevated plus-maze test in rats. Pharmacol Biochem Behav 77: 361-364.
47. Sano A, Sei H, Seno H, Morita Y, Moritoki H (1998) Influence of cedar essence on spontaneous activity and sleep of rats and human daytime nap. Psychiatry Clin Neurosci 52: 133-135.
48. Saiyudthong S, Marsden CA (2011) Acute effects of bergamot oil on anxiety-related behaviour and corticosterone level in rats. Phytother Res 25: 858-862.
49. Komori T, Matsumoto T, Motomura E, Shiroyama T (2006) The sleep-enhancing effect of valerian inhalation and sleep-shortening effect of lemon inhalation. Chem Senses 31: 731-737.
50. Hirokawa K, Nishimoto T, Taniguchi T (2012) Effects of lavender aroma on sleep quality in healthy Japanese students. Percept Mot Skills 114: 111-122.
51. Chien LW, Cheng SL, Liu CF (2012) The effect of lavender aromatherapy on autonomic nervous system in midlife women with insomnia. Evid Based Complement Alternat Med 2012: 740813.
52. Moeini M, Khadibi M, Bekhradi R, Mahmoudian SA, Nazari F (2010) Effect of aromatherapy on the quality of sleep in ischemic heart disease patients hospitalized in intensive care units of heart hospitals of the Isfahan University of Medical Sciences. Iran. J. Nurs. Midwifery Res 15: 234-239.
53. Hudson R (1996) The value of lavender for rest and activity in the elderly patient. Complement. Ther. Med 4: 52-57.
54. Stringer J, Donald G (2011) Aromasticks in cancer care: an innovation not to be sniffed at. Complement Ther Clin Pract 17: 116-121.
55. Cannard G (1996) The effect of aromatherapy in promoting relaxation and stress reduction in a general hospital. Complement Ther Nurs Midwifery 2: 38-40.
56. Goel N, Lao RP (2006) Sleep changes vary by odor perception in young adults. Biol Psychol 71: 341-349.
57. Raudenbush B, JerrodSmith, JeffreyZoladz, Phillip (2003) Effects of Odorant Administration on Objective and Subjective Measures of Sleep Quality, Post-Sleep Mood and Alertness, and Cognitive Performance. North Am. J. Psychol 5: 181.
58. Gao L, Zhang M, Gong H, Bai L, Dai XJ, et al. (2014) Differential activation patterns of FMRI in sleep-deprived brain: restoring effects of acupuncture. Evid Based Complement Alternat Med 2014: 465760.
59. Huang LS, Wang DL, Wang CW, Hu YP, Zhou JW, et al. (2009) The needle-rolling therapy for treatment of non-organic chronic insomnia in 90 cases. J Tradit Chin Med 29: 19-23.

60. Chen HY, Shi Y, Ng CS, Chan SM, Yung KK, et al. (2007) Auricular acupuncture treatment for insomnia: a systematic review. J Altern Complement Med 13: 669-676.

61. Cheuk DKL, Yeung WF, Chung KF, Wong V (2012) Acupuncture for insomnia. Cochrane Database Syst. Rev 9 :CD005472.

62. Huang W, Kutner N, Bliwise DL (2009) A systematic review of the effects of acupuncture in treating insomnia. Sleep Med Rev 13: 73-104.

63. Yeung WF, Chung KF, Leung YK, Zhang SP, Law ACK (2009) Traditional needle acupuncture treatment for insomnia: a systematic review of randomized controlled trials. Sleep Med 10: 694-704.

64. Chun-I Fan (2015) The Efficacy of Using an Auricular Acupressure Program to Improve Sleep Disturbance in Cancer Patients [Chinese]. J. Nurs. Healthc. Res 11: 3-12.

65. Wang H, Yeh ML, Chung U, Yang CH (2008) Improving sleep quality: The efficacy of auricular acupressure. J. Evid.-Based Nurs 4: 243-250.

66. Chang WL, Ko SH, Chang TH, Hung LC (2010) Effect of auricular acupressure on improving sleep quality in nurses [Chinese]. J. Nurs. Healthc. Res 6: 261-270.

67. Sok SR, Erlen JA, Kim KB (2003) Effects of acupuncture therapy on insomnia. J Adv Nurs 44: 375-384.

68. Gao QW (1997) Acupuncture treatment of insomnia: clincial observation of 288 cases. Int. J. Clin. Acupunct 8: 183-185.

69. Shang YI (2000) Ear pressing for insomnia: observation of 82 cases. Int. J. Clin. Acupunct 11: 65-67.

70. Wang Y (1992) An observation on the therapeutic effect of acupuncture in treating 50 cases of insomnia. Int. J. Clin. Acupunct 3: 91-93.

71. Cabýoglu MT, Ergene N, Tan U (2006) The mechanism of acupuncture and clinical applications. Int J Neurosci 116: 115-125.

72. Faraguna U, Vyazovskiy VV, Nelson AB, Tononi G, Cirelli C (2008) A causal role for brain-derived neurotrophic factor in the homeostatic regulation of sleep. J Neurosci 28: 4088-4095.

73. Giese M, Unternährer E, Hüttig H, Beck J, Brand S, et al. (2014) BDNF: an indicator of insomnia? Mol Psychiatry 19: 151-152.

74. Zuppa C, Prado CH, Wieck A, Zaparte A, Barbosa A, et al. (2015) Acupuncture for sleep quality, BDNF levels and immunosenescence: a randomized controlled study. Neurosci Lett 587: 35-40.

75. Borbély AA (1982) A two process model of sleep regulation. Hum Neurobiol 1: 195-204.

76. Hoyt BD (2005) Sleep in patients with neurologic and psychiatric disorders. Prim Care 32: 535-548.

77. Rosenthal NE, Joseph-Vanderpool JR, Levendosky AA, Johnston SH, Allen R, et al. (1990) Phase-shifting effects of bright morning light as treatment for delayed sleep phase syndrome. Sleep 13: 354-361.

78. Watanabe T, Kajimura N, Kato M, Sekimoto M, Takahashi K (1999) Effects of phototherapy in patients with delayed sleep phase syndrome. Psychiatry Clin Neurosci 53: 231-233.

79. Cole RJ, Smith JS, Alcalá YC, Elliott JA, Kripke DF (2002) Bright-light mask treatment of delayed sleep phase syndrome. J Biol Rhythms 17: 89-101.

80. Akyar I, Akdemir N (2013) The effect of light therapy on the sleep quality of the elderly: an intervention study. Aust. J. Adv. Nurs 31: 31-38.

81. Lack L, Bramwell T, Wright H, Kemp K (2007) Morning blue light can advance the melatonin rhythm in mild delayed sleep phase syndrome. Sleep Biol. Rhythms 5.

82. Lack L, Wright H (1993) The effect of evening bright light in delaying the circadian rhythms and lengthening the sleep of early morning awakening insomniacs. Sleep 16: 436-443.

83. Lack L, Wright H, Kemp K, Gibbon S (2005) The treatment of early-morning awakening insomnia with 2 evenings of bright light. Sleep 28: 616-623.

84. Demirbag B, Erci B (2012) The effects of sleep and touch therapy on symptoms of fibromyalgia and depression. Iran J Public Health 41: 44-53.

85. Richards KC (1998) Effect of a back massage and relaxation intervention on sleep in critically ill patients. Am J Crit Care 7: 288-299.

86. Engle VF, Graney MJ (2000) Biobehavioral effects of therapeutic touch. J Nurs Scholarsh 32: 287-293.

87. McCaffrey R (2008) Music listening: its effects in creating a healing environment. J Psychosoc Nurs Ment Health Serv 46: 39-44.

88. Bernatzky G, Presch M, Anderson M, Panksepp J (2011) Emotional foundations of music as a non-pharmacological pain management tool in modern medicine. Neurosci Biobehav Rev 35: 1989-1999.

89. Beccaloni AM (2011) The medicine of music: a systematic approach for adoption into perianesthesia practice. J Perianesth Nurs 26: 323-330.

90. Pittman S, Kridli S (2011) Music intervention and preoperative anxiety: an integrative review. Int Nurs Rev 58: 157-163.

91. Engwall M, Duppils GS (2009) Music as a nursing intervention for postoperative pain: a systematic review. J Perianesth Nurs 24: 370-383.

92. Jespersen KV, Vuust P (2012) The Effect of Relaxation Music Listening on Sleep Quality in Traumatized Refugees: A Pilot Study. J. Music Ther 49: 205-229.

93. Ryu MJ, Park JS, Park H (2012) Effect of sleep-inducing music on sleep in persons with percutaneous transluminal coronary angiography in the cardiac care unit. J Clin Nurs 21: 728-735.

94. Bloch B, Reshef A, Vadas L, Haliba Y, Ziv N, et al. (2010) The effects of music relaxation on sleep quality and emotional measures in people living with schizophrenia J Music Ther 47: 27-52.

95. Deshmukh AD, Sarvaiya AA, Seethalakshmi R, Nayak AS (2009) Effect of Indian classical music on quality of sleep in depressed patients: A randomized controlled trial. Nord. J. Music Ther 18: 70-78.

96. Harmat L, Takács J, Bódizs R (2008) Music improves sleep quality in students. J Adv Nurs 62: 327-335.

97. Lai HL, Good M (2005) Music improves sleep quality in older adults. J Adv Nurs 49: 234-244.

98. Hernández-Ruiz E (2005) Effect of music therapy on the anxiety levels and sleep patterns of abused women in shelters. J Music Ther 42: 140-158.

99. Johnson JE (2003) The use of music to promote sleep in older women. J Community Health Nurs 20: 27-35.

100. Kullich W, Bernatzky G, Hesse HP, Wendtner F, Likar R, et al. (2003) [Music therapy--effect on pain, sleep and quality of life in low back pain]. Wien Med Wochenschr 153: 217-221.

101. Renzi C, Peticca L, Pescatori M (2000) The use of relaxation techniques in the perioperative management of proctological patients: preliminary results. Int J Colorectal Dis 15: 313-316.

102. Zimmerman L, Nieveen J, Barnason S, Schmaderer M (1996) The effects of music interventions on postoperative pain and sleep in coronary artery bypass graft (CABG) patients. Sch Inq Nurs Pract 10: 153-170.

103. Nilsson U (2011) Music: a nursing intervention. Eur J Cardiovasc Nurs 10: 73-74.

104. Lai HL (2004) Music preference and relaxation in Taiwanese elderly people. Geriatr Nurs 25: 286-291.

105. Manjunath NK, Telles S (2005) Influence of Yoga and Ayurveda on self-rated sleep in a geriatric population. Indian J Med Res 121: 683-690.

106. Kudesia RS, Bianchi MT (2012) Decreased nocturnal awakenings in young adults performing bikram yoga: a low-constraint home sleep monitoring study. ISRN Neurol 2012: 153745.

107. Hariprasad VR, Sivakumar PT, Koparde V, Varambally S, Thirthalli J, et al. (2013) Effects of yoga intervention on sleep and quality-of-life in elderly: A randomized controlled trial. Indian J Psychiatry 55: S364-368.

108. Halpern J, Cohen M, Kennedy G, Reece J, Cahan C, et al. (2014) Yoga for improving sleep quality and quality of life for older adults. Altern Ther Health Med 20: 37-46.

109. Irwin MR, Olmstead R, Motivala SJ (2008) Improving sleep quality in older adults with moderate sleep complaints: A randomized controlled trial of Tai Chi Chih. leep 31: 1001-1008.

110. Li F, Fisher KJ, Harmer P, Irbe D, Tearse RG, et al. (2004) Tai chi and self-rated quality of sleep and daytime sleepiness in older adults: a randomized controlled trial. J Am Geriatr Soc 52: 892-900.

15

Pilot Study of a Nasal Airway Stent for the Treatment on Obstructive Sleep Apnea

Yumi Hirata[1*] **and Makoto Satoh**[2,3*]

[1]*Division of Sleep Medicine, Graduate School of Comprehensive Human Sciences, University of Tsukuba, Japan*

[2]*International Institute for Integrative Sleep Medicine, University of Tsukuba, Japan*

[3]*Ibaraki Prefectural Center for Sleep Medicine and Sciences, Japan*

***Corresponding author:** Makoto Satoh and Yumi Hirata, International Institute for Integrative Sleep Medicine, University of Tsukuba, 1-1-1 Tennodai, Tsukuba, Ibaraki 305-8575, Japan, E-mail: yumi.h.n.19811013@gmail.com, satoh@md.tsukuba.ac.jp

Abstract

Study background: Obstructive sleep apnea (OSA) is a common disease characterized by repetitive upper airway obstruction during sleep. OSA is associated with an increased risk of cardiovascular morbidity. Continuous positive airway pressure (CPAP) has been established as a standard therapy for OSA, but it is not always tolerated by OSA patients.

Objective: In a pilot study, we evaluated the therapeutic effects of the nasal airway stent (NAS), a new nasopharyngeal device placed in the nasopharynx, on OSA and snoring.

Methods: Six subjects with OSA were enrolled. The apnea-hypopnea index, oxygen desaturation index, lowest oxygen saturation, and snore index were analyzed before and during treatment with the NAS.

Results: All subjects tolerated the NAS, with good compliance. Treatment with the NAS ameliorated apnea and hypopnea events and improved oxygen saturation in subjects with mild to moderate OSA. Snoring in all subjects was improved by the NAS.

Conclusions: The NAS stent is a readymade device that could be an alternative therapy for patients with mild to moderate OSA who cannot tolerate CPAP or for subjects with snoring.

Keywords: Nasal airway stent; Obstructive sleep apnea; Sleep medicine; Snoring

Abbreviations:

AHI: Apnea Hypopnea Index; BMI: Body Mass Index; CPAP: Continuous Positive Airway Pressure; HI: Hypopnea Index; NAS: Nasal Airway Stent; ODI: Oxygen Desaturation Index; OSA: Obstructive Sleep Apnea; s-NAS: Single NAS; SpO_2: Oxygen Saturation With Pulse Oximetry

Introduction

Obstructive sleep apnea (OSA) is a common public health problem that affects as much as 4% of the adult population [1,2]. Because OSA is associated with recurrent hypoxia and apnea during sleep, patients are exposed to decreased oxygen saturation, leading to the potential development and exacerbation of not only cardiovascular and cerebrovascular, but also metabolic diseases [3-6]. Several therapies have been developed to treat OSA, including surgery and continuous positive airway pressure (CPAP) [7]. CPAP has been established as a standard therapy for patients with OSA [7-9]. However, although it is effective, low patient tolerance remains an obstacle to be overcome [10,11]. Moreover, patients with OSA may have difficulties with both poor portability of CPAP machines (which can be large and heavy) and lack of availability of electrical power supply during travel. Alternative therapeutic devices that could replace CPAP for short or long periods are therefore required. Some previous studies have reported oral or nasopharyngeal appliances as non-surgical alternatives to CPAP for OSA patients who do not tolerate CPAP treatment [12-18]. Although the concept of nasopharyngeal tube insertion to maintain airflow through the upper airway during sleep was proposed in the 1980s and has been reviewed before [7,12,18], such devices are not currently in common use. The nasal trumpet has been used successfully to decrease airway obstruction in the short term, such as immediately after surgery for OSA [18]. However, the stiffness, length, and consequent discomfort of nasal trumpets mean that they need to be improved for long-term tolerability [18].

We developed a nasal airway stent (NAS), which is a ready-made, non-invasive, and tolerated treatment device for subjects with OSA or snoring. The NAS is specifically designed as a nasopharyngeal stent that maintains the patency of the nasal airway through to the nasopharynx and retropalatal oropharynx during sleep. Although we have developed three kinds of NAS—single NAS (s-NAS), double NAS, and expandable NAS [19] these devices have not yet been manufactured commercially. Here, we performed a pilot study to assess the therapeutic efficacy of the s-NAS on OSA and snoring in subjects with varying degrees of severity of OSA. We verified that the use of the s-NAS is feasible as a supportive therapy for mild to moderate OSA and snoring.

Materials and Methods

Subjects

The subjects were six male subjects (age, 42.1 ± 8.9 years; body mass index (BMI), 26.6 ± 2.1) who had been previously diagnosed as having OSA by polysomnography. All subjects provided written informed consent after receiving a full explanation of the procedures involved. This study was approved by the University of Tsukuba institutional review committee and was performed in accordance with the recommendations in the Helsinki Declaration.

The s-NAS

The s-NAS is specially designed as a nasopharyngeal stent that maintains the patency of the nasal airway through to the nasopharynx and retropalatal oropharynx by mechanically preventing the upper airway obstruction by the movement and vibration of soft palate during sleep. Unlike currently available nasopharyngeal appliances, the s-NAS is constructed of resilient silicone rubber for the purpose of maintaining the patency of the upper airway by insertion into the nasal cavity. The device consists of a tube-shaped shaft (4.4 mm internal diameter) encapsulated by a water-soluble gel as a lubricant, and a proximal nose clip to fix the device in the appropriate position for optimal treatment efficacy (Figure 1a). The shaft of s-NAS is designed to maintain not to collapse by a pressure of more than 20 cm H_2O in an airflow of 0.1 to 0.51 L/sec—approximately the maximum speed of inspiration under normal breathing conditions. s-NAS devices with a variety of lengths (120 to 145 mm) were manufactured to enable appropriate treatment efficacy for all subjects (Figure 1b) [12]. The distal end of the s-NAS is inserted via the nostril into the nasal cavity until it reaches the retropalatal oropharynx (Figure 1c). Each device comes singly wrapped in a sterile bag. All manufacturing processes were kindly performed by Seven Dreamers Laboratories, Inc., Tokyo, Japan.

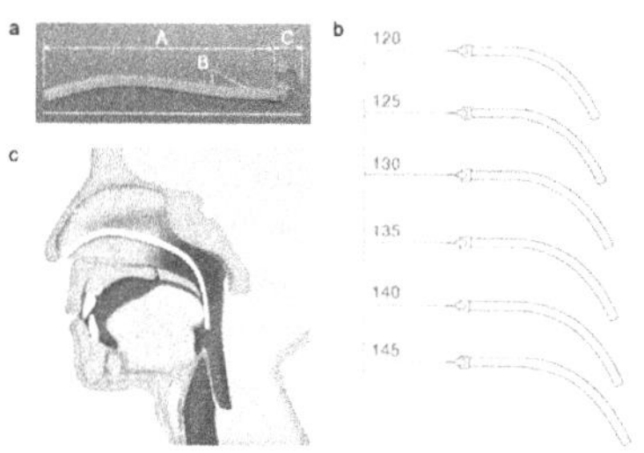

Figure 1: Diagrams of the single nasal airway stent (s-NAS). (a) Overview. A, tube; B, air holes; C, nose clip. White scale bar, 120 to 145 mm. (b) Schematic diagram of s-NAS devices of various lengths. (c) Schematic diagram of nasopharyngeal insertion of the s-NAS. The device is inserted via a nostril into the nasal cavity until it reaches the retropalatal oropharynx.

Study design

Nocturnal respiratory events in all subjects, including oxygen saturation, snoring, and apnea and hypopnea events, were recorded by portable monitoring during treatment with the s-NAS. Physicians determined the appropriate length of the s-NAS for each subject and then instructed and trained all subjects on how to insert the s-NAS into the nasal cavity by themselves to maintain patency of the upper airway. Respiratory events in subjects using the s-NAS were recorded no more than 1 month after the first recording without the s-NAS.

Measurements

Each subject wore a 4-channel portable device (SAS-2100 for airflow, snoring, oxygen desaturation, and heart rate; Nihon Kohden, Tokyo, Japan); this device is categorized as a Level 4 device by the American Academy of Sleep Medicine [20]. Nasal flow, oxygen saturation with pulse oximetry (SpO_2), and snoring were recorded for at least 4 h at night by portable monitoring with the SAS-2100. The apnea-hypopnea index (AHI) and 3% oxygen desaturation index (ODI) were analyzed manually with the QP-021W software (Nihon Kohden). On the basis of the respiratory event scoring of the American Academy of Sleep Medicine [21], apnea was defined as a reduction in amplitude of airflow by more than 90% from the pre-event baseline for no less than 10 sec. Hypopnea was defined as a reduction in amplitude of the airflow by more than 30% from the pre-event baseline for no less than 10 sec, in association with a drop of 3% or more in oxygen saturation. The AHI was calculated as the total number of apnea events per hour (apnea index; AI) plus hypopnea events per hour (hypopnea index; HI) in nocturnal recording periods. The 3% ODI was defined as the total number of 3% desaturations of oxyhemoglobin divided by the total number of nocturnal recording hours; it was represented as the number of events per hour. Snores were analyzed automatically by using the QP-021W software. The snore index was calculated as the number of snores per hour during nocturnal recording periods.

Results

The s-NAS is specifically designed as a nasopharyngeal stent that maintains the patency of the nasal airway through to the nasopharynx and retropalatal oropharynx during sleep (Figure 1). Although nasopharyngeal appliances are currently available, unlike those appliances, the s-NAS is constructed of resilient silicone rubber that enables the upper airway to maintain the patency. The silicone-made shaft of the device is designed to have a resistant to collapse by a pressure of the maximum speed of inspiration under normal breathing conditions. Furthermore, as compared with many of conventional nasopharyngeal appliances, another important feature of the s-NAS is a readymade device that patients readily insert it into the nasal cavity by themselves, leading to the better compliance for patients with OSA and subjects with snoring than currently available nasopharyngeal appliances.

Six male subjects with varying severities of OSA were enrolled in the study. To assess the therapeutic effects of the s-NAS on mild ($5 \leq AHI < 15$), moderate ($15 \leq AHI < 30$), and severe ($30 \leq AHI$) OSA, and on snoring, we evaluated AHI, 3% ODI, the lowest SpO_2, and the snore index before and during treatment with the s-NAS by portable monitoring (Table 1).

Subject		Length of s-NAS (mm)	Sex	Age	BMI (kg/m2)	AHI (/hr)	3% ODI	Lowest SpO2	Snore index
A	Pretreatment		Male	39	24.7	12.7	10.6	88	0.7
	Treatment	135				4.6	5.0	93	0.4
B	Pretreatment		Male	37	25.9	13.1	11.0	73	9.8
	Treatment	130				12.0	11.5	79	0.3
C	Pretreatment		Male	34	26.9	18.5	17.0	85	104.7
	Treatment	130				9.0	9.0	89	24.7
D	Pretreatment		Male	39	24.1	19.8	16.3	82	25.5
	Treatment	130				7.4	6.9	92	5.8
E	Pretreatment		Male	45	29.6	22.4	21.8	70	129.4
	Treatment	130				10.1	10.5	79	93.3
F	Pretreatment		Male	59	28.4	30.4	30.4	77	368.2
	Treatment	130				19.1	17.1	88	18.4

Table 1: Summary of subjects enrolled in the study. (Age, BMI, AHI, 3% ODI, lowest SpO_2, and snore index before and during treatment with the single nasal airway stent (s-NAS) were recorded overnight by portable monitoring with an SAS-2100 monitor and were analyzed with QP-021W software. Respiratory events in subjects using the s-NAS were recorded no more than 1 month after the first recording without the s-NAS).

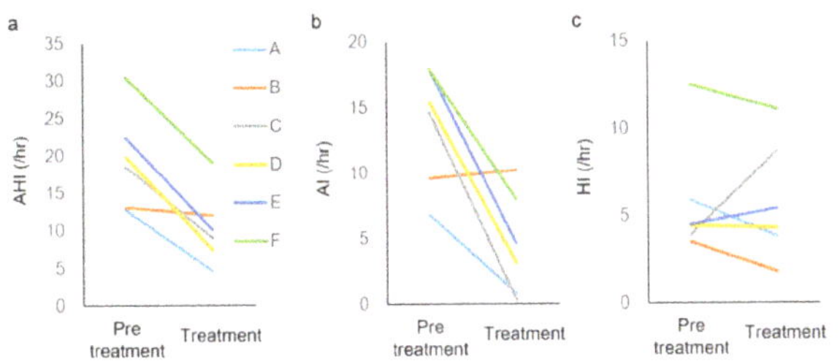

Figure 2: Therapeutic effect of the single nasal airway stent (s-NAS) on apnea-hypopnea index, (AHI), apnea index (AI), and hypopnea index (HI). (a) AHI, (b) AI, and (c) HI before treatment and during treatment with the s-NAS are shown. Subjects A and B had mild OSA, subjects C, D, and E had moderate OSA, and subject F had severe OSA (Table 1).

All subjects tolerated the use of the s-NAS, and compliance of all subjects with the device for a month was confirmed. Treatment with the s-NAS obviously ameliorated mild and moderate OSA, as confirmed by the decrease in 3% ODI, AHI, and AI and the improvement in the lowest SpO_2 (Table 1, Figure 2a and 2b); the device had limited therapeutic impact on HI (Figure 2c). However, the s-NAS had no effect on hypoxic events in one subject with tonsillar hypertrophy (subject B), even though this subject had only mild OSA.

The therapeutic impact of the s-NAS was also limited in subjects with severe OSA, although there was some improvement in their apneic events. Remarkably, s-NAS treatment had a marked therapeutic impact on snoring in all subjects, regardless of the severity of OSA (Table 1). Throughout the clinical trial, no adverse effects, such as nosebleed, pain, discomfort, infection, or allergic responses, were reported following insertion of the s-NAS.

Discussion

In this pilot study we examined the effectiveness of the s-NAS for treating OSA, as determined by the AHI and oxygen desaturation, as well as snoring. We verified the therapeutic efficacy of the device in mild to moderate OSA and in snoring, with good compliance for a month. The s-NAS could be useful as not only a ready-made tool for subjects with OSA or snoring, or both, when traveling, but also as an alternative for OSA patients who cannot tolerate CPAP. Unlike oral appliances the device is immediately available [16]. The s-NAS is designed to maintain airflow through the nasopharynx and retropalatal oropharynx by mechanically preventing the upper airway obstruction by the movement and vibration of soft palate during sleep, but it does not ameliorate the hypopharyngeal airway obstruction theoretically. Thus, the device has a therapeutic effect on the movement and vibration of soft palate during sleep anatomically. Although we did not classified our patients in accordance to the Fujita classification, all subjects who showed ameliorated OSA and snoring by using the s-NAS would be classified in Fujita type I [22]. As we expected, on the basis of features of the s-NAS (length, structure, and design), the device was not effective in one subject with mild OSA and tonsillar hypertrophy and it was unable to normalize the AHI in severe OSA; these findings were consistent with those in previous studies of nasal and oral appliances [12,14,17,18]. Intriguingly, the device improved the number of apnea events, rather than the number of hypopnea events, in subjects with varying degrees of severity of OSA (Figure 2). The precise mechanism by which the device was especially effective in treating apnea events remains undetermined. The s-NAS may ameliorate episodes of apnea by shifting a total obstruction to a partial obstruction, whereas hypopnea events could be curable, resulting in a decrease in the total AHI. Further randomized clinical trials with a larger number of subjects are required to precisely validate the feasibility of the s-NAS in patients with OSA.

A further structural modifications, such as the production of an expandable NAS with an attachment for expandable parts on its distal end [19], could improve the device's efficacy in treating both apnea and hypopnea events, as well as snoring. The NAS should be beneficial as a tool for OSA therapy in combination with CPAP, oral appliances, surgical approaches, or weight loss programs.

Acknowledgments

We thank Dr. Tsukasa Nabekura (University of California, San Francisco, U.S.A.) for critical comments on the manuscript. We also thank the staff of the Division of Sleep Medicine at the Tsukuba University Hospital for their technical help. This research was supported by grants from the Ministry of Health, Labour and Welfare of Japan.

Conflict of Interest

Seven Dreamers Laboratories, Inc. was not involved in any part of the study apart from the manufacture and provision of the s-NAS.

References

1. Young T, Palta M, Dempsey J, Skatrud J, Weber S, et al. (1993) The Occurrence of Sleep-Disordered Breathing Among Middle-Aged Adults. N Engl J Med 328: 1230-1235.
2. Strollo PJ Jr, Rogers RM (1996) Obstructive sleep apnea. N Engl J Med 334: 99-104.
3. Peppard PE, Young T, Palta M, Skatrud J (2000) Prospective study of the association between sleep-disordered breathing and hypertension. N Engl J Med 342: 1378-1384.
4. Somers VK, White DP, Amin R, Abraham WT, Costa F, et al. (2008) Sleep Apnea And Cardiovascular Disease: An American Heart Association/American College of Cardiology Foundation Scientific Statement from the American Heart Association Council for High Blood Pressure Research Professional Education Committee, Council on Clinical Cardiology, Stroke Council, and Council on Cardiovascular Nursing. J Am Coll Cardiol 52: 686-717.
5. Somers VK, White DP, Amin R, Abraham WT, Costa F, et al (2008) Sleep apnea and cardiovascular disease: an American Heart Association/american College Of Cardiology Foundation Scientific Statement from the American Heart Association Council for High Blood Pressure Research Professional Education Committee, Council on Clinical Cardiology, Stroke Council, and Council On Cardiovascular Nursing. In collaboration with the National Heart, Lung, and Blood Institute National Center on Sleep Disorders Research (National Institutes of Health). Circulation 118: 1080-1111.
6. Vgontzas AN, Papanicolaou DA, Bixler EO, Hopper K, Lotsikas A, et al. (2000) Sleep apnea and daytime sleepiness and fatigue: relation to visceral obesity, insulin resistance, and hypercytokinemia. J Clin Endocrinol Metab 85: 1151-1158.
7. Liistro G, Aubert G, Rodenstein DO (1995) Management of sleep apnoea syndrome. Eur Respir J 8: 1751-1755.
8. Sullivan CE, Issa FG, Berthon-Jones M, Eves L (1981) Reversal of obstructive sleep apnoea by continuous positive airway pressure applied through the nares. Lancet 1: 862-865.
9. McDaid C, Durée KH, Griffin SC, Weatherly HL, Stradling JR, et al. (2009) A systematic review of continuous positive airway pressure for obstructive sleep apnoea-hypopnoea syndrome. Sleep Med Rev 13: 427-436.
10. Kohler M, Smith D, Tippett V, Stradling JR (2010) Predictors of long-term compliance with continuous positive airway pressure. Thorax 65: 829-832.
11. Weaver TE, Grunstein RR (2008) Adherence to continuous positive airway pressure therapy: the challenge to effective treatment. Proc Am Thorac Soc 5: 173-178.
12. Nahmias JS, Karetzky MS (1988) Treatment of the obstructive sleep apnea syndrome using a nasopharyngeal tube. Chest 94: 1142-1147.
13. Colrain IM, Brooks S, Black J (2008) A pilot evaluation of a nasal expiratory resistance device for the treatment of obstructive sleep apnea. J Clin Sleep Med 4: 426-433.
14. Rossi VA, Winter B, Rahman NM, Yu LM, Fallon J, et al. (2013) The effects of Provent on moderate to severe obstructive sleep apnoea during continuous positive airway pressure therapy withdrawal: a randomised controlled trial. Thorax 68: 854-859.
15. Tsuiki S, Isono S, Minamino O, Maeda K, Kobayashi M, et al. (2012) Tongue position controller as an alternative treatment for obstructive sleep apnea. Sleep Breath 16: 957-960.
16. Lazard DS, Blumen M, Lévy P, Chauvin P, Fragny D, et al. (2009) The tongue-retaining device: efficacy and side effects in obstructive sleep apnea syndrome. J Clin Sleep Med 5: 431-438.
17. Barthlen GM, Brown LK, Wiland MR, Sadeh JS, Patwari J, et al. (2000) Comparison of three oral appliances for treatment of severe obstructive sleep apnea syndrome. Sleep Med 1: 299-305.
18. Kumar AR, Guilleminault C, Certal V, Li D, Capasso R, et al. (2015) Nasopharyngeal airway stenting devices for obstructive sleep apnoea: a systematic review and meta-analysis. J Laryngol Otol 129: 2-10.
19. Satoh M (2012) Effect Of Nasal Airway Stent (NAS) On Obstructive Sleep Apnea. Proceedings of the American Thoracic Society International Conference published in American Journal of Respiratory and Critical Care Medicine.
20. Chesson AL Jr, Berry RB, Pack A; American Academy of Sleep Medicine; American Thoracic Society, et al. (2003) Practice parameters for the use of portable monitoring devices in the investigation of suspected obstructive sleep apnea in adults. Sleep 26: 907-913.
21. Berry RB, Brooks R, Gamaldo CE, Harding SM, Lloyd RM, Marcus CL and Vaughn BV for the American Academy of Sleep Medicine (2013) The AASM Manual for the Scoring of Sleep and Associated Events: Rules, Terminology and Technical Specifications, Version 2.0.2. www.aasmnet.org, American Academy of Sleep Medicine, Darien, Illinois.
22. Fairbanks DN, Fujita S, Ikematsu T (1987) Snoring and Obstructive Sleep Apnea. Raven Press, New York, New York.

16

Pilot Study of Oral Negative Pressure Therapy for Obstructive Sleep Apnea-Hypopnea Syndrome

Yuji Yamaguchi* and Masako Kato

Sleep Disorders Center at Fukuoka, Fukuoka Urasoe Clinic, Japan

***Corresponding author:** Yuji Yamaguchi, Sleep Disorders Center at Fukuoka, Fukuoka Urasoe Clinic, 2-12-19-9F Ropponmatsu, Chuo-ku, Fukuoka-8100044, Japan, E-mail: yuujiya1124@kde.biglobe.ne.jp; yuujiya@poppy.ocn.ne.jp

Abstract

Background: Although the continuous positive airway pressure is the gold standard therapy for patients with moderate to severe obstructive sleep apnea-hypopnea syndrome (OSAHS), there are several treatment options such as mandibular advancement devices, tongue-retaining devices, and nasal airway stent devices. Recently, newly developed intraoral pressure gradient therapy system, iNAP® Sleep Therapy System, was introduced as an alternative treatment for OSAHS patients.

Purpose: This feasibility study explored the effectiveness of the iNAP® device for patients with mild to moderate OSAHS.

Materials and Methods: The iNAP® device consisted of an oral interface, a tube set with a saliva container, and a negative pressure console. Negative pressure is introduced directly from the oral interface and the pressure pulls the tongue anteriorly, resulting in improving the obstruction or narrowing of the upper airway. A total of 5 male and 4 female patients with mild to moderate OSAHS, aged between 32 and 62, with 50.6 years+11.7 years were recruited in the study.

Results: The baseline apnea-hypopnea index (AHI) was 17.2 events per hour+4.7 events per hour, while AHI with the iNAP® device was 12.7+5.4 ($p<0.01$). Regarding the sleep architecture, a significant reduction in wakefulness after sleep onset (WASO) on the initial night of treatment from 97 min+50.0 min to 70.7 min+36.9 min ($p<0.05$) was observed; however, other sleep parameters was not.

Conclusion: This study demonstrated that negative pressure therapy with the iNAP® device improved the apnea severity in patients with mild to moderate OSAHS, the degree of whose amelioration of AHI was marginal but significant. Although the number of patients recruited was small, this study is the first report on the effectiveness of the intraoral pressure gradient therapy.

Keywords: Obstructive sleep apnea-hypopnea syndrome; Intraoral pressure gradient therapy; iNAP® Sleep Therapy System

Introduction

Obstructive sleep apnea-hypopnea syndrome (OSAHS) is a common condition characterized by repetitive obstruction of the upper airway resulting in daytime sleepiness due to sleep fragmentation caused by an airway obstruction. There are several papers on the prevalence of OSAHS showing that 7% to 26% of men and 2% to 13% of women have an apnea-hypopnea index (AHI) of more than 15 events per hour [1-5].

In Japan, the prevalence of OSAHS in the male working population has increased over the past decade, being estimated at 22.3% in patients with moderate to severe sleep-disordered breathing (SDB) [6]. It is significantly correlated with cardiovascular morbidity and mortality [7-8]. For patients with moderate to severe OSAHS, standard treatment is the continuous positive airway pressure (CPAP) ventilation. Compliance with and tolerance of CPAP are not always favourable, whose adherence rate is low, being 40% to 83% [9-10].

In Japan, CPAP treatment is not covered by health insurance for OSAHS patients with AHI of less than 20 events per hour. Consequently, one of the oral appliances (OA), prosthetic mandibular advancement (PMA), is a solid alternative to manage patients with mild to moderate OSAHS.

PMA causes protrusion of the mandible and tongue and enlarges and stabilizes the upper airway during sleep. Although the PMA has been shown to be effective for patients with mild to moderate OSAHS, adherence is poor [11,12]. Studies on PMA treatment have indicated that about 75% of patients remained adherent after 12 months of treatment, which may decrease to 50% after 5 years. In the PMA treatment, there are several side effects including tooth pain, pain of the temporomandibular joint (TMJ), gum disease, and dry mouth. Therefore, PMA treatments are not indicated for use in all patients who prefer PMA to CPAP, who do not respond to CPAP, or who show failed treatment attempts with CPAP. It is consequently important to develop other treatment options besides PMA for sleep apnea.

A newly developed intraoral pressure gradient therapy system (IPGT), the iNAP® Sleep Therapy System (Somnics Inc., Hsinchu, Taiwan), was introduced as an alternative treatment for OSAHS [13].

The feasibility study explored the abilities and safety of the new device, the iNAP®Sleep Therapy System, for patients with OSAHS in our clinical sleep laboratory using full-night polysomnography.

Materials and Methods

Participants

A total of 5 males and 4 females' patients with mild to moderate OSAHS aged between 32 and 62 years visiting the Fukuoka Urasoe Clinic were recruited. The chief complaint of each patient was daytime sleepiness, witnessed apnea, and/or loud snoring.

All the patients were required to undergo diagnostic polysomnography (PSG). Patients with no history of cardiovascular diseases, cerebrovascular diseases, or diabetes mellitus (DM) were enrolled in this study.

This study was approved by the Institutional Ethics Committee at the Nakamura Clinic, Urasoe, and Okinawa, Japan. Informed consent was obtained from all patients before enrollment in this study, which was performed in accordance with the Helsinki Declaration.

Protocol design and device description

This study was a single-center, non-controlled, non-randomized, proof-of-concept, single-treated night study in which subjects underwent a non-treatment PSG followed by a second PSG with the iNAP® Lite Sleep Therapy System.

The device, the intraoral pressure gradient therapy system, consisted of an oral interface, a tube set with a saliva container and a negative pressure console (Figure 1A).

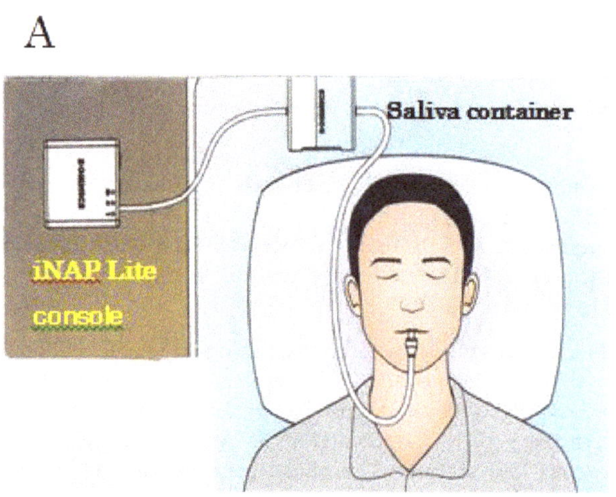

Figure 1A: The intraoral pressure gradient therapy system, iNAP® Lite, consists of a console containing a pump, a saliva container, and oral interface connected with a flexible tube.

Negative pressure is introduced from the oral interface and the pressure pulls the tongue, soft palate, and uvula formed in order to keep the oropharynx stable during sleep (Figure 1B). The device detects the air pressure within the oral cavity and automatically adjusts the pressure gradient applied to the airway as needed.

The system in a console provides the negative pressure with 2 AA-sized batteries, which have a running life of approximately 7 days.

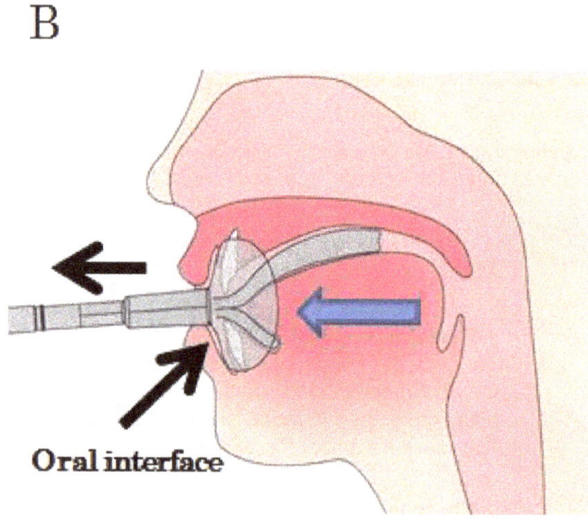

Figure 1B: With the oral interface in place, the lip shield is located between the teeth and lips, and keeps the mouth closed. A gentle oral vacuum produces a pressure gradient intended to pull the soft palate forward, resulting in opening the airway during sleep. (From the instruction book of iNAP® Lite with permission from Mr. Chung-Chu Chen, CEO, Somnics Inc.)

Polysomnography

As shown in our previous study, standard overnight PSG included continuous monitoring with a central electroencephalogram (EEG), electrooculogram (EOG), submental and anterior tibial electromyogram (EMG), and electrocardiogram (ECG) using conventional leads. Airflow was monitored with oral and nasal thermistors, and respiratory effort by respiratory inductance plethysmography with transducers placed around the chest and abdomen. Oxyhemoglobin saturation was continuously recorded with a pulse oximeter (3900P, Datex-Ohmeda Co., Louisville, CO, USA). All variables were continuously recorded using REMbrandt™ version 8.0 (Embla, Broomfield, CO, USA) and RemLogic™ version 3.2 (Embla, Thornton, CO, USA). All recordings were scored directly on the screen by polysomnographers certified by the Japanese Society of Sleep Research using the 2014 guidelines from the American Academy of Sleep Medicine (AASM) [13]. Apneas were defined as >90% reduction in tidal volume lasting >10 seconds. Hypopneas were defined as >30% reduction of the pre-event baseline using nasal pressure lasting >10 seconds with a >3% oxygen desaturation from the pre-event baseline or an event associated with an arousal.

Statistical analysis

All subjects who had an AHI greater than 5 events per hour during the baseline night were included in the data analysis. A paired t-test was used to test the change from the baseline to treatment within each patient. Statistical analyses were performed using StatMate ver. 5.01 (Atoms, Tokyo).

Results

Patient characteristics

Five men and four women were included in the study, whose ages ranged from 32 years to 62 years with a mean+standard deviation (SD) of 50.6 years+11.7 years. The body mass index (BMI) ranged from 21.3 kg/m^2 to 31.8 kg/m^2 with a mean+SD of 24.6 kg/m^2 ± 3.4 kg/m^2. No patients enrolled in the study were refused, and all subjects tolerated the use of the iNAP® device.

The effectiveness of iNAP® therapy

The baseline AHI was 17.2 events per hour+4.7 events per hour (mean+SD), while AHI with the iNAP® device was 12.7+5.4 ($p<0.01$) (Figure 2).

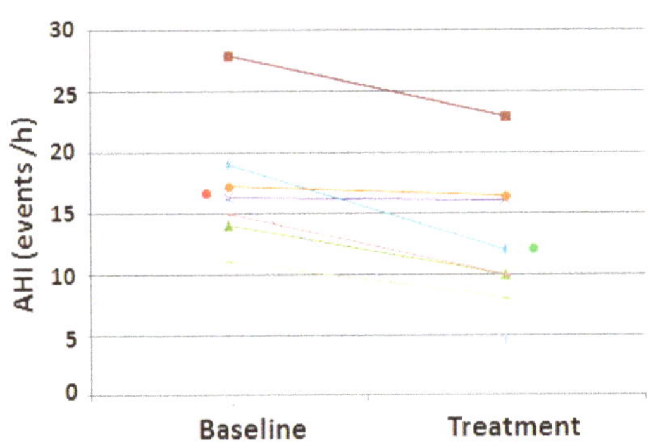

Figure 2: Individual effects of intraoral pressure gradient therapy on the apnea-hypopnea severity in the obstructive sleep apnea-hypopnea syndrome (OSAHS) patients. The apnea-hypopnea index (AHI) at baseline and on the first treatment night of iNAP® therapy in 9 patients with mild to moderate OSAHS with PSG is presented.

Regarding sleep architecture, a significant reduction in wakefulness after sleep onset (WASO) on the initial night of treatment from 97.0 min+50.0 min to 70.7+36.9 min ($p<0.05$) was observed. However, other sleep parameters including sleep efficiency, stage N1, arousal index, and desaturation was not (data not shown). There were no serious adverse events in the 9 subjects who used the device during PSG.

Discussion

Our study confirmed that intraoral pressure gradient therapy (IPGT) study is well tolerated by OSAHS patients. In addition, the results of the present study show the improvement of apnea severity and WASO in patients with mild to moderate OSAHS. However, the improvement of AHI in patients with AHI of less than 30 events per hour was only 26%, with a decrease from the baseline AHI of 17.2 to treatment AHI of 12.7, which was marginal but significant.

In our data, the improvement rate of AHI in patients between those younger than 50 years and older than 50 years was 40 and 17.6%, respectively. Although the number of patients analysed in our study was small, the IPGT might appear to be more effective in younger rather than elderly patients.

In this study, the subset of OSAHS patients who were strong responders to the IPGT could not be clarified. However, in those who showed a clinically significant effect, the benefits were observed on the first night of treatment. In the future, more studies should be conducted to further define patients who can be managed successfully. How to select appropriate patients for IPGT has been an on-going clinical challenge.

As the present study was a clinical feasibility research, there are important limitations that should be recognized for evaluating this study and in planning future studies. With data from only a single night of treatment for each patient, the durability of the treatment effect cannot be evaluated and a study of long-term treatment is needed. Whether or not long-treatment with IPGT leads to the reduction of daytime sleepiness should be investigated,

It is difficult to establish a treatment control (sham oral device) because subjects are aware of the sensation of oral negative pressure produced by the iNAP® device. In addition, each patient feels differently with the oral interface. Accordingly, one of the reasons why responses to IPGT in patients are different might be due to the unfavourable positioning of the mouthpiece in the oral cavity relative to the tongue. Optimizing the oral interface shape, size, and applied negative pressure might increase comfort. It is important to further define what subset of OSAHS patients are most indicative for the negative pressure therapy.

In this study, the first PSG was carried out in order to study the AHI severity at the baseline, and the second PSG was performed to evaluate it on treatment. In consequence, concern about a potential "first-night effect" might be raised regarding the effectiveness for apnea severity. Based on the fact that several studies have uniformly reported no first-night effect on respiratory parameters [14-16], it has been considered that the improvement of apnea severity with the iNAP® device is not likely to be due to the first-night effect. However, the amelioration of WASO with the iNAP® device might be due to the first-night effect.

The main limitation factors of this study were the small number of patients recruited. The study was not supported by any corporate sponsors and a large number of patients with OSAHS could not be enrolled because of economic limitations in our clinic. However, the data from this study are the first report showing the role of iNAP® device to treat patients with mild to moderate OSAHS.

Another device that reduces airway obstruction and airflow during sleep by moving the soft palate anteriorly with negative pressure produced by the pump in the console via a mouthpiece, oral pressure therapy (OPT) (ApniCare, Inc., Redwood City, CA, USA) was recently developed [17]. There are several advantages of negative pressure therapy using iNAP® compared with OPT. iNAP® can still be used for edentulous patients or those with poor dentition. In addition, iNAP® is light, small, and compact, and can work with 2 AA batteries for 7 days. Therefore, this device is very travel-friendly, and can be used on a long-distance airplane or coach travel.

In conclusion, this study demonstrated that the negative pressure therapy using the iNAP® Sleep Therapy System improved the apnea severity in patients with mild to moderate OSAHS, whose degree of amelioration of apnea severity was marginal but significant. In the study, although the number of patients recruited was small, this paper is the first to report on the effectiveness and safety of IPGT. Future studies should be carried out with more patients with mild to severe OSAHS, and the daytime sleepiness or quality of life should be evaluated by long-term treatment with the device.

Acknowledgment

We would like to express our deepest thanks to the excellent sleep technologists in our clinic for their technical assistance.

Conflict of Interest

Somnic Inc. was not involved in any part of the study. We declare conflict of interest related to this study.

References

1. Young T, Palta M, Dempsey J, Skatrud J, Weber S, et al. (1993) The occurrence of sleep-disordered breathing among middle-aged adults. New Engl J Med 328: 1230-1235.
2. Redline S, Kump K, Tishler PV, Browner I, Ferrette V (1994) Gender differences in sleep disordered breathing in a community-based sample. Amer J Respir Crit Care Med 149: 722-726.
3. Bixler EO, Vgontzas AN, Ten Have T, Tyson K, Kales A (1998) Effects of age on sleep apnea in men. I. Prevalence and severity. Amer J Respir Crit Care Med 157: 144-148.
4. Duran J, Esnaoda S, Rubio R, Iztueta A (2001) Obstructive sleep apnea-hypopnea and related clinical features in a population-based sample of subjects aged 30 to 70 yr. Amer J Respir Crit Care Med 163: 685-689.
5. Peppard PE, Young T, Barnet JH, Palta M, Hagen EW, et al. (2013) Increased prevalence of sleep-disordered breathing in adults. Amer J Epidemiology 177: 1006-1014.
6. Nakayama-Ashida Y, Takegami M, Chin K, Sumi K, Nakamura T, et al. (2008) Sleep-disordered breathing in the usual lifestyle setting as detected with home monitoring in a population of working men in Japan. Sleep 31: 419-425.
7. Young T, Finn L, Peppard PE, Szkio-Coxe M, Austin D, et al. (2008) Sleep disordered breathing and mortality. eighteen-year follow-up of the Wisconsin sleep cohort. Sleep 31: 1071-1078.
8. Levy P, Pepin JL, Arnaud C, Baguet JP, Dematteis M, et al. (2009) Obstructive sleep apnea and atherosclerosis. Prog Cardiovas Dis 51: 400-410.
9. Powell ED, Gay PC, Ojile JM, Litinski M, Malhotra A (2010) A pilot study assessing adherence to auto-bilevel following a poor initial encounter with CPAP. J Clin Sleep Med 8: 43-47.
10. Aloia MS, Stanchina M, Arnedt JT, Malhotra A, Millman RP (2005) Treatment adherence and outcomes in flexible vs. standard continuous positive pressure therapy. Chest 127: 2085-2093.
11. Marlund M, Stenlund H, Franklin KA (2004) Mandibular advancement devices in 630 men and women with obstructive sleep apnea and snoring: Tolerability and predictors of treatment success. Chest 125: 1270-1278.
12. Attali V, Chaumereuil C, Arnulf I, Golmard J, Tordjman F, et al. (2016) Predictors of long-term effectiveness to mandibular repositioning device treatment in obstructive sleep apnea patients after 1000 days. Sleep Med 27-28: 107-114.
13. Berry RB, Brooks R, Gamaldo CE, Harding SM, Lloyd RM, et al. (2014) The AASM manual for the scoring of sleep and associated events: Rules, terminology, and technical specifications, version 2.1. AASM.
14. Hutchison KN, Song Y, Wang L, Mallow BA (2008) Analysis of sleep parameters in patients with obstructive sleep apnea studied in a hospital vs. a hotel-based sleep center. J Clin Sleep Med 4: 119-122.
15. Selwa LM, Marzec ML, Chervin RD, Weatherwax KJ, Vaughn BV (2008) Sleep staging and respiratory events in refractory epilepsy patients: Is there a first night effect? Epilepsia 49: 2063-2068.
16. Gouveris H, Selivanova O, Bausmer U, Goepel B, Mann W (2010) First-night effect on polysomnographic respiratory sleep parameters in patients with sleep-disordered breathing and upper airway pathology. Eur Arch Otorhinolaryngol 267: 1449-1453.
17. Farid-Moayer M, Siegel LC, Black J (2013) Oral pressure therapy for treatment of obstructive sleep apnea: Clinical feasibility Nat Sci Sleep 5: 53-59.

Prenatal Stress and Sleep Quality Influence on Antenatal Women Psychological Capital in Mother/Child Hospital in Akure, Ondo State

Ajele Kenni Wojujutari*, Oladejo Teslim Alabi and Olasupo Matthew

Department of Psychology, Obafemi Awolowo University, Ile-Ife, Osun State, Nigeria

***Corresponding author:** Ajele Kenni Wojujutari, Department of Psychology, Obafemi Awolowo University, Ile-Ife, Osun State, Nigeria, E-mail: kennyajele@yahoo.com

Abstract

The study examined the influence of prenatal stress and sleep quality on pregnant women psychological capital before birth. A cross-sectional survey was used in the study. Convenience sampling technique was used to select 238 antenatal women attending Mother/Child clinic in Ondo State. The result showed significant relationship between prenatal stress and psychological capital among antenatal women. Also sleep quality had a significant influence on psychological capital among antenatal women. It was concluded that inadequate sleep and prenatal stress affect psychological capital. Based on the study findings, it was recommended that health practitioners and maternal health policy makers and nongovernmental agencies should provide adequate prenatal stress management training for antenatal women and maternal health care providers should also provide important information about good sleep quality in relations to their conditions to enhance their psychological capital.

Keywords: Psychological capital; Prenatal stress; Quality sleep

Introduction

Antenatal women positive psychological resources of hope, efficacy, resilience, and optimism could be affected by prenatal stress and inadequate sleep quality. Antenatal period is a supportive stage whereby pregnant women receiving instrumental, emotional, and informational supports from professionals, colleagues and family members to improve psychological capital for their safe delivery. Antenatal Women psychological capital is their positive psychological state of development that is characterized by having confidence (self-efficacy) to take on and put in the necessary effort to succeed at challenging task, making a positive attribution (optimism) about succeeding now and in the future, persevering toward goals and, when necessary, redirecting paths to goals (hope) in order to succeed, and when beset by problems and adversity, sustaining and bouncing back and even beyond (resilience) to attain success in delivery [1].

Pregnancy is unavoidable for women and associated with physiological, psychological and social challenges that could affect their psychological capital [2]. The main reason to provide antenatal care for pregnant women is to manage the intensive effect of prenatal stress on their psychological resources such as hope, efficacy, resilience, and optimism for safe delivery. Prenatal stress can change the metabolic environment of the fetus and accounts for some of these early programming effects on brain development of the conceived the child. Prenatal stress can associated with premature delivery, reduced birth weight and smaller head circumference in humans.

Studies show that unmanaged prenatal stress that leads to miscarriages, and child lost during birth can be associated with later neurodevelopmental affective disorders that may affect the psychological resources such as hope, efficacy, resilience, and optimism. Such disorders include attention and temperament disorders, schizophrenia, autism, and anxiety disorders [3,4]. In addition, elevated prenatal cortisol is associated with aborted fetuses, hyperactive fetuses, delayed fetal growth and development, premature birth, low birth weight, and chronic adult illnesses [5]. Prenatal administration of exogenous, synthetic GCs such as dexamethasone has been linked to a higher prevalence of infection, most likely due to the immunosuppressive role of GCs [6].

Rodent studies of prenatal stress revealed various stressors that associated pregnant barriers. Kofman, study shows that severe stressors include restraint stress, cold exposure, and electric shock will associate with complications during child delivery. Wilson, Koenig et al. studies show that offspring's whose mothers were exposed to prenatal stress show significantly higher corticosterone levels than undressed after mothers were exposed to an intense acute stressor. However, most of those emerging evidence that indicated prenatal stress has negative effect on pregnant women psychological capital are conducted on animals [7,8].

Sleep is an inevitable daily activity that cans affact physiological, psychological and social well-being individuals if not properly observed. Therefore, sleep quality can affect the psychological capital of antenatal woman which is their ability develop positive psychological state. Actual definition of sleep is the state of the organism, in which its environmental interaction is reversible, partially and periodically lost and can be revoked by various external stimuli. Sleep quality is an essential factor for health and well-being. Good sleep quality buffered better health, less daytime sleepiness, greater well-being and better psychological functioning. Poor sleep quality is one of the defining features of chronic insomnia. WHO described the consequences of inadequate sleep quality into three categories such as physical effects (sleepiness, fatigue, hypertension), cognitive impairment (deterioration of performance, attention and motivation), and diminishment of mental (concentration and intellectual capacity and increase of the likelihood of accidents at work and during stimuli and mental health complications) [9-14].

Emerging evidence indicates that inadequate sleep quality is the major problems experiencing by pregnant women which some time affect their psychological capital. Also numbers of empirical evidence revealed those inadequate sleep quality factors that affect pregnant women psychological capital such as sleep loss such as short sleep duration poor sleep quality [15-20].

Objective of the Study

The main of objectivity of study was to assess pregnant women psychological capital before birth. These specific objectives are to examine the influence of prenatal stress on antenatal women psychological capital; and investigate the influence of Sleep quality has no antenatal women psychological capital.

Method

Research design

A cross-sectional survey design was used to examine the influence of prenatal stress, sleep quality on antenatal women psychological.

Participants

The study population consisted of pregnant women attending antenatal clinic at Akure, mother/child clinic hospital in Akure, Ondo State. The study used convenient sampling technique; where by available potential respondents were approached individually on their antenatal clinic days to select 238 participants.

Research instruments

Psychological Capital Questionnaire (PCQ): Psychological Capital Questionnaire was developed by the Luthans, Avolio, Avey & Norman. PCQ consists of 24 items. The PCQ comprises four subscales with equal weight: (1) hope, (2) optimism, (3) self-efficacy and (4) resilience. Each of these subscales consists of six items with response options on a six-point Likert scale ranging from 1 ('strongly disagree') to 6 ('strongly agree'). Good internal consistency for the respective subscales (hope: 0.72, 0.75, 0.80, 0.76; optimism: 0.74, 0.69, 0.76, 0.79; self-effcacy: 0.75, 0.84, 0.85, 0.75; and resilience: 0.71, 0.71, 0.66, 0.72) on the four samples utilised in the Luthans, Avolio, Avey, & Norman study were reported. Also Görgens-Ekermans & Herbert reported reliability Cornbrash's alpha coefficients 0.70 on optimism, self-efficacy and resilience.

The A–Z Stress Scale: A to Z stress scale developed by Kazi. The A–Z Stress Scale consists of 30 items which measure pregnancy related stress. The A–Z Stress Scale containing three subscales measuring family-related concerns (husband, children, in-laws and parents), socioeconomic concerns and pregnancy-related concerns. The A–Z Stress Scale using Thurstone scaling, items were ranked 0–10 scale of severity (0 as "no stress" and 10 as "maximum stress"). The reliability of scale is 0.91 (inter rater) and validity of the scale used in Cronbach method is 0.82 reported by Kazi.

Pittsburgh Sleep Quality Index: The Pittsburgh Sleep Quality Index (PSQI) was used to assess the antenatal women sleep quality. The PSQI is based on eighteen self-reported questions; measuring the components of: (1 subjective sleep quality), (2 sleep latency), (3 sleep duration), (4 habitual sleep efficiency), (5 sleep disturbances), (6 use of sleeping medication), and (7 daytime dysfunction). Based on the responses to the questions, each sub-score will be calculated on a scale of 0 to 3, with a score of 0 indicating no presence of the habit and 3 indicating a high presence of the habit. All sub-scores are totaled forming a global score, which ranges from 0-21. A cutoff score of 5 or above is indicative of a sleep disturbance. The PSQI has been shown to be reliable (Interclass correlation (r)=0.87) between test and re-test sessions.

Procedure: Ethical was sought and obtained from research committee of Mother/Child clinic Akure, Ondo State. The questionnaires were administered individually to the respondents by the researcher on their antenatal clinic days (Thursdays and Fridays) within the hospital premises. All respondents were been instructed to fill the questionnaire privately, and to submit to the researcher the same day. This is to guarantee the respondents confidentially and privacy.

Analysis of data: Data collected were analyzed using regression and One-Way Analysis of Variance was used to test the hypotheses. All analyses were carried out with the programme of the Statistics Package for Social Sciences (SPSS Version 22.0) [21-23].

Results

A total of 238 participants were included in the study. The Table 1 presented that age of the respondents ranged between 29 - 46 years with the Mean and SD ($\bar{x}$=31.53; SD=6.78). Most 37.5% had tertiary educational level, 28.2% were civil servants, 45.8% of the respondents already had children between 3 to 6, and only 55.5% of the respondents were Christian.

Characteristics	Groups	Frequency	Percentages (%)	Mean(σ)
Age				31.53 (6.78)
Educational Level	Primary	34	14.3	
	Secondary	71	29.8	
	Tertiary	89	37.4	
	No formal Education	44	18.5	
Occupation	Civil Servants	67	28.2	
	Farmer	18	7.6	

	Tailor	37	15.5	
	Trader	62	26.1	
	Unemployed	22	9.2	
	Others jobs	32	13.4	
Number(s) of Children	1-3	82	34.5	
	3-6	140	58.8	
	7 and above	16	6.7	
Religion	Christianity	132	55.5	
	Islam	96	40.3	
	Traditional	10	4.2	

Table 1: Socio-demographic characteristics of the respondents (N=238).

Hypothesis 2 stated that sleep quality has no significant influence on psychological capital among Antenatal Women in Mother/Child Clinic Akure, Ondo State. This hypothesis was test with ANOVA was presented. The result showed that sleep quality has significant influence on psychological capital F (2,235) 32.040, $p<0.05$. The alternative was accepted while the Null hypothesis was rejected. Hypothesis 1 stated that there is no significant relationship between prenatal stress and psychological capital among antenatal women in mother/child clinic Akure Ondo state. This hypothesis was test with Pearson simple correlation which presented in Table 2. The result showed that there is significant relationship between prenatal stress and psychological capital $r=0.257$, $p<0.05$. The alternative was accepted while the Null hypothesis was rejected.

Variables	**M**	**SD**	**R**	**P**
Psychological Capital	35.7353	11.60393	0.257	0.002
Prenatal Stress	31.8235	9.79636		

Table 2: Pearson simple moment correlation analysis between prenatal stress and psychological capital among antenatal women in mother/child clinic Akure, Ondo State (N=238).

The Table 3 presented the Post Hoc analysis comparison of psychological capital by sleep quality groups among antenatal women. The result showed that antenatal who experience good sleep quality ($x=41.75$) where more significant than poor (Mean=29.56, Std. Error=1.69, MD=12.19, $p<0.05$) on psychological capital. The result also showed that antenatal who experience moderate sleep quality ($x=38.99$) where more significant than poor (Mean=29.56, Std. Error=1.57, MD=9.42, $p<0.05$) on psychological capital (Table 4).

Source	**df**	**SS**	**MS**	**F**	**p**
Between Groups	2	6837.385	3418.693	32.040	0.000
Within Groups	235	25074.938	106.702		
Total	237	31912.324			

Table 3: One-way analysis of variance of psychological capital by sleep quality among antenatal women in mother/child clinic Akure, Ondo State.

Group1	**Group2**	**M1**	**2**	**Std. Error**	**MD**	**p**
Good Sleep Quality	Poor Sleep Quality	41.75	29.56	1.69	12.19	0.000
Moderate Sleep Quality	Poor Sleep Quality	38.99	29.56	1.57	9.42	0.000

Table 4: Post hoc multiple comparison analysis of psychological capital sleep quality groups.

Discussion

The study examined the prenatal stress and sleep quality on psychological capital among antenatal women. The study results affiliated previous studies that showed prenatal stress is associated with later neurodevelopmental affective disorders that impair the ability to cope with stress and hope, efficacy, resilience, and optimism. Such disorders include attention and temperament disorders, schizophrenia, autism, and anxiety disorders. This result supported studies conducted on animal's prenatal stress such as rodent studies of prenatal stress expose pregnant barriers to various stressors. Mild to moderate stressors include saline injections and unpredictable noise. Severe stressors include restraint stress, cold exposure, and electric shock. Exposure to prenatal stress results in offspring that have similar baseline corticosterone levels as control rodents. Prenatal stress offspring show significantly higher corticosterone levels than unstressed control offspring after exposed to an intense acute stressor.

The result of the study confirmed recent studies individual that always had good sleep quality have less and no complications in child delivery while those also showed that worker who have always adequate sleep quality perform better than their counterparts that who experience inadequate sleep quality. Large numbers of empirical evidence revealed that inadequate sleep quality factor that affects pregnant women psychological capital such as sleep loss such as short sleep duration, poor sleep quality, poor sleep efficiency with an increase in time spent awake during the night.

Those bodies literature on the area of prenatal stress were conducted on animals and not properly linked to psychological capital of pregnant women. Also sleep quality studies were directed to job performance, work engagement, and less attention was paid to sleep quality effect pregnancy but was not adequately linked with antenatal psychological capital. Therefore, this study has played significant role by provided the insight of the existing relationship between prenatal stress and psychological capital and the influence of good sleep on psychological capital among antenatal women.

Conclusion

The study conducted the inadequately managed prenatal stress and poor sleep quality associated with antenatal women negative psychological capital and may led to complications during child delivery. Since psychological capital of pregnant women is the development of positive psychological state, experience deep happiness, resilience, hope, optimism, self-efficacy.

Recommendations

Based on the study findings, it was recommended that health practitioners and maternal health policy makers, nongovernmental agencies should provide adequate prenatal stress management training for antenatal women and maternal health care providers should also provide important information about good sleep quality in relations to their conditions to enhance their psychological capital.

References

1. Allison GH, Kathleen S, Katriina LW, Damian M, Harvinder V (2008) The subjective meaning of sleep quality: A comparison of individuals with and without insomnia. Sleep 31: 383-393.
2. Backhaus J, Junghanns K, Broocks A, Riemann D, Hohagen F (2002) Testretest reliability and validity of the Pittsburgh Sleep Quality Index in primary insomnia. J Psychosom Res 53: 737-740.
3. Buysse DJ, Reynolds CF, 3rd Monk TH, Berman SR, Kupfer DJ (1989) The Pittsburgh Sleep Quality Index: A new instrument for psychiatric practice and research. Psychiatry Res 28: 193-213.
4. Christoph A (2011) Associations of subjective sleep quality with depression score, anxiety, physical symptoms and sleep onset latency in students. Cent Eur J Public Health, 19: 115-117.
5. Edinger JD, Bonnet MH, Bootzin RR (2004) Derivation of research diagnostic criteria for insomnia: Report of an American Academy of Sleep Medicine Work Group. Sleep 27: 1567-1596.
6. Field T, Diego M, Hernandez-Reif M, Figueiredo B, Deeds O (2008) Prenatal dopamine and neonatal behaviour and biochemistry. Infant Behav Dev 31: 590-593.
7. Görgens-Ekermans G, Herbert M (2013) Psychological capital: Internal and external validity of the Psychological Capital Questonnaire (PCQ-24) on a South African sample. South Africa J Indus Psych 39: 1-12.
8. Greenwood KM, Hazendonk KM (2004) Self-reported sleep during the third trimester of pregnancy. Behavioral Sleep Medicine 2: 191-204.
9. Han KS, Kim L, Shim I (2012) Stress and sleep disorder. Exp Neurobiol 21: 141-150.
10. Hunter LP, Rychnovsky JD, Yount SM (2009) A selective review of maternal sleep characteristics in the postpartum period. J Obstet Gynecol Neonatal Nurs 38: 60-68.
11. Kazi A (2009) Development of a stress scale for pregnant women in the south Asian contact the A-Z stress scale. East Mediterr Health J 15: 350-361.
12. Kempler L, Sharpe L, Bartlett D (2012) Sleep education during pregnancy for new mothers. BMC Pregnancy Childbirth 12: 155.
13. Kızılırmak A, Timur S, Kartal B (2012) Insomnia in pregnancy and factors related to insomnia. Scient World J 32: 63-71.
14. Knowlton AR, Hua W, Latkin C (2005) Social support networks and medical service use among HIV-positive injection drug users: Implications to intervention. AIDS Care 17: 479-492.
15. Koenig LJ, Moore J (2000) Women, violence and HIV: A critical evaluation with implications for HIV services. Matern Child Health J 4: 103-109.
16. Luthans F, Youssef CM, Avolio BJ (2007) Psychological capital: Developing the human compettve edge. Oxford, UK: Oxford University Press.
17. Naud K, Ouellet A, Brown C, Pasquier JC, Moutquin JM (2010) Is sleep disturbed in pregnancy? J Obstet Gynaecol Can 32: 28-34.
18. Niederhofer H, Reiter A (2000) Maternal stress during pregnancy, its objectivation by ultrasound observation of fetal intrauterine movements and child's temperament at 6 months and 6 years of age: A pilot study. Psychological Reports 86: 526-528.
19. Palagini L, Bruno RM, Gemignani A, Baglioni C, Ghiadoni L, et al. (2013) Sleep loss and hypertension: A systematic review. Curr Pharm Des 19: 2409-2419.
20. Pien GW, Schwab RJ (2004) Sleep disorders during pregnancy. Sleep 27: 1405-1417.
21. Sevil U, Bakıcı A (2002) Identification of the physical health problems and affecting factors in pregnancy. Health Social J 12: 56-62.
22. WHO (2004) WHO technical meeting on sleep and health.
23. Wilson CA, Vazdarjanova A, Terry AV Jr (2013) Exposure to variable prenatal stress in rats: Effects on anxiety-related behaviors, innate and contextual fear, and fear extinction. Behav Brain Res 238: 279-288.

Quality of Life and Affective Health of Patients with Vitiligo

Nermin Almomani[1], **Imad Abdulmajeed**[2*], **Saeed Ur Rahman**[3] **and Amal Alakkam**[1]

[1]*Family Medicine Consultant, NGHA-Riyadh, Saudi Arabia*

[2]*Public Health Specialist, NGHA-Riyadh, Saudi Arabia*

[3]*Community Medicine Dept. DED, NGHA-Riyadh, Saudi Arabia*

[*]**Corresponding author:** Imad Abdulmajeed, Khashmalaan Road, P.O.Box 22490, NGHA, KAMC-Riyadh, Family Medicine Dept. Admin Building, Mail code -2330, Central Region, Riyadh-11426, Saudi Arabia, E-mail: dr.imadyaseen@gmail.com

Abstract

Background: Vitiligo is a common hypopigmentary skin disease that can affect the quality of life and has an impact on the psychological health of the patient. Unfortunately these aspects are usually missed in the care process and underestimated in the assessment and management of vitiligo patients.

Aim of the Study: To determine the quality of life and assess the psychological impact of Vitiligo among Saudi patients, to understand the variables which may influence their psychological wellbeing and to assess the association between the quality of life and psychological morbidity.

Methods: Using cross sectional design, 234 adult patients were recruited from different hospitals in Saudi Arabia between October 2010 and February 2011. Quality of life and psychological health were assessed by Dermatological Quality of life Index and Hospital Anxiety and Depression scale respectively, which are well known, widely accepted questionnaires.

Results: Quality of life was more affected in females, age group (21 -30) years, low income patients and patients with generalized vitiligo. Anxiety was noticed more in females and in patients with jobs which required dealing with people on daily basis. Depression was higher in less educated and low income patients. DQLI score positively correlated with the HAD scale.

Conclusion: Vitiligo has a large impact on quality of life and mental health. Psychosocial history should be assessed and considered in any patient with Vitiligo.

Keywords: Quality of life; Depression; Anxiety; Primary health Care

Introduction

Our skin influences our appearance, and plays a major role in our social interactions [1]. Disfiguring of the skin due to any reason could be a potential source of emotional distress and mental illness [2]. It is a chronic, progressive hypopigmentary skin disorder. Many theories have been proposed for causality implicating immune, genetic, and environmental factors but none of them proven [3].

Vitiligo does not result in a direct physical impairment but it can influence the patient's quality of life and psychological wellbeing [4].

Vitiligo patients suffer from poor body images, low self-esteem and sever social impairment [5], especially if the lesion is found in exposed areas such as face, hands or feet [3]. Due to its chronic nature, unpredictable course of remissions and relapses, long term treatment, and no curable therapy, its often affects the patient's quality of life in different aspects of social activities, work, study and marriage [5]. In addition, it has an impact on patients' feelings including embarrassment, shame, anxiety, depression and feeling of stigmatization because of their skin condition.

Many studies have been conducted worldwide demonstrating effects of vitiligo on quality of life and psychological health [1,3,4,6,7]. Homan, et al. [8] in 2009 found that dark skin and vitiligo on exposed body parts are associated with adverse psychological impact compared to patient with fair skin and lesions in non-exposed areas. Psamponga, et al. [9] showed very strong association between quality of life and psychological problems in vitilgo patients including worries of being worse with time, feeling of anger, embarrassment and shame. Dolatshahi, et al. [10] described a significant relationship between DQLI score and marital status especially among married women. Also they found DQLI score associated with disease of extended duration. Saleh, et al. [1] found that 24% of vitiligo patients have significant suicidal thoughts.

In Saudi Arabia Robaee et al. [3], conducted a study in AlQassim in 2007 shows that vitiligo has a severe impact on quality of life specially among those who are on light therapy and with a generalized involvement.

The purpose of this study was to measure the quality of life of patients with vitiligo and the effects of the disease on their mental health and its relationship with variables such as gender, age, education, and income and skin color.

Methods

Using a cross sectional study design, the study was conducted in dermatology clinics in both governmental and private sectors. From governmental sector the following centers were engaged: King AbdulAziz Medical City, National Guard (KAMC), Security Forces Hospital Program, and King Saud Medial Complex. From private sector the National Center for Vitiligo and Psoriasis (Light Clinics) participated. Data collected between October 2010 and February 2011.

Subjects were all adult patients' ≥18 years who had vitiligo, of any type, and on topical or light therapy. We excluded patients who were diagnosed with any psychiatric illnesses before having vitiligo, patients who had any skin disease other than vitiligo, and patients with chronic illnesses.

The sample size was calculated using open epi epidemiologic calculator. Based on the assumption of a 15% prevalence of affective disorders among primary care visitors, the calculated sample size was 255, with 95% Confidence interval and margin of error ±5%. Subjects who presented to the primary care clinics during the period between october 2011 and February 2011 and met the inclusion criteria were recruited to the study by convenience untill the required sample size was satisfied.

Research assistants were trained on the study objective and questionnaire. They distributed the questionnaires and helped the patients understand and fill the survey form properly.

The questionnaire

The questionnaire composed of 4 parts: Socio demographic data, Information about vitiligo, Dermatology Quality of Life Index (DQLI) and Hospital Anxiety and Depression Scale (HAD) [11-13].

The DQLI was first described by Finally and Khan in 1994; it is composed of 10 questions the 1st and 2nd about the sign and symptoms of the dermatological disease, 3rd and 4th about daily activities, 5th and 6th about leisure, 7th about work and school, 8th and 9th about personal relationships, and the 10th question about the treatment. It gives the range from 'no effect' to 'extremely large effect' on the patient's life with score of 0-3. We calculated the answers of all questions, so the total in minimum is 0 and the maximum is 30.

The HAD scale is composed of 14 questions, 7 to assess depression, and 7 to assess Anxiety. Each question is given a score of 0-3. The total minimum score is 0 and the maximum is 21 with a range from (0-7) normal, (8-11) patients are at risk and should be of concern to the doctors, and (12-21) patients need to be assessed by a psychiatrist.

Data analysis

Data entry, Statistical analysis and statistical tests were done using SPSS package version 20.

Data was analyzed descriptively with mean, median, modes, standard deviations, frequencies and percentages. Further analysis was carried out using chi square, t-test, ANOVA and linear regression.

P value was considered to be significant at ≤ 0.05.

Ethical Approval: Ethical approval was obtained from the Institutional review board of King Abdullah International Medical Research Center (KAIMRC).

Results

Two hundred and thirty four Saudi patients were involved in our study. Seventy-four percent were from Riyadh and rest from Abha and Jeddah. The age range was (18–66) years (mean: 30.8 SD ±11.23). Twenty-one percent were under the age of 20 years, 39% of patients were between 21- 30 year old and only 17.5% older than 40 year. The mean age of having vitiligo found to be 21.4 years (±SD 12.98). The mean duration of vitiligo was 9.5 years (± SD 8.09), and the mean of duration of vitiligo treatment was 5.92 years (SD ± 5.99). 52% were males. Single patients were 51.6% and 48.4% were married. Above 41% were found to have a university degree and above. About 45% had income less than 5000 SR / month (Table 1).

Characteristic	Frequency	Percentage
Location		
Inside Riyadh	173	73.9
Outside Riyadh	61	26.1
Institution		
Governmental Sector	106	45.3
Private Sector	120	54.7
Gender		
Male	123	52.6
Female	111	47.4
Age Groups (years)		
≤20	49	20.9
(21-30)	91	38.9
(31-40)	53	22.6
>40	41	17.5
Marital Status		
Single	115	51.6
Married	108	48.4
Educational Level		
Elementary and Intermediate	53	23
High School or Diploma	82	35.7
University or above	95	41.3
Monthly Income (SAR)		
≤5000	106	45.3
5001-10.000	73	31.2
>10.000	55	23.5
Public job		
Yes	134	57.3
Sometimes	45	19.2
No	55	23.5

Type of Family		
Alone	14	6
Nuclear Family	199	85
Extended Family	21	9

Table 1: Characteristics of the Study Subjects

Majority of the patients (59.8%) had a medium skin color. Positive family history of vitiligo was in 38.9%, with 72.2% first degree relatives (Table 2).

Disease Characteristic	Frequency	Percentage
Skin Color		
Fair	53	22.6
Medium	140	59.8
Dark	41	17.5
Family history of Vitiligo		
Yes	91	38.9
No	143	61.1
Type of relationship of positive family history		
First Degree	65	27.8
Second Degree	25	10.7

Table 2: Disease related characteristics

The mean percentage of affected area was 27.66% (±SD 21.55) and 88.5% of the patients had 50% involvement of their body. Involvement of the face was in 38%, hands 62.4%, feet 56.8% and only 12% of the whole body. Among single patients, 29% reported that vitiligo is the cause of being unmarried and for 42% it was not an issue for being unmarried. 19.2% of married people admitted that vitiligo caused some marital problems. Regarding their experience with other people, 32.3% suffered from strange looks from others due to their skin condition, 35.6% would avoid marriage in families that had someone with vitiligo. 15.4% thought it was an infectious disease, 42% consider it as an inherited disease (Table 3).

Social effect	Frequency	Percentage
Cause of being unmarried		
Yes	36	29
No	52	41.9
I Don't Know	36	29
Cause of marital problems		
Yes	24	19.2
No	87	69.6
I Don't Know	14	11.2
Strange looks		
Yes	75	32.3
No	103	44.4
I Don't Know	54	23.3
Avoid marriage from families with Vitiligo		
Yes	77	35.6
No	44	20.4
Sometimes	95	44
Vitiligo is Infectious Disease		
Yes	36	15.4
No	130	55.6
Some people	68	29.1
Vitiligo is Inherited Disease		
Yes	98	41.9
No	48	20.5
Some People	88	37.6

Table 3: Social effects of vitiligo

The mean score of DQLI for all cases was 8.72 (±SD 6.09) and 33.8% of the patients had 'very large' to 'extreme' effect on their quality of life. Physical symptoms like itching were reported in more than 60% of the patients with about 14% reporting it as severe. Near 80% admitted that they feel embarrassed because of their skin with almost half of those report the feelings as extreme. Over 17% said that their personal relationships were extremely affected. Choosing of clothes was 'very much' affected in almost 40% of the patients. Vitiligo treatment affected the patient's life in nearly 84% (Tables 4 and 5).

Parameter	Extremely affected (%)	A Little (%)	Not at All/ Not relevant (%)
Symptoms	33(14.1)	110(47)	91 (38.9)
Feelings	90(38.5)	96 (41)	48 (20.5)
Shopping	39(16.6)	57 (24.4)	138 (59)
Clothes	91(38.9)	46(19.7)	97 (41.4)
Social	38(16.2)	50 (21.4)	146 (62.4)
Sport	37(15.8)	42 (17.9)	155 (66.3)
Working or Studying	17 (8.5)	72 (35.8)	112 (55.7)
Relationships	41(17.5)	68 (29.1)	125 (53.4)
Sexual	30(12.8)	26(11.1)	178 (76.1)
Treatment	135(57.7)	61 (26.1)	38 (16.3)

Table 4: Distribution of patients related to Dermatology Quality of Life Index

Factors	No or Small effect {No (%)}	Moderate effect {No (%)}	V. large/ extreme effect {No (%)}	Chi sq (P value)
Gender				
Male	58 (64.4)	39 (6.0)	26 (32.9)	18.77(0.00)
Female	32 (35.6)	26 (40)	79 (67.1)	
Age group (years)				
≤ 20	15 (16.7)	12 (18.5)	22 (27.8)	13(0.04)
21- 30	36 (40.0)	28 (43.1)	27 (34.2)	
31-40	15 (16.7)	18 (27.7)	20 (25.3)	
> 40	24 (26.7)	7 (10.8)	10 (12.7	
Marital status				
Single	42(47.7)	29(46.8)	44(60.3)	3.3(0.19)
Married	46 (52.3)	33(53.2)	29 (39.7)	
Education				
1ry/ 2ry school	19(21.3)	9 (14.1)	25 (32.5)	8.4(0.76)
High school or diploma	30(33.7)	24(37.5)	28(36.4)	
University	40(44.9)	31 (48.4)	24(31.2)	
Public job				
Yes	57(63.3)	38(58.5)	39(49.4)	6.5(0.15)
Sometimes	14(15.6)	16(24.6)	15(19)	
No	19(21.1)	11(16.9)	25(31.6)	
Monthly Income (SR)				
≤5000	27(30)	29(44.6)	50(63.3)	21(0.00)
5001-10.000	32(35.6)	23(35.4)	18(22.8)	
>10.000	31 (34.4)	13(20)	11 (13.9)	
Skin color				
Fair	23 (25.6)	11(16.9)	19(24.1)	3.65(0.45)
Medium	55(61.1)	42 (64.6)	43(54.4)	
Dark	12(13.3)	12(18.5)	17(21.5)	

Table 5: Relationship of DQLI with variables

DQLI

DQLI was worse in female where 47.7% of them had 'very large' to 'extreme' effect while in males this effect was seen only in 21.1% (chi-sq.=18.77, p<0.001). Higher DQLI score was seen in age group (21-30 years) compared to other age groups (chi- sq.=13, p=0.043). DQLI score was higher among low income patients compared to high income patients (chi sq.=21, p<0.001).

Involvement of the neck had a significant impact on quality of life rather than other parts of the body (mean DQLI score t-test=2.21, p<. 028, mean diff.=2.2).

Patients who had involvement of >50% of body surface had more effect on quality of life index (t-test=2.15, P=0.013).

The difference of DQLI among marital status, educational level, skin color or for those in public jobs dealing with people, was found to be statistically insignificant.

HAD scale

Regarding anxiety the mean score of HAD scale was 5.94 (± SD 4.51) and mean score for depression was 4.90 (±SD 4.06). Anxiety was common among females with 62.7% having 'high' score while only 37.3% in males had 'high' score (chi sq. 10.27, p<0.001). Anxiety was higher in patients dealing with people on daily basis (chi sq. 10.12, p= 0.006), in contrast to HAD scale for depression, where dealing with people had no significant effect.

Vitiligo on the face has been associated with significant anxiety than any other part of the body (mean HAD anxiety score t-test=2.31, p=0.022, mean diff.=1.382) (Table 6).

	Variable	HAD scale for Anxiety			HAD scale for Depression		
		Normal {No (%)}	High {No (%)}	Chi sq (p)	Normal {No (%)}	High {No (%)}	Chi sq (p)
Gender	Male	95 (59.7)	28 (37.3)	10.3 (0.00)	96 (56.5)	27(42.2)	3.8 (0.05)
	Female	64 (40.3)	47(62.7)		74(43.5)	37(57.8)	
Age group	≤20	30 (18.9)	19(25.3)	3.72 (0.29)	38(22.4)	11(17.2)	1.8 (0.61)
	21- 30	68(42.8)	23(30.7)		67(73.6)	24(37.5)	
	31-40	33(20.8)	20(26.7)		35(20.6)	18(28.1)	
	>40	28(17.6)	13(17.3)		30(17.6)	11(17.2)	
Marital Status	Single	74 (48.1)	41(59.4)	2.4 (0.12)	85(51.8)	30(50.8)	0.17 (0.89)
	Married	80(51.9)	28(40.6)		79(48.2)	29(49.2)	
Education	Primary/Secondary school	32(20.3)	21(29.2)	5.26 (0.07)	32(19.2)	21(33.3)	6.6 (0.037)
	High school or diploma	53(33.5)	29(40.3)		59(35.3)	23(36.5)	
	University	73(46.2)	22(30.6)		76(45.5)	19(30.2)	
Public job	Yes	102(64.2)	32(42.7)	10.1 (0.00)	105(61.8)	29(45.3)	5.4 (0.065)
	Sometimes	24(15.1)	21(28.0)		28(16.5)	17(26.6)	
	No	33(20.8)	22(29.3)		37(21.8)	18((28.1)	
Monthly income (SR)	≤ 5000	66(41.5)	40(53.3)	3 (0.22)	68(40.0)	38(59.4)	7.1 (0. 028)
	5001-10.000	54(34)	19(25.3)		59(34.7)	14(21.9)	
	>10.000	39(24.5)	16(21.3)		43(25.3)	12(18.8)	
Skin color	Fair	34(21.4)	19(25.3)	0.46 (0.79)	37(21.8)	16(25)	0.39 (0.819)
	Medium	97(61)	43(57.3)		102(60)	38 (59.4)	
	Dark	28(17.6)	13(17.3)		31(18.2)	10(15.6)	

Table 6: Relationship of HAD scale with variables

No difference was noted in Anxiety score between different age groups, marital status, income, educational level, skin color or extended duration of the disease.

In HAD scale for depression we found a higher score in females 57.8% compared to 42.2% in males but this difference was borderline insignificant (chi sq. 3.8, p=0.051).

Over 45.5% of 'normal' depression scale was seen in high educational level (university and above) while 19.2% of normal scale seen in low educational level (chi-sq. 6.6, p=0.037).

Nearly 60% of 'higher' depression score was seen in patients with low income while only 18.8% of 'high' score was noted in the high income bracket (chi-sq. 7.15, p=0.028.)

We did not find a significant association between the HAD for Depression and physical distribution of vitiligo.

Similar to HAD scale for anxiety, no effect was seen on depression scale for skin color, marital status, different age groups or extension of the disease.

There was a significant difference between 'high' scores in both scales (DQLI and HAD for both Anxiety and Depression) and frustration of treatment, (t-test 5.77, 7.58 and 3.827 respectively, p <0.001).

For suicidal thoughts both DQLI and HAD for Anxiety (t test 4.2 and 4.7, p<0.001 respectively) and for HAD scale for Depression

(t test=2.31, p=0.022,).

The mean score for DQLI of suicidal attempts was 21.67 (SD + 4.93) which was significantly higher from those who did not attempt suicide (t test=3.8, p<0.001), as well for HAD scale where the mean score for Anxiety was 15.33 (SD + 4.04) and for Depression was 9.67 (SD + 3.21), (p<0.001, t test=3.733 and p=0.041 t test=2.06 respectively).

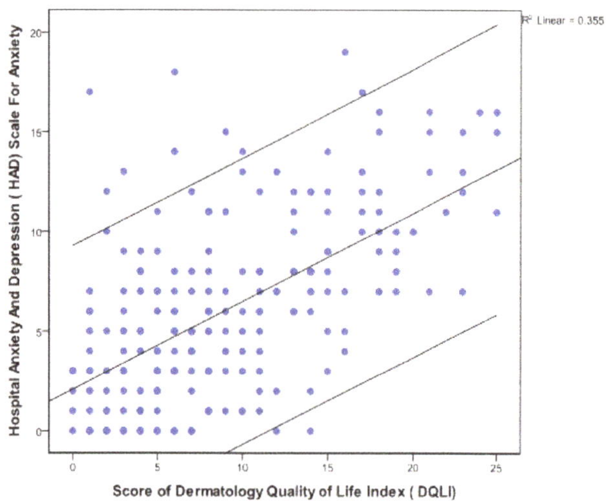

Figure 1: Relationship of Score of DQLI and HAD Anxiety Scale, Adjusted R2=35.2%, F=127.5, p<0.001, Simple Linear Regression Equation: (y=a + bx), HAD Anxiety=2.09 + 0.44 DQLI (Higher DQLI predicts Higher HAD Anxiety)

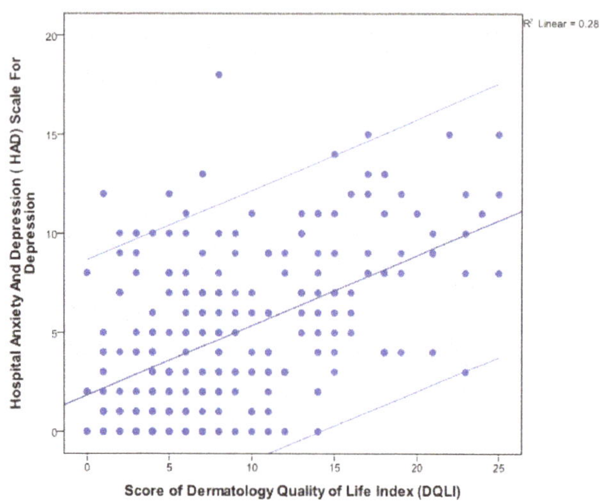

Figure 2: Relationship of Score of DQLI and HAD Depression Scale, Adjusted R2=27.7%, F=90.4, p<0.001, Simple Linear Regression Equation: (y=a + bx), HAD Depression=1.82 + 0.35 DQLI, (Higher DQLI predicts Higher HAD depression)

A moderately positive correlation was noted between the DQLI and HAD scale for anxiety, where the patients with poorer quality of life had a higher HAD anxiety score (R2=0.35, p<0.001). The same for HAD scale for Depression (R2=0.28, p<0.001). (Figures 1 and 2).

Discussion

Vitiligo has a very large effect on quality of life and psychological wellbeing. In most skin conditions psychiatric morbidity was strongly associated with poorer quality of life [7]. The mean DQLI in this study was 8.72(±SD 6.09) which was less than the score reported in 109 patients by AlRobaee in alQassim study, i.e. 14.72 [3], Compared to international studies we have a higher score than Kent et al. Abadie [14], where they found score of 4.82 in UK, as well in Ongenae et al. [4] study in Belgian patientswho had a mean total score of 4.95. Our findings are near the results of Finaly and Khan [15] who had a DQLI score of 7.3 in UK study, and in the same category 10.67 reported by Parased et al. [16] in India.

In our study we found females more affected than males with higher DQLI score, unlike the AlRobaee [3], Parsad et al. [16], and Kent and Abadie [14] who did not report any gender difference in score, while Ongenae et al. [4], Do Young Kim et al. [6] and Sampogna et al. [9] found that women overall had a higher score than men. We expected this finding as women are more concerned about her skin and beauty. Age also influenced DQLI where the highest effect about 34.2% was seen in age group of 21-30 years while this effect decreased to 12.7% in patients older than 40 years. This is expected as younger people are usually more concerned about their appearance.

Other factors found to have a significant effect on the quality of life was income, where 63.3% of 'very large' or 'extreme' effect was seen in low income category while 13.9% of the same effect seen in high income group. Low income patients have more life stressors beside vitiligo which can be a burden on opportunities. We found that involvement of the neck has been associated with a significant impact on quality of life more than any other part of the body. This may be due to cultural differences. In other studies like in Tunisia, they found that exposed areas have a higher impact on quality of life than non-exposed parts of the body [5].

Interestingly we found no effect of skin color on quality of life. Linborst Homan et al. In Amesrtdam reported that subjects with darker skin are more anxious about their appearance [8].

As expected we found that patients with generalized and more body surface involvement have more impact on their quality of life, the same seen in previous studies [3,4].

Although Vitiligo is considered to be idiopathic, there some theories saying that stress is one of the causes, [2,7,8]. We assessed our patients for the possibility of psychiatric illness using the HAD scale, which can differentiate between people who are normal and who need to have further evaluation and assessment.

The mean score for HAD scale for Anxiety was 5.94 (±4.51 SD), and for depression was 4.90 (±4.06 SD) where we found that 62.7% of high anxiety seen in females comparing to 37.3% in males (p<0.001) as well in depression scale a 57.8% of high reading was in female and 42.2% in male (p=0.51) even this difference was insignificant, but we think that female have a higher potential to have anxiety as well as depression more than males [2].

As in DQLI, we found that income had a psychological impact where HAD scale for Depression was high on patients with low income with a 59.4% as compared to 18.8% in patient with low income. While Anxiety scale was not affected by the income, on the other hand, it was high in patients who were dealing with people on a daily basis as job requirement.

This interaction with other people perhaps puts vitiligo patients under stress due to different reactions that are expressed towards them. Over 32.3% of people get strange looks due to their skin condition and 14.5% of people think that vitilgo is an infectious disease all of these factors may cause burden on patients and increase their level of anxiety, interestingly DQLI and Depression scale were not affected by public dealing jobs.

In contrast to both DQLI and Anxiety scale we noticed that depression scale was associated with educational level as 45.5% of those with university degree were normal on depression scale compared to only 19.2% of those who had a low educational level (p=. 037), this can be explained by assuming that more educated people can understand their disease and its chronic nature which may help them in the acceptance and compliance of long treatment regimen.

HAD for anxiety as well as for depression didn't report any significant association with age, but we noticed some pattern where high scores were reported with age group 21-30 years, as same category where DQLI showed a significant effect. This is supported by Ijaz Ahmed study were they report that psychiatric illness was predominant in patients below 30 years of age [2].

Surprisingly we found no association with marital status or skin color with either DQLI or HAD scale for both Depression and Anxiety. On the contrary, literature reported higher psychological problems seen in unmarried subjects [2]. In our study 46.2% were married and 53.8% were single, among those singles 41% thought that vitiligo is not a cause of being unmarried. Family history of vitiligo was seen in 38.9%, and only 35.6% believed that people avoid marriage from families that have vitiligo. Nearly 70% of the married patients said that vitiligo was not a cause of any marital problems and 87.2% stated it has no sexual difficulties due to their disease.

Regarding the skin color 60% had a medium skin color, most of the literature indicates that darker skin color had more stress on patients with vitiligo, however that was not noticed in our study, perhaps because only 17% reported their skin as 'dark' and they did not express higher impairment.

Patients with face involvement were found to be suffering from anxiety rather than depression, in the literature it was reported that patients with exposed area affected have more psychiatric disorders [2].

We found that the patients who had a large effect on 'quality of life' scale had an abnormal HAD score for both Depression and Anxiety. The higher the quality of life impairment, the higher will be the chance of developing psychological problems as depression or anxiety. This association was seen also in Sampogana et al. Study 2004 [7], Mechri et al. in Tunisia 2006 [17] and HananSaleh study in Egypt 2008 [1].

Limitation

The DQL index assesses the effect of any dermatological disease during the last 2 weeks and might not reflect the long term implications of the disease.

Conclusion

This study demonstrates that vitiligo has a negative effect on quality of life and it can be a probable cause of psychological diseases. More attention should be focused on female, low income patients as they may have a more severe impairment. Patients who have a poor quality of life should be screened for depression and anxiety as there is an association between them.

Patients with vitiligo need more attention from both dermatologist as well as family physician, even its not a serious or life threatening disease but it has large effect on quality of life, its psychological and psychiatric consequences need to be evaluated and proper action should be taken, especially in low income, low educational level, and young age group.

Involving a psychiatrist or psychologist may be appropriate step in management of high risk patients. Having patient support groups may be a good forum for exchanging their experiences with other patients locally or internationally.

References

1. Saleh HM, Salem S, El-Sheshetawy RS, El-Samei M (2007) Comparative study of psychiatric morbidity and quality of life in psoriasis, vitiligo and alopecia areata. Egyptian Dermatology Online Journal. 4: 2-28.
2. Ahmed I, Ahmed S, Nasreen S (2007) Frequency and pattern of psychiatric disorders in patients with vitiligo. J Ayub Med Coll Abbottabad 19: 19-21.
3. Al Robaee AA (2007) Assessment of quality of life in Saudi patients with vitiligo in a medical school in Qassim province, Saudi Arabia. Saudi Med J 28: 1414-1417.
4. Ongenae K, Van Geel N, De Schepper S, Naeyaert JM (2005) Effect of vitiligo on self-reported health-related quality of life. Br J Dermatol 152: 1165-1172.
5. Jalel A, Soumaya GS, Hamdaoui MH (2009) Dermatology life quality index scores in vitiligo: reliability and validity of the Tunisian version. Indian J Dermatol 54: 330-333.
6. Kim do Y, Lee JW, Whang SH, Park YK, Hann SK, et al. (2009) Quality of life for Korean patients with vitiligo: Skindex-29 and its correlation with clinical profiles. J Dermatol 36: 317-322.7.
7. Sampogna F, Picardi A, Sampogna F, Picardi A, Chren MM, Melchi CF, Pasquini P, et al. (2004) Association between poorer quality of life and psychiatric morbidity in patients with different dermatological conditions. Psychosom Med 66: 620-624.
8. Linthorst Homan MW, Spuls PI, de Korte J, Bos JD, Sprangers MA, et al. (2009) The burden of vitiligo: patient characteristics associated with quality of life. J Am Acad Dermatol 61: 411-420.
9. Sampogna F, Raskovic D, Guerra L, Pedicelli C, Tabolli S, et al. (2008) Identification of categories at risk for high quality of life impairment in patients with vitiligo. Br J Dermatol 159: 351-359.
10. Dolatshahi M, Ghazi P, Feizy V, Hemami MR (2008) Life quality assessment among patients with vitiligo: comparison of married and single patients in Iran. Indian J Dermatol Venereol Leprol 74: 700.
11. Basra MK, Fenech R, Gatt RM, Salek MS, Finlay AY (2008) The Dermatology Life Quality Index 1994-2007: a comprehensive review of validation data and clinical results. Br J Dermatol 159: 997-1035.
12. Bjelland I, Dahl AA, Haug TT, Neckelmann D (2002) The validity of the Hospital Anxiety and Depression Scale. An updated literature review. J Psychosom Res 52: 69-77.
13. Malasi TH, Mirza IA, el-Islam MF (1991) Validation of the Hospital Anxiety and Depression Scale in Arab patients. Acta Psychiatr Scand 84: 323-326.

14. Kent G, al-Abadie M (1996) Factors affecting responses on Dermatology Life Quality Index items among vitiligo sufferers. Clin Exp Dermatol 21: 330-333.
15. Finlay AY, Khan GK (1994) Dermatology Life Quality Index (DLQI)--a simple practical measure for routine clinical use. Clin Exp Dermatol 19: 210-216.
16. Parsad D, Pandhi R, Dogra S, Kanwar AJ, Kumar B (2003) Dermatology Life Quality Index score in vitiligo and its impact on the treatment outcome. Br J Dermatol 148: 373-374.
17. Mechri A, Amri M, Douarika AA, Ali Hichem BH, Zouari B, et al. (2006) [Psychiatric morbidity and quality of life in Vitiligo: a case controlled study]. Tunis Med 84: 632-635.

19

Sadly Awake: Short Sleep Duration and Depressive Symptoms among Adolescents

Samuel Reisman*

Department of Medicine, Suny Downstate School of Medicine, USA

Abstract

Background: Inappropriate sleep duration has been showed to be associated with increased suicidality among high school students in the United States. An association between inappropriate sleep duration and general depressive symptoms among this population has not been reported.

Methods: The biennial Youth Risk Behavior Surveillance System uses national and local school-based surveys to measure the prevalence of health-risk behaviors among youth and young adults. Students reported how many hours a night they get on an average school night and whether their daily routine was altered for two consecutive weeks due to sadness or hopelessness. We analyzed whether 8-10 hours of sleep was associated with depressive symptoms. Covariates included sex, race, BMI, bullying, abuse, smoking, alcohol use, and drug use.

Results: Students who reported <8 or ≥ 10 hours of sleep had an odds ratio of 1.66(1.49, 1.86) of concurrent depressive symptoms.

Conclusion: Routine adolescent depression surveillance may be enhanced by sleep duration assessments.

Keywords: Insomnia; Depression; Sleep medicine

Introduction

Insomnia is a risk factor for depression [1]. Meta-analysis demonstrates a two-fold increase in risk for depression among non-depressed individuals with insomnia [2], an association validated with as few as two weeks of sleep data [3]. Increased depression risk can persist for 30 years [4]. There is significant heterogeneity in how studies measure insomnia. Insomnia symptoms, insomnia symptoms with daytime consequences, insomnia diagnosis, and sleep dissatisfaction have been used to measure insomnia [5]. Current diagnostic criteria for insomnia include prolonged dissatisfaction with sleep quantity or quality coupled with difficulty initiating or maintaining sleep and functional impairments [6].

Insomnia implies poor sleep quantity or quality [7]. The definition of sleep quality may be subjective [8] and difficult to define [9]. Systematic deficiencies exist in the understanding and measurement of sleep quality [8-10]. Sleep quality-related complaints and diagnosis often are not correlated with objective sleep measurements, including electroencephalogram [11] and polysomnography [12]. Polysomnography is considered the "gold standard" of sleep measurement [13] but is expensive and impractical to use in large studies. The most commonly used standardized measurement of sleep quality is the Pittsburgh Sleep Quality Index (PSQI) [14], a survey-based measurement. PSQI is valid and reliable across heterogeneous populations13. PSQI incorporates sleep quantity and daily functioning into its measurement of sleep quality and cannot establish the validity or reliability of self-reported sleep quantity or quality alone.

In contrast to sleep quality, sleep quantity is essentially an objective measure. When measured subjectively through self-reporting, respondents tend to underestimate sleep duration [15]. A recent meta-analysis showed a moderate to strong correlation between self-reported and objectively measured sleep duration [16], consistent with previous studies [15,17-19]. Adolescents' estimates of sleep duration are strongly correlated with objective measurement in weekday sleep reports, and only moderately correlated in weekend sleep reports [15,16]. Self-report validity may be significantly enhanced by daily diary entries [20].

Multiple studies have reported associations between sleep duration and depression . A recent analysis of 22, 281 adult participants in the US National Health and Nutrition Examination Surveys showed a significant association between sleep duration and depression [21]. Less than seven hours of sleep is associated with incident mood-related risks, including tension, depression, and dissatisfaction with life [22]. A longitudinal study of 2,259 students found that less than six hours of sleep per night predicts depressive symptoms and low self-esteem [23]. A recent cross-sectional study of 894 pairs of twins found an association between depressive symptoms and less than seven or greater than nine hours of sleep [24]. Insufficient sleep duration among adolescents is estimated at one-fourth to one-fifth of the population and predicts depressed mood and poor quality of life [7].

Despite conflicting evidence [25], sleep quality [4,22,26] seems to be more significantly correlated with poor emotional functioning than sleep quantity. Regardless of their relative importance, both sleep quantity and sleep quality are independently associated with depression [24] and poor depression outcomes [27,28]. Sleep duration data are simpler to define and tabulate than insomnia or sleep quantity data. Many large surveys routinely collect sleep duration data with a single question. If sleep duration is associated with depression, it can be an important mental health surveillance tool. We used a recent, large, representative study of US high school student to test the hypothesis that sleep duration predicts depression.

***Corresponding author:** Samuel Reisman, Department of Medicine, Suny Downstate School of Medicine, USA;
E-mail: samuel.reisman@downstate.edu

Methods

The biennial Youth Risk Behavior Surveillance System (YRBS) uses national and local school-based surveys to measure the prevalence of health-risk behaviors among youth and young adults [29]. The survey is directed by the Centers for Disease Control and Prevention. In 2013, the response rate was 77% among schools and 88% among students, with an overall response rate of 68%. Weighted adjustments were used to adjust for non-response rates and oversampling. The survey collected data on 99 questions related to individual characteristics and health-risk behaviors. A total of 13,583 usable questionnaires were completed by students in grades 9-12.

Our exposure variable of sleep duration is assessed by the survey question, "On an average school night, how many hours of sleep do you get?" Fixed-choice responses are, in hours, ≤ 4, 5, 6, 7, 8, 9, and ≥ 10. The American Academy of Sleep Medicine (AASM) recommends 8-10 hours of sleep for adolescents [30]. To best match these recommendations, students who reported<8 hours or ≥ 10 of sleep on school nights are compared with those who reported 8 or 9 hours of sleep. Combining appropriate (=10) and inappropriate (>10) durations of sleep into a single level was unavoidable, but thought to be important to report upon.

Variables	1	2	3	4
Intercept	-1.267*** (0.041)	-1.835*** (0.143)	-2.376***(0.157)	-2.401*** (0.168)
<8 or ≥10 Hours of sleep	0.592*** (0.047)	0.597*** (0.050)	0.517*** (0.054)	0.507*** (0.057)
Female		0.872*** (0.043)	0.704*** (0.046)	0.793*** (0.050)
Age		-0.000561	0.002 (0.019)	-0.026 (0.020)
BMI		0.013*** (0.004)	0.010** (0.004)	0.010** (0.005)
Black		-0.240*** (0.079)	-0.133 (0.085)	-0.078 (0.090)
Hispanic		0.203*** (0.075)	0.283*** (0.081)	0.281*** (0.086)
White		-0.008307	-0.164** (0.077)	-0.242*** (0.081)
Bullied in school			0.808*** (0.060)	0.834*** (0.064)
Bullied online			0.763*** (0.067)	0.775*** (0.072)
Physically assaulted			0.285*** (0.080)	0.238*** (0.099)
Sexually assaulted			0.215*** (0.030)	0.191*** (0.032)
Rape victim			0.732*** (0.089)	0.666*** (0.098)
Smoking				0.461*** (0.094)
Alcohol use				0.046*** (0.013)
Recreational Injectable drug use				-0.079 (0.144)
Recreational Prescription drug use				0.156*** (0.025)
N	12,264	11,277	10,839	9,901
Log Likelihood	-7,452.611	-6,610.11	-5,901.61	-5,257.017
Akaike Inf. Crit.	14,909.220	13,236.22	11,829.22	10,548.030

***Significant at the 1% level.
**Significant at the 5% level.
*Significant at the 10% level.

Table 1: Summary of logistic regression analysis for variables predicting depressive symptoms.

Models	Odds Ratio	Lower Limit	Upper Limit
Model 1	1.81	1.65	1.98
Model 2	1.82	1.65	2.01
Model 3	1.68	1.51	1.86
Model 4	1.66	1.49	1.86

Table 2: Odds ratio and 95% CI of depressive symptoms with <8 hours of sleep.

Variables	Odds Ratio	Lower Limit	Upper Limit	p-value
<8 or ≥10 Hours of sleep	1.66	1.49	1.86	5.67E-19
Age	0.97	0.94	1.01	
Female	2.21	2.01	2.45	1.12E-56
BMI	1.01	1	1.02	3.50E-02
Black	0.93	0.76	1.1	
Hispanic	1.32	1.12	1.57	1.09E-03
White	0.78	0.67	0.92	2.90E-03
Bullied in school	2.3	2.03	2.61	1.50E-38
Bullied online	2.17	1.89	2.5	3.19E-27
Physically assaulted	1.27	1.05	1.54	1.66E-02
Sexually assaulted	1.21	1.14	1.29	3.67E-09
Rape victim	1.94	1.61	2.36	1.26E-11
Smoking	1.59	1.32	1.9	1.07E-06
Alcohol use	1.05	1.02	1.07	3.23E-04
Injectable drug abuse	0.92	0.7	1.23	
Prescription drug abuse	1.17	1.11	1.23	2.98E-10

Table 3: Odds ratio and 95% CI of depression (Model 4).

Our outcome variable of depression is assessed by the yes/no question, "During the past 12 months, did you ever feel so sad and hopeless almost every day for two weeks or more in a row that you stopped doing some usual activities?" Depressed mood or loss of interest in activities for two weeks or more are the cardinal criteria for major depressive disorder (MDD) [31] and are necessary but not sufficient conditions for diagnosis [32]. The YRBS also contains data on suicidality, another major depressive disorder symptom. Our analyses do not include suicidality because it is a restrictive criterion for depression; half or more of those with MDD do not consider suicide [33,34], while a study of patients with MDD found the prevalence of depressed mood and loss of interest in activities to be 93.7% and 82.2%, respectively [34]. Fitzgerald et al. [35] previously found inappropriate sleep duration to be associated with suicide ideation in YRBS survey data. This study analyzes whether that finding can be extended to depressive symptoms.

Logistic regression was used to measure the association between sleep duration and depressive symptoms, adjusting for possible confounders including age, sex, race, body mass index (BMI), physical assault victim, sexual assault victim, rape victim, smoking, alcohol use, recreational injectable drug use and recreational prescription drug use (survey items listed in Appendix A). Four logistic regression models were used. The first contained no covariates. The second model added gender, race, and BMI. The third model added bullying- and abuse-related covariates. The fourth model added smoking, alcohol use, and drug use.

Results

Logistic regression revealed a strong and consistent correlation between<8 or ≥ 10 hours of sleep and depressive symptoms across all models (Table 1).

In our initial model, <8 or ≥ 10 hours of sleep had an odds ratio of 1.71 for depressive symptoms. The correlation remained significant through all our models with odds ratios ranging from 1.66 to 2.01 (Table 2).

Female sex (OR=2.21 in model 4), physical bullying (2.30), online bullying (2.17), and rape (1.95) were the strongest correlates of depressive symptoms across our models. The level of correlation with depressive symptoms was similar for smoking (1.59) and <8 or ≥ 10 hours of sleep (1.66). Physical assault (1.27) and sexual assault (1.21) were associated to a lesser degree. The individual associations of physical and online bullying, as well as rape and sexual assault, may be underestimated due to collinearity. Hispanics had greater odds of depressive symptoms (OR=1.32) while Whites had lower odds (OR=0.78). Alcohol use (1.05) showed only a small association with depressive symptoms (Table 3).

Discussion

Analysis of survey data from a nationally representative sample of high school students shows a significant association between<8 or ≥ 10 hours of sleep and depressive symptoms. This association remains statistically and practically significant after controlling for confounders. The results suggest that sleep duration may be an important indicator of depression. Fitzgerald et al. [35] found, using YRBS survey data, that sleep duration predicts suicide ideation, and should be a routine component of suicide surveillance efforts in adolescents. Our findings suggest that sleep duration should be used routinely in general depression surveillance efforts as well.

Our results suggest that Hispanic adolescents may have greater odds of depression than other racial groups, a finding consistent with previous studies [36,37]. The stress of immigrant acculturation may cause increased risk of depression and suicide ideation [38]. These findings suggest that identifying effective school interventions for adolescent Hispanics may be of particular importance [39].

Many covariates had the expected positive correlation with depressive symptoms predicted by previous research. Female sex has been widely shown to be a risk factor for depression [40]. Bullying has been associated with depression and suicidility [41]. Physical assault [42], sexual assault [43], smoking [44], and alcohol and drug abuse [45] have also been associated with depression. The YRBS data additionally supports the need to focus intervention efforts on these at-risk populations.

This study has several limitations. First, YRBS data is cross-sectional and can only establish associations, not longitudinal risk. Second, the discrete, 7-level classification of sleep duration can hide important intragroup differences, as each level contains individuals with different sleep durations. In addition, the variable level of ≥ 10 hours of sleep combines appropriate and inappropriate 30 levels of sleep. Third, the survey contains numerous data, and can be analyzed using many different groups of covariates. We did not perform stepwise analysis of possible confounders, but rather decided on a set of confounders prior to data analysis. Nevertheless, there are other survey data that can be reasonably included in the analysis. Thus our results can be due to an unknown confounder or group of confounders. Fourth, the survey data are subjective, and not corroborated with objective measurement. The possibility remains that depression is correlated with self-reported but not objective sleep durations.

Conclusion

In conclusion, Data from the 2013 YRBS survey of high school students indicates that sleep durations of <8 or ≥ 10 hours of sleep is associated with a significantly increased odds of depression. Routine adolescent depression surveillance may be enhanced by sleep duration assessment. Future studies should look for causal associations between sleep duration and depressive symptoms.

References

1. Sivertsen B, Salo P, Mykletun A, Hysing M, Pallesen S, et al. (2012) The bidirectional association between depression and insomnia: The HUNT Study. Psychosom Med 74: 758-765.
2. Baglioni C, Battagliese G, Feige B, Spiegelhalder K, Nissen C, et al. (2011) Insomnia as a predictor of depression: a meta-analytic evaluation of longitudinal epidemiological studies. J Affect Disord 135: 10-19.
3. Riemann D, Voderholzer U (2003) Primary insomnia: A risk factor to develop depression? J Affect Disord 76: 255-259.
4. Chang PP, Ford DE, Mead LA, Cooper-Patrick L, Klag MJ (1997) Insomnia in young men and subsequent depression. The Johns Hopkins Precursors Study. Am J Epidemiol 146: 105-114.
5. Ohayon MM (2002) Epidemiology of insomnia: what we know and what we still need to learn. Sleep Med Rev 6: 97-111.
6. Association AP (2003) Sleep-wake disorders. Diagnostic and Statistical Manual of Mental Disorders. 5th edtn. Washington, DC 2013.
7. Roberts RE, Roberts CR, Duong HT (2009) Sleepless in adolescence: prospective data on sleep deprivation, health and functioning. J Adolesc 32: 1045-1057.
8. Akerstedt T, Hume K, Minors D, Waterhouse J (1994) The meaning of good sleep: a longitudinal study of polysomnography and subjective sleep quality. J Sleep Res. 3: 152-158.
9. Harvey AG, Stinson K, Whitaker KL, Moskovitz D, Virk H (2008) The subjective meaning of sleep quality: a comparison of individuals with and without insomnia. Sleep 31: 383-393.
10. Krystal AD, Edinger JD (2008) Measuring sleep quality. Sleep Med 9: 10-17.
11. Rosa RR, Bonnet MH (2000) Reported chronic insomnia is independent of poor sleep as measured by electroencephalography. Psychosom Med 62: 474-482.
12. Moul DE, Nofzinger EA, Pilkonis PA, Houck PR, Miewald JM, et al. (2002) Symptom reports in severe chronic insomnia. Sleep 25: 553-563.
13. Beck SL, Schwartz AL, Towsley G, Dudley W, Barsevick A (2004) Psychometric evaluation of the Pittsburgh Sleep Quality Index in cancer patients. J Pain Symptom Manage 27:140-148.
14. Grandner MA, Kripke DF, Yoon IY, Youngstedt SD (2006) Criterion validity of the Pittsburgh Sleep Quality Index: Investigation in a non-clinical sample. Sleep Biol Rhythms 4:129-139.
15. Wolfson AR, Carskadon MA, Acebo C, Seifer R, Fallone G, et al. (2003) Evidence for the validity of a sleep habits survey for adolescents. Sleep 26: 213-216.
16. Nascimento FMV, Collese TS, de Moraes ACF, Rendo UT, Moreno LA, et al. (2016) Validity and reliability of sleep time questionnaires in children and adolescents: A systematic review and meta-analysis. Sleep medicine reviews 30: 85-96.
17. Monk TH, Buysse DJ, Kennedy KS, Pods JM, DeGrazia JM, et al. (2003) Measuring sleep habits without using a diary: The sleep timing questionnaire. Sleep 26: 208-212.
18. Lauderdale DS, Knutson KL, Yan LL, Liu K, Rathouz PJ. (2008) Sleep duration: How well do self-reports reflect objective measures? The CARDIA Sleep Study. Epidemiology (Cambridge, Mass) 19: 838-845.
19. Cespedes EM, Hu FB, Redline S, Rosner B, Alcantara C, et al. (2016) Comparison of self-reported sleep duration with actigraphy: Results from the hispanic community health study/study of Latinos Sueno Ancillary Study. Am J Epidemiol 183: 561-573.

20. Arora T, Broglia E, Pushpakumar D, Lodhi T, Taheri S (2013) An investigation into the strength of the association and agreement levels between subjective and objective sleep duration in adolescents. PLoS One 8: e72406.

21. Cepeda MS, Stang P, Blacketer C, Kent JM, Wittenberg GM (2016) Clinical relevance of sleep duration: Results from a cross-sectional analysis using NHANES. J Clin Sleep Med 12: 813-819.

22. Pilcher JJ, Ginter DR, Sadowsky B (1997) Sleep quality versus sleep quantity: Relationships between sleep and measures of health, well-being and sleepiness in college students. J Psychosom Res 42: 583-596.

23. Fredriksen K, Rhodes J, Reddy R, Way N (2004) Sleepless in Chicago: Tracking the effects of adolescent sleep loss during the middle school years. Child Dev 75: 84-95.

24. Watson NF, Harden KP, Buchwald D, Vitiello MV, Pack AI, et al. (2014) Sleep duration and depressive symptoms: A gene-environment interaction. Sleep 37: 351-358.

25. Vriend JL, Davidson FD, Corkum PV, Rusak B, McLaughlin EN, et al. (2012) Sleep Quantity and Quality in Relation to Daytime Functioning in Children. Children's Health Care 41: 204-222.

26. Augner C. (2011) Associations of subjective sleep quality with depression score, anxiety, physical symptoms and sleep onset latency in students. Cent Eur J Public Health 19: 115-117.

27. Troxel WM, Kupfer DJ, Reynolds CF, Frank E, Thase ME, et al. (2012) Insomnia and objectively measured sleep disturbances predict treatment outcome in depressed patients treated with psychotherapy or psychotherapy-pharmacotherapy combinations. J Clin Psychiatry 73: 478-485.

28. Blasco FH, Alegria AA, Lopez CJ Legido-Gil T, Saiz-Ruiz J, et al. (2011) Short self-reported sleep duration and suicidal behavior: a cross-sectional study. J Affect Disord 133: 239-246.

29. Youth Risk Behavior Surveillance System. 2016.

30. Paruthi S, Brooks LJ, Ambrosio C, Hall WA, Kotagal S, et al. (2016) Consensus Statement of the American Academy of Sleep Medicine on the Recommended Amount of Sleep for Healthy Children: Methodology and Discussion. J Clin Sleep Med 12: 1549-1561.

31. Richardson L, McCauley E, Katon W (2009) Collaborative care for adolescent depression: a pilot study. Gen Hosp Psychiatr 31: 36-45.

32. Association AP (2003) Depressive Disorders. Diagnostic and Statistical Manual of Mental Disorders. 5th edtn. Washington, DC.

33. Nyer M, Holt DJ, Pedrelli P, Fava M, Ameral V et al. (2013) Factors that distinguish college students with depressive symptoms with and without suicidal thoughts. Ann Clin Psychiatry 25: 41-49.

34. Zimmerman M, Ellison W, Young D (2015) Chelminski I, Dalrymple K. How many different ways do patients meet the diagnostic criteria for major depressive disorder? Compr Psychiatry 56: 29-34.

35. Fitzgerald CT, Messias E, Buysse DJ (2011) Teen sleep and suicidality: Results from the youth risk behavior surveys of 2007 and 2009. J Clin Sleep Med 7: 351-356.

36. Cespedes YM, Huey SJ (2008) Depression in Latino adolescents: A cultural discrepancy perspective. Cultur Divers Ethnic Minor Psychol 14:168-172.

37. Potochnick SR, Perreira KM (2010) Depression and anxiety among first-generation immigrant Latino youth: Key correlates and implications for future research. J Nerv Ment Dis 198: 470-477.

38. Hovey JD, King CA (1996) Acculturative stress, depression, and suicidal ideation among immigrant and second-generation Latino adolescents. J Am Acad Child Adolesc Psychiatry 35: 1183-1192.

39. Bandy T, Moore KA (2016) What works for Latino/Hispanic children and adolescents: Lessons from experimental evaluations of programs and interventions.

40. Burt VK, Stein K (2002) Epidemiology of depression throughout the female life cycle. J Clin Psychiatry. 63: 9-15.

41. Brunstein KA, Marrocco F, Kleinman M, Schonfeld IS, Gould MS. (2007) Bullying, depression, and suicidality in adolescents. J Am Acad Child Adolesc Psychiatry 46: 40-49.

42. Duncan RD, Saunders BE, Kilpatrick DG, Hanson RF, Resnick HS (1996) Childhood physical assault as a risk factor for PTSD, depression, and substance abuse: findings from a national survey. Am J Orthopsychiatry 66: 437-448.

43. Burnam MA, Stein JA, Golding JM, Siegel JM, Sorenson SB, et al. (1988) Sexual assault and mental disorders in a community population. J Consult Clin Psychol 56: 843-850.

44. Fergusson DM, Goodwin RD, Horwood LJ (2003) Major depression and cigarette smoking: Results of a 21-year longitudinal study. Psychol Med 33:1357-1367.

45. Deykin EY, Levy JC, Wells V (1987) Adolescent depression, alcohol and drug abuse. Am J Public Health 77: 178-182.

20

Rehabilitation or Recovery Sleep: A Future Potential Therapeutic Target for Sleep Deprivation

Reena Chittora, Durgesh Sharma and Maheep Bhatnagar*

Department of Zoology, Mohan Lal Sukhadia University, Udaipur, India

***Corresponding author:** Bhatnagar M, Department of Zoology, Mohan Lal Sukhadia University, Udaipur, India, Tel: 0294-2470918; E-mail: mbhatnagar@yahoo.com

Abstract

Sleep is a period of relaxation and repair. During sleep, waste products of brain metabolism are removed. It plays central role in maintenance of physiological homeostasis and psychological balance. Sufficient sleep helps us think more clearly, complete complex tasks better and more consistently. One of the important function of sleep is to promote synaptic plasticity and neuronal recovery for proper brain functioning. Memory consolidation, brain growth and repair are other functions proposed for sleep. Problems related to sleep deprivation are being increased in today's modern society. Every day there seems to be twice as much work and half as much time to complete it, this results in a decrease in sleep or extended periods of wakefulness. Sleep deprived individuals may not have difficulty of verbal disturbances but research studies have shown that individuals have more difficulty in reacting well, to taking biological discussion and implementing the task with efficiency of action. Although day time performance due to sleep loss is experienced universally but in professionals such as paramilitary forces, army personals, who work under stressful conditions are more vulnerable to the sleep deprivation. These conditions become more stressful during emergencies and war because, after periods of extended wakefulness neurons may begin to malfunction, visibly affecting person's behavior. Rapid eye movement (REM) sleep plays a role in learning due to an activation of the hippocampus involved in encoding new memories. Many experiments have shown that the day after a good night's sleep, one may retain newly acquired knowledge or a newly learned skill more effectively. An enriched environment (EE) which is a complex combination of social, cognitive, and physical stimulation, improves learning and memory. Many changes such as increased brain weight, synaptic plasticity, gliogenesis, growth of dendritic spine as well as change in neurotransmitter content, up regulation of neuronal signaling molecules, neurotrophin levels and adult hippocampal neurogenesis have been reported.

Keywords: Sleep; Recovery; Wakefulness; Brain; Memory

Introduction

In this fast moving world, money is earned by sacrificing the basic needs of the body i.e. sleep. Sleep is one of the important needs like oxygen for survival and nutrition for health. Sufficient sleep helps us think more clearly, complete complex tasks better, more consistently. It is a state characterized by absence of consciousness, deferred sensory activity, and inactivity of voluntary muscles. In other words, it is a heightened anabolic state, accentuating the growth and rejuvenation of the immune, nervous, skeletal and muscular systems [1]. Sleep depends on two major factors: A circadian regulator and a homeostatic regulator. Homeostatic regulation means that sleep is delayed and often become more intense after extended waking, thus also called recovery sleep [2]. Xie et al. reported that during sleep, waste products of brain metabolism are removed; this is due to change in milieu of the brain's extracellular space between sleep and waking states [3]. Besides, sleep plays important role to promote synaptic plasticity and neuronal recovery for proper brain functioning [4]. Memory consolidation, brain growth and repair are other functions proposed for sleep [5].

The timing of sleep is organized by the circadian clock and sleep-wake homeostasis. The circadian clock works in association with the neurotransmitter adenosine, that inhibits wakefulness associated processes and cause sleepiness [6].

According to National sleep foundation and National Institutes of Health (NIH), National Center on Sleep Disorders Research and Office of Prevention, Education, and Control, USA 7-9 hours' sleep is necessary for adults or elderly.

Although sleep occupies approximately a one third of the human lifespan, the amount of time humans spend awake has increased over the years. Problems of sleep deprivation (SD) are being increased in today's modern society. SD results in either extended periods of wakefulness or a decrease in sleep over an extended period of time. Sleep deprived individuals though do not have difficulty of verbal disturbances but research studies have shown more difficulty in reacting well, to taking biological discussion and implementing them as well with efficiency of action. Day time effects due to sleep loss are experienced universally but in professionals belonging to paramilitary forces, army personals etc. who work under stressful conditions are more vulnerable to the sleep deprivation as conditions become more stressful during emergencies and war. After periods of extended wakefulness or reduced sleep, neurons may begin to malfunction, visibly affecting a person's behavior [7]. Sleep deprivation ensue mental fatigue, impaired learning, decision-making, epileptic attacks and heightened risk of migraine. Chronic or complete insomnia, which may ultimately, results in death [8].

It has been also evident that sleep deprivation is responsible for the induction and worsening of various neurological disorders. Sleep disorders include the circadian rhythm sleep disorders, narcolepsy, periodic limb movement disorder (PLMD), restless leg syndrome

(RLS), obstructive sleep apnea in which major pauses in breathing occur during sleep. Anxiety is also one of the most important neurobehavioral consequences of rapid eye movement (REM) sleep deprivation and total Sleep deprivation (both REM+NREM) [9,10]. SD also impairs cognition either by adversely affecting the encoding or initial learning of memories (referred to as acquisition) or by affecting memory consolidation. Studies in human subjects, suggested that insomnia markers are possible biomarkers for depression [11].

Recovery Sleep: The Potential Role of Enriched Environment

The old assumption that connections in the adult brain are rigid and no longer modifiable is luckily not true. Indeed, the brain is capable to adapt to new demands the whole life long, which is essential for learning processes and to adapt to our environment as a result of active training, passive exposure or if we suffer from a brain injury. That is what we call neuronal plasticity- the ability of the brain to adapt in response to modified inputs from the environment both structurally and functionally.

Environmental enrichment involves changes to an animal's home cage or secondary exploratory area which provide enhanced sensory, motor, cognitive and potentially social opportunities [12]. Rosenzweig et al. established EE (Environment enrichment) as a scientific concept (Figure 1) [13].

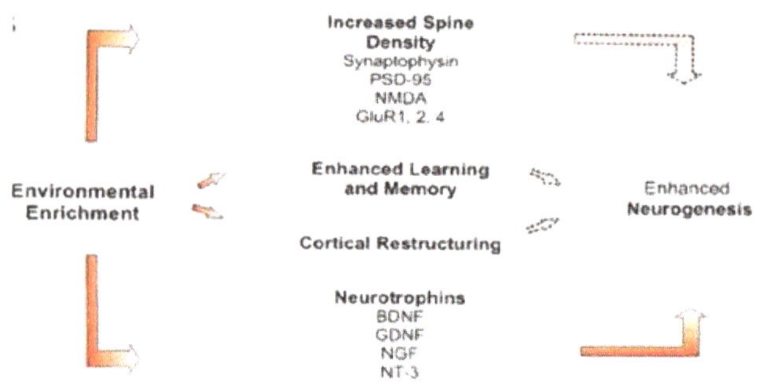

Figure 1: Effect of environmental enrichment on enhanced learning and memory & neurogenesis.

The purpose of EE is to provide possibilities for enhanced voluntary physical exercise, social interactions, multi-sensory and cognitive stimulation. Wakefulness and sleep deprivation are both characterized by increased activity of neuronal cells and increased consumption of ATP while in recovery sleep neuronal activity reduced and decrease consumption of ATP [14].

EE has profound effects on the developing and the adult brain, spanning from the molecular to the anatomical and behavioral level [15,16]. EE increases adult hippocampal neurogenesis by means of survival of new cells in the Dentate gyrus (DG) and involves cortical restructuring and affect different phases of the neurogenic process in distinct ways which improve spatial learning ability [16].

In adult animals, EE leads to better performance in various learning and memory tasks like the Morris-water-maze, the novel object recognition task and fear-conditioning task [17].

EE is also capable of delaying the progression and reducing provoked deficits of various neurological pathologies, including neurodegenerative diseases and stroke [18]. This is possibly due to increased levels of BDNF [19,20] and insulin-like growth factor 1 (IGF-1) [21], enhanced maturation of the inhibitory GABAergic system and accelerated CRE/CREB (cAMP response element-binding protein)-mediated gene expression [19].

In the adult rodent visual cortex, EE increase levels of BDNF (Brain derived neurotrophic factor) [22] and serotonin. Decrease GABA (Gamma amino butyric acid) levels and release [23] and number of GAD67+ interneurons [22,24].

Moreover, EE also increase levels of histone acetylation in the hippocampus and neocortex [25]. Rather, EE exposure actually converses already established long term potentiation (LTP) thus affects dendritic spine density, synaptic proteins receptors expression as well as expression of neurotrophins [26].

Sleep Deprivation and Rehabilitation (Recovery Sleep)

Recovery sleep induce by EE also induces various molecular and structural changes in the brain, contributing to the changes in neuronal functions and ultimate, in behavior. These mechanisms are thought to trigger EE-induced neural plasticity. Social contact and play behavior is important for normal development. The enriched social housing condition has compensated for the adverse effects of SD. Recovery sleep or rehabilitation by an enriched environment helps in removal of toxic by-products of wakefulness and redirects the regenerative power of sleep [27,28].

Effect of Recovery Sleep on Sleep Deprivation Induced Neurodegeneration

The harmful cellular consequences of prolonged waking may result from excitotoxicity and oxidative mechanisms which sensitize the brain to neurodegeneration [29,30]. Morrisey et al. (2003) reported that SD led to decreased brain mass, an increase in expression of apoptotic proteins in the cerebral cortex and, subsequently changes in behavior of adults [31]. EE induced recovery sleep improves neuronal survival, enhances neurogenesis and decreases apoptotic cell death. The survival-promoting effect of enrichment is expressed independently of the cell lineage, resulting in a net increase in both neuronal and glial cells in the dentate gyrus, although proportionally most of these new cells are neurons [32]. Shehata and Rizk reported that the recovery sleep led to ameliorative effects on cognition especially on memory and learning in 3 days sleep deprived rats. This might be due to the regenerative effects of sleep [28]. Wu et al. (2008) showed that the 24 hours of sleep could not reversed the deterioration caused by SD in the pre-frontal cortex, BAX (Bcl-2-associated X protein or a proapoptotic protein), Bcl-2 and the Bcl-2/BAX ratio not returning to basal levels. A possible explanation of this result is that effects of SD on the prefrontal cortex are long-lasting and more time is required for complete recovery [33].

Montes-Rodrı´guez et al. reported that the Bcl-2/BAX ratio increases during recovery sleep following SD and showed that the hippocampus seems to benefit from sleep [34]. An earlier study on p53 and Bcl-2 protein levels (pro- and anti-apoptosis proteins, respectively) after 6 hours of sleep deprivation and 2 hours of post-deprivation sleep (PDS) in the rat hypothalamus revealed an increase in Bcl-2 and p53 after SD and after PDS, the high levels of p53 and Bcl-2 being preserved [35].

Effect of Recovery Sleep on Neurogenesis

Sleep loss is reported to inhibit neurogenesis and cell proliferation in hippocampus, processes involved in learning and memory [36]. Mirescu et al. (2006) found that SD reduces adult neurogenesis and cell proliferation in the hippocampus by elevations in Glucocorticoid level.

The survival of the newborn cells and their neuronal differentiation, appear to be stronger stimulated by environmental enrichment [37,38]. In support of this explanation, previous studies showed that environmental enrichment promote hippocampal neurogenesis and may even decrease or reverse earlier brain deficits [18,39]. Study also suggested that 4 weeks of sleep restriction did not appear to affect the differentiation of new cells into neurons as double cortin (DCX) labeling in the outer granule cell layer (GCL) and subgranular zone (SGZ) of the DG did not differ between the control and sleep restricted groups. However, data showed that recovery sleep caused a significant increment in cell proliferation in the SGZ [40]. Exposure of animals to an EE led to enhanced neurogenesis specifically in the hippocampus and showed improvement in performance of several learning tasks [32]. One study concluded that in addition to increased neurogenesis by enrichment, enhanced synaptogenesis has also been observed in the CA3 and CA1 areas of the dentate gyrus in hippocampus. Hence it is proved that EE enhances proliferation, survival and maturation of neuronal cells, leading to improved cognition [33,34].

EE further modifies the expression of several enzymes, growth factors and transcription factors that are involved in the stimulation of neural stem cells (NSCs). Enhanced neurogenesis associates with improved synaptic plasticity and memory [41]. Hence, approaches aimed towards a better understanding of the modulation and control of neurogenesis, e.g. using peripheral or environmental factors, could have important clinical benefits in sleep disorders.

Effect of Recovery Sleep on Nitrergic Neurotransmitter Level

Sleep homeostasis is the process by which recovery sleep is spawned by prolonged wakefulness. Sleep loss, induced by prolonged wakefulness, produces a decline in cognitive and motor performance, mood disturbances, memory deficits and effects on immune function [42]. These effects are restored by recovery sleep, which is characterized by extension and intensification of both non-rapid eye movement (NREM) and rapid eye movement (REM) components. The possible role of nitric oxide (NO) in the regulation of behavioral state and specifically in the induction of recovery sleep suggesting that NO may have a role as a sleep facilitating agent. Neuronal NO neurotransmitter produced by inducible nitric oxide synthase (iNOS) is an important homeostatic factor in promoting recovery sleep after SD [43]. nNOS is co-localized with acetylcholine (ACh) in most of the basal forebrain (BF) nuclei, as well as in the laterodorsal tegmental (LDT) and pedunculopontine tegmental (PPT) nuclei that project to the BF and is involved in the regulation of the sleep–wake cycle. Study conducted in male rats assigned to EE for 1 year, showed that NO production decreased by 47% in hippocampal submitochondrial membranes of EE rats as compared with control animals [44]. The EE-induced structural and functional changes which include increase cell proliferation, and enhance the number and stability of synapses, occur through molecular cascades that include neurotransmitter levels, improved expression of regulatory proteins and increases in neurotrophic factor that promote neurotransmitter release, [45].

Effect of Recovery Sleep on Cholinergic Neurotransmitter Level

The neurodegeneration caused by SD may spread throughout the brain or affect prevalently specific types of neurons such as the cholinergic neurons. EE also reduces the effects of stress on acetylcholine concentrations. Studies suggested that EE increases the acetylcholine level thus reduces the reactivity of the cholinergic system to stress in the prefrontal cortex [46]. Levels of other neurotransmitters also increase following EE which are associated with synaptic plasticity [47]. EE-induced changes in neurotransmitter levels and excitatory activity also shifts following EE housing, due to an enhanced expression of AMPA and NMDA receptors with increase in hippocampal extracellular glutamate levels [46]. The effects of EE on the increase of acetylcholine in the pre-frontal cortex (PFC) could lead to differences in behavioral parameters such as consolidation of aversive memories and working memory [48].

Effect of Recovery Sleep on Sleep Deprivation Induced Behavioral Changes

Adults with chronic sleep loss report excess mental distress, depressive symptoms, anxiety, and alcohol use [49]. SD is being considered a trait marker for predicting anxiety. Anxiety has been recognized as one of the most important neurobehavioral consequences of rapid eye movement (REM) in sleep deprivation and in total SD (both REM+NREM) [50]. The mechanistic approach to SD induced anxiety is oxidative stress, nitric oxide (NO) stress, neuroinflammation as well as cholinergic signaling.

ROS production and clearance by endogenous antioxidant defense system [51]. The mechanism by which SD induces anxiety may be hypothesized as being linked with elevated oxidative stress in sleep-deprived subjects. Early studies in animals showed that the enhanced stimulation of recovery sleep induces by enriched environment produces many extraordinary benefits at anatomical, molecular as well as at behavioral levels. Exposure to an enriched environment, providing more opportunity for learning and social interaction than standard laboratory living conditions, has been shown to enhance behavioural performance in various learning tasks [52]. One study concluded that the EE mice showed decreased anxiety-like behavior and higher activity, revealed by the increased number of entries and by a greater percentage of time spent into the open arms of the elevated plus maze in comparison to standard animals. EE reduces fearfulness, as suggested by reduction of defecation in open field tests [53]. At the neurochemical level, earlier study Brenes et al., showed that overall 1 month exposure of EE was enough to produce strong behavioral and neurochemical effects. Social isolation increase 5-HT or serotonin turnover without affecting the tissue levels of 5-HT and norepinephrine (NE), a stress hormone in rats [54]. Nitric oxide synthase (NOS) enzyme is also involved in the regulation of anxiety, sleep and aggressive behavior.

Effect of Recovery Sleep on Cognitive Performance

Many studies have shown that acute sleep deprivation affects cognitive performance and emotionality. Previous experimental studies in healthy human subjects showed that successive nights of restricted sleep resulted in a gradually accruing decline in cognitive function [55]. Another study conducted by Franzen et al. compared a group of 15 healthy, young human adults following one night of sleep deprivation with 14 who had normal sleep and concluded that sleep deprivation led to performance and mood deficits [56]. Study by Lim and Dinges suggested that sleep deprivation leads to a general slowing in response time, an increase in incorrect responses, and time-on task effect. Sustained attention deficits are responsible for many of the performance deficits in memory and executive functioning tasks following sleep deprivation [57].

The recovery processes of cognitive deficits after sleep loss are still obscure. Recovery sleep is different from normal sleep. Evidence suggested that one sleep period (at least eight hours) can reverse the adverse effects of total SD on cognition [58]. After chronic partial sleep restriction, it seems to take longer the recovery process of cognitive functioning than after acute total SD. One study observed that after one week of sleep restriction, three 8 h recovery nights were not enough to restore performance even in the group that spent 7 hrs in bed [59]. Thus concluded that the brain adapted to a stressful condition, during mild and moderate chronic partial SD, yet at a reduced level to maintain performance in humans. This adaptation process was obviously so challenging that it postponed the restoration of normal functioning. One recovery night is enough to restore cognitive performance and daytime sleepiness deficits induced by acute or chronic sleep deprivation [60]. A study investigating recovery after a period of chronic sleep restriction suggested that a single recovery night of up to 10 hrs time in bed is insufficient for some behavioral functions to return to prerestriction levels and deficits were reversed by repeated nights of recovery sleep [61]. Rehabilitation in traumatic brain injury (TBI) patients based on EE principles results in improved cognitive and motor skills [62]. A number of studies have also shown that by increasing the duration and intensity of exposure to rehabilitative therapy results in improved recovery times.

Conclusion

"Sleep is in essential, food for the brain. Insufficient sleep can be harmful, even life threatening. Sleep is thus an essential element, in learning and memory which allows us to perform critical daily functions at peak optimization when obtaining the correct amount. Sleep is important because it has a determining role in mental and physical health of individual, along with quality of life. In conclusion, sleep deprivation is a biological stress condition for the brain. All physiological and neurological changes due to SD ultimately lead to physical/cellular stress or oxidative stress, a condition which is a major cause of neurodegeneration [63]. SD cause hippocampal volume to be reduced because of neuronal cell death, diminished arborization in dendrites, slowed neurogenesis and a decreased number of glial cells.

An enriched environment (EE) which is a complex combination of social, cognitive, and physical stimulation has shown improvement in learning and memory in rodents housing in an EE. In particular, changes in neurotransmitter content, gliogenesis, synaptic plasticity and dendritic spine growth, increased brain weight, as well as up regulation of neurotransmitters, neurotrophin levels and adult hippocampal neurogenesis have been associated with cognitive enhancement.

By providing the environment necessary for neuronal maintenance and repair, it has been proposed that recovery sleep with novel and complex multisensory environments should result in enhancement in neural plasticity as well as various neurological and behavioral changes also occur. Current body of literature on the effects of rehabilitation by means of recovery sleep in neurological disease indicates that Environmental Enrichment represents significant therapeutic potential, on its own and in combination with pharmacological treatments. This is by inducing neuroprotective mechanisms and behavioral outcomes underlying molecular mechanisms of experience-induced plasticity that possibly can be used to identify new therapeutic targets.

Competing Interests

The authors declare that they have no competing interests.

References

1. Stenberg D (2007) Neuroanatomy and neurochemistry of sleep. Cell Mol Life Sci 64: 1187-1204.
2. Lack LC, Wright HR (2007) Chronobiology of sleep in humans. Cell Mol Life Sci 64: 1205-1215.
3. Xie L, Kang H, Xu Q, Chen MJ, Liao Y, et al. (2013) Sleep drives metabolite clearance from the adult brain. Science 342: 373-377.
4. Torabi-Namia M, Nasehie M, Zarrindasta MR (2013) Sleep loss and the brain vulnerability to neurodegeneration: behavioral, biochemical and neuro-histopathological observations in a rat model. J Excli 12: 347-372.
5. Kumar VM (2008) Sleep and sleep disorders. Indian J Chest Dis Allied Sci 50: 129.
6. Wyatt JK, Ritz-De Cecco A, Czeisler CA, Dijk DJ (1999) Circadian temperature and melatonin rhythms, sleep, and neurobehavioral function in humans living on a 20-h day. Am J Physiol Regul Integr Comp Physiol 277: R1152-R1163.
7. Ledoux S (2008) The Effects of Sleep Deprivation on Brain and Behavior. http://serendip.brynmawr.edu/exchange/node/1690.
8. Herculano-Houzel S (2013) Sleep it out. Science 342: 316-317.
9. Hagewoud R, Havekes R, Novati A, Keijser JN, Van der Zee EA, et al. (2010) Sleep deprivation impairs spatial working memory and reduces hippocampal AMPA receptor phosphorylation. J Sleep Res 19: 280-288.
10. Martins PJ, Nobrega JN, Tufik S, D'Almeida V (2008) Sleep deprivation-induced gnawing-relationship to changes in feeding behavior in rats. Physiol Behav 93: 229-234.
11. Szklo-Coxe M, Young T, Peppard PE, Finn LA, Benca RM (2010) Prospective associations of insomnia markers and symptoms with depression. Am J Epidemiol 454: 709-720.
12. Reynolds S, Lane SJ, Richards L (2010) Using animal models of enriched environments to inform research on sensory integration intervention for the rehabilitation of neurodevelopmental disorders. J Neurodev Disord 2: 120-132.
13. Rosenzweig I, Glasser M, Polsek D, Leschziner GD, Williams SC, et al. (2015) Sleep apnoea and the brain: A complex relationship. Lancet Respir Med 3: 404-414.
14. Dworak M, McCarley RW, Kim T, Kalinchuk AV, Basheer R (2010) Sleep and brain energy levels: ATP changes during sleep. J Neurosci 30: 9007–9016.
15. Van Praag H, Kempermann G, Gage FH (2000) Neural consequences of environmental enrichment. Nat Rev Neurosci 1: 191-198.
16. Baroncelli L, Braschi C, Spolidoro M, Begenisic T, Sale A, et al. (2010a) Nurturing brain plasticity: Impact of environmental enrichment. Cell Death Differ 17: 1092-1103.
17. Rampon C, Tsien JZ (2000) Genetic analysis of learning behavior-induced structural plasticity. Hippocampus 10: 605-609.
18. Nithianantharajah J, Hannan AJ (2006) Enriched environments, experience-dependent plasticity and disorders of the nervous system. Nat Rev Neurosci 7: 697-709.
19. Cancedda L, Putignano E, Sale A, Viegi A, Berardi N, et al. (2004) Acceleration of visual system development by environmental enrichment. J Neurosci 24: 4840-4848.

20. Sale A, Putignano E, Cancedda L, Landi S, Cirulli F, et al. (2004) Enriched environment and acceleration of visual system development. Neuropharmacology 47: 649-660.

21. Maya-Vetencourt JF, Baroncelli L, Viegi A, Tiraboschi E, Castren E, et al. (2012) IGF-1 restores visual cortex plasticity in adult life by reducing local GABA levels. Neural Plast 2012: 250421.

22. Tognini P, Manno I, Bonaccorsi J, Cenni MC, Sale A, et al. (2012) Environmental enrichment promotes plasticity and visual acuity recovery in adult monocular amblyopic rats. PLoS ONE 7: e34815.

23. Baroncelli L, Bonaccorsi J, Milanese M, Bonifacino T, Giribaldi F, et al. (2012) Enriched experience and recovery from amblyopia in adult rats: impact of motor, social and sensory components. Neuropharmacology 62: 2388-2397.

24. Scali M, Baroncelli L, Cenni MC, Sale A, Maffei L (2012) A rich environmental experience reactivates visual cortex plasticity in aged rats. Exp Gerontol 47: 337-341.

25. Fischer A, Sananbenesi F, Wang XY, Dobbin M, Tsai LH (2007) Recovery of learning and memory is associated with chromatin remodelling. Nature 447: 178-182.

26. Olson AK, Eadie BD, Ernst C, Christie BR (2006) Environmental enrichment and voluntary exercise massively increase neurogenesis in the adult hippocampus via dissociable pathways. Hippocampus 16: 250-260.

27. He Y, Jones CR, Fujiki N, Xu Y, Guo B, et al. (2009) The transcriptional repressor DEC2 regulates sleep length in mammals. Science 325: 866-870.

28. Shehata AM, Rizk HA (2015) Total sleep deprivation compromises blood–brain barrier integrity and impairs learning and memory: A protective effect of glibenclamide and recovery sleep. J Global Biosci 4: 1971-1981.

29. Cirelli C, Shaw PJ, Rechtschaffen A, Tononi G (1999) No evidence of brain cell degeneration after long-term sleep deprivation in rats. Brain Res 840: 184-193.

30. Vyazovskiy VV, Olcese U, Hanlon EC, Nir Y, Cirelli C, et al. (2011) Local sleep in awake rats. Nature 472: 443-447.

31. Morrissey MJ, Duntley SP, Anch AM, Nonneman R (2004) Active sleep and its role in the prevention of apoptosis in the developing brain. Med Hypotheses 62: 876-879.

32. Bruel-Jungerman E, Laroche S, Rampon C (2005) New neurons in the dentate gyrus are involved in the expression of enhanced long-term memory following environmental enrichment. Eur J Neurosci 21: 513-521.

33. Wu H, Zhao Z, Stone WS, Huang L, Zhuang J, et al. (2008) Effects of sleep restriction periods on serum cortisol levels in healthy men. Brain Res Bull 77: 241-245.

34. Montes-Rodríguez CJ, Alavez S, Soria-Gómez E, Rueda-Orozco PE, Guzman K, et al. (2009) BCL-2 and BAX proteins expression throughout the light–dark cycle and modifications induced by sleep deprivation and rebound in adult rat brain. J Neurosci Res 87: 1602-1609.

35. Artamokhina IV, Belova VA, Romanova IV (2011) Immunohistochemical investigation of Bcl-2 and p53 levels in rat hypothalamus after sleep deprivation. J Evol Biochem Physiol 47: 391-395.

36. Alkadhi K, Zagaar M, Alhaider I, Salim S, Aleisa A (2013) Neurobiological consequences of sleep deprivation. Curr Neuropharmacol 11: 231.

37. Mirescu C, Peters JD, Noiman L, Gould E (2006) Sleep deprivation inhibits adult neurogenesis in the hippocampus by elevating glucocorticoids. Proc Natl Acad Sci 103: 19170-19175.

38. Bolijn S, Lucassen PJ (2015) How the body talks to the brain; peripheral mediators of physical activity-induced proliferation in the adult hippocampus. Brain Plast 1: 5-27.

39. Fabel K, Wolf S, Ehninger D, Babu H, Galicia P, et al. (2009) Additive effects of physical exercise and environmental enrichment on adult hippocampal neurogenesis in mice. Front Neurosci 3: 2.

40. Novati A, Hulshof HJ, Granic I, Meerlo P (2012) Chronic partial sleep deprivation reduces brain sensitivity to glutamate N-methyl-d-aspartate receptor-mediated neurotoxicity. J Sleep Res 21: 3-9.

41. Rampon C, Tang YP, Goodhouse J, Shimizu E, Kyin M, et al. (2000) Enrichment induces structural changes and recovery from nonspatial memory deficits in CA1 NMDAR1-knockout mice. Nat Neurosci 3: 238-244.

42. Valero J, España J, Parra-Damas A, Martín E, Rodríguez-Álvarez J, et al. (2011) Short-term environmental enrichment rescues adult neurogenesis and memory deficits in APP (Sw, Ind) transgenic mice. PloS one 6: e16832-e16832.

43. Voss MW, Vivar C, Kramer AF, van Praag H (2013) Bridging animal and human models of exercise-induced brain plasticity. Trends Cogn Sci 17: 525-544.

44. Faraut B, Boudjeltia KZ, Vanhamme L, Kerkhofs M (2012) Immune, inflammatory and cardiovascular consequences of sleep restriction and recovery. Sleep Med Rev 16: 137-149.

45. Kalinchuk AV, McCarley RW, Porkka-Heiskanen T, Basheer R (2010) Sleep deprivation triggers inducible nitric oxide-dependent Nitric oxide production in wake–active basal forebrain neurons. J Neurosci 30: 13254-13264.

46. Lores-Arnaiz S, Arnaiz ML, Czerniczyniec A, Cuello M, Bustamante J (2010) Mitochondrial function and nitric oxide production in hippocampus and cerebral cortex of rats exposed to enriched environment. Brain Res 1319: 44-53.

47. Alonso-Alconada D, Álvarez A, Arteaga O, Martínez-Ibargüen A, Hilario E (2013) Neuroprotective effect of melatonin: A novel therapy against perinatal hypoxia-ischemia. Int J Mol Sci 14: 9379-9395.

48. Segovia G, Del Arco A, Garrido P, de Blas M, Mora F (2008) Environmental enrichment reduces the response to stress of the cholinergic system in the prefrontal cortex during aging. Neurochem Int 52: 1198-1203.

49. Garrido P, De Blas M, Ronzoni G, Cordero I, Antón M, et al. (2013) Differential effects of environmental enrichment and isolation housing on the hormonal and neurochemical responses to stress in the prefrontal cortex of the adult rat: relationship to working and emotional memories. J Neural Transm 120: 829-843.

50. Hasler G, Buysse DJ, Gamma A, Ajdacic V, Eich D, et al. (2005) Excessive daytime sleepiness in young adults: A 20-year prospective community study. J Clin Psychiatry 66: 521-529.

51. Pires GN, Tufik S, Andersen ML (2013) Grooming analysis algorithm: Use in the relationship between sleep deprivation and anxiety-like behavior. Prog Neuropsychopharmacol Biol Psychiatry 41: 6-10.

52. Gopalakrishnan A, Ji LL, Cirelli C (2004) Sleep deprivation and cellular responses to oxidative stress. Sleep 27: 27-35.

53. Benaroya-Milshtein N, Hollander N, Apter A, Kukulansky T, Raz N, et al. (2004) Environmental enrichment in mice decreases anxiety attenuates stress responses and enhances natural killer cell activity. Eur J Neurosci 20: 1341-1347.

54. Brenes JC, Padilla M, Fornaguera J (2009) A detailed analysis of open-field habituation and behavioral and neurochemical antidepressant-like effects in postweaning enriched rats. Behav Brain Res 197: 125-137.

55. Dinges DF, Rogers NL, Baynard MD (2005) Chronic sleep deprivation. Principles and practice of sleep medicine.

56. Franzen PL, Siegle GJ, Buysse DJ (2008) Relationships between affect, vigilance, and sleepiness following sleep deprivation. J Sleep Res 17: 34-41.

57. Lim J, Dinges DF (2008) Sleep deprivation and vigilant attention. Ann N Y Acad Sci 1129: 305-322.

58. Kendall AP, Kautz MA, Russo MB, Killgore WD (2006) Effects of sleep deprivation on lateral visual attention. Int J Neurosci 116: 1125-1138.

59. Belenky G, Wesensten NJ, Thorne DR, Thomas ML, Sing HC, et al. (2003) Patterns of performance degradation and restoration during sleep restriction and subsequent recovery: A sleep dose-response study. J Sleep Res 12: 1-12.

60. Philip P, Sagaspe P, Prague M, Tassi P, Capelli A, et al. (2012) Acute versus chronic partial sleep deprivation in middle-aged people: Differential effect on performance and sleepiness. Sleep 35: 997.

61. Goel N, Basner M, Rao H, Dinges DF (2013) Circadian rhythms, sleep deprivation, and human performance. Prog Mol Bio Transl Sci 119: 155-190.

62. Alwis DS, Rajan R (2014) Environmental enrichment and the sensory brain: The role of enrichment in remediating brain injury. Front Syst Neurosci 8.

63. Chittora R, Jain A, Suhalka P, Sharma C, Jaiswal N, et al. (2015) Sleep deprivation: Neural regulation and consequences. Sleep Biol Rhythms 13: 210-218.

Relation of Snoring Habits with Body Mass Index and Neck Circumference among Adult Population

Biswas RSR[1*], Rahman MH[2] and Fazlee Kibria Chowdhury Md[1]

[1]*Department of Medicine, Chattagram Maa O Shishu Hospital Medical College, Agrabad, Chittagong, Bangladesh*

[2]*Department of Medicine, Chittagong Medical College, Chittagong, Bangladesh*

[*]**Corresponding author:** Biswas RSR, Assistant Professor, Department of Medicine, Chattagram Maa O Shishu Hospital Medical College, Agrabad, Chittagong, Bangladesh, E-mail: rajatbiswas76@yahoo.com

Abstract

Objective: To observe the frequency of snoring and its relation with body mass index (BMI) and neck circumference (NC) among Bangladeshi adult Population.

Method: A cross sectional study was designed among 119 adult healthy Bangladeshi population who were the accompanying persons of patients visiting the medicine outdoors of a tertiary care hospital, Chittagong, Bangladesh. A 'Snore Survey' questionnaire based on Berlin Questionnaire was used to find the snoring frequency. BMI was calculated as weight in kg/height^2 and NC was measured by placing a measuring tape just below the Adam's apple and extending the tape horizontally around the neck. Data was analyzed by SPSS 20.

Results: With a valid response rate of 88.1%, 63 (52.94%) male and 56 (47.06%) female were recruited. Frequency of snoring was 28 (23.5%) of total subjects where male snorer was 33.3% and female snorer was 12.5%. Snoring distributed from daily to monthly phenomenon. Some had very loud (25.0%) snoring and others also had variable loudness. Snorers had statistically significant higher level of body weight and NC ($P<0.001$) but statistically insignificant height and BMI differences ($P>0.05$).

Conclusion: Snoring is more common in males and those having higher body weight and neck circumference among Bangladeshi adult population.

Keywords: Neck circumference; BMI; Snoring

Introduction

Snoring is regarded as a common condition nowadays. Years ago it was regarded as a social nuisance and was thought as a harmless matter for the victim but now it is a matter of medical importance and related with many adverse health consequences. Frequency of snoring is 16%-89% in general populations, about 50% adult male and 24%-50% adult female are snorer with male to female ratio is 2.35: 1 [1,2]. It is a common condition, caused by movement of air across soft tissues of mouth and throat. Snoring is one end of the spectrum of sleep disordered breathing with Obstructive Sleep Apnea (OSA) at the other end. Snoring can be considered as a predecessor of OSA and needs to be evaluated and managed at an early stage. There is a close relationship between body anthropometry and snoring. Overweight induces multiple physiologic changes at the respiratory and circulatory system level. 24% of overweight men, 9% of women have Sleep Disordered Breathing compared with 1%-4% of total population. It may lead to obstructive sleep apnea (OSA) which requires an overnight PSG, which is an expensive test with limited availability. If we can predict sleep apnea early it will be great in a resource poor setting like Bangladesh. Neck circumference (NC), body mass index (BMI), snoring with pauses and excessive daytime sleepiness are simple some inexpensive simple tools which can be used for this prediction. So the present study was designed to see the relation of snoring habit with NC and BMI in the context of Bangladeshi populations.

Method

This study was conducted in a tertiary care hospital of Bangladesh, among 119 healthy persons. During consulting the diseased person, the accompanying attendant who carried the patients were explained about the study and after an informed written consent from him/her, a structured questionnaire were introduced. Subjects were interviewed face to face using 'snore survey' questionnaire which was adopted from the Berlin questionnaire. Detailed information regarding snoring like snoring loudness, snoring frequency, bothersome snoring and non-bothersome snoring were recorded. BMI was calculated as weight in kg/height^2 and NC was measured by placing a measuring tape just below the Adam's apple and extending the tape horizontally around the neck. Data was analyzed by SPSS 20.

Results

Among the 119 respondents frequency of snoring was 23.5% (28). Where male snorer was 33.3% and female snorer was 12.5%. Snoring distributed from daily to monthly attacks. Some had very loud (25.0%) snoring and others also had variable loudness (Table 1). Among all 52.94% (63) male and 47.06% (56) female subjects were recruited. Male to female ratio was 1: 0.88 (Table 2). Snorers had statistically significant higher level of body weight and NC (P<0.001) but statistically insignificant height and BMI differences (P>0.05) (Table 3).

Snoring characteristics		Frequency	Percentage (%)
Snoring Status	1. Snorers	28	23.5
	2. Non snorers	84	70.6
	3. Not known	7	5.9
Snoring frequency	1. Almost every day	7	25
	2. 1-2 times per week	6	21.4
	3. 3-4 times per week	7	25
	4. 1-2 times per month	8	28.6
Snoring loudness	1. Loud as breathing	8	28.6
	2. Loud as talking	8	28.6
	3. Louder than talking	5	17.8
	4. Very loud	7	25
Snoring bothers others	1. Yes	15	53.6
	2. No	13	46.4

Table 1: Snoring characteristics of study subjects.

Gender		Frequency	Percentage (%)
Male	Present	21	33.3
	Absent	35	55.6
	Unknown	7	11.1
	Total	63	100
Female	Present	7	12.5
	Absent	49	87.5
	Total	56	100

Table 2: Gender distribution with snoring among the study subjects.

Snoring		N	Mean	Std. Deviation	P value*
Height in meter	Present	28	1.6804	0.09343	0.569
	Absent	84	1.6394	0.37456	
Body weight in Kg	Present	28	67.3214	7.49347	0.001
	Absent	84	61.4286	7.59087	
BMI	Present	28	23.7903	0.92233	0.983
	Absent	84	23.8066	4.01783	
Neck circumference	Present	28	36.75	2.63347	0.001
	Absent	84	34.3333	2.6083	
*p value is calculated by independent sample t test					

Table 3: Relation of snoring with height, weight, BMI and neck circumferences.

Discussion

With a valid response rate of 88.1%, 63 (52.94%) male and 56 (47.06%) female were recruited. Frequency of snoring was 28 (23.5%) of total subjects where male snorer was 33.3% and female snorer was 12.5%. In an Indian Study found 24%-50% of men, 14%-30% of women are snorer [3]. Snoring distributed from daily to monthly attacks. Some had very loud (25.0%) snoring and others also had variable loudness. A study done in India on apparently healthy attendants of patients in whom snoring was found in 31.1%. In another Indian study done by Udwadia et al. who found the prevalence of snoring of about 26% in middle-aged urban community [4].

Snorers had statistically significant higher level of body weight and NC ($P<0.001$) but statistically insignificant height and BMI differences ($P>0.05$). Body mass index was found uninfluenced in relation with snoring frequency which subsequently may lead to OSA. As the higher NC and BMI are on the higher side in the middle-aged population, there is greater prevalence of snoring and severe OSA in this age group. According to Bixler et al. the average BMI did increase with age for subjects with OSA [5]. As the present study is done on a small sample size (n=119) further large scale study is needed to explore whether these anthropometric variables actually has any influence in snoring status and also to have a strong conclusion. From this study it was found that snoring is not an uncommon medical condition among healthy young people. Considering the large population of Bangladesh these data may be poor and it needs a large scale study for the awareness among the patients as well as health professionals about this neglected but very significant health problem.

References:

1. Jones TM, Swift AC (2000) Snoring: Recent developments. Hospital Medicine 61: 330-334.
2. Koskenvuo M, Partinen M, Kaprio J (1994) Snoring and cardiovascular risk factors. Ann Med 26: 371-376.
3. Prasad R, Garg R, Verma RK, Agarwal SP, Ahuja RC (2006) A study on snoring habits in healthy population of Lucknow. J Sleep Med 1: 37-40.
4. Udwadia ZF, Doshi AV, Lonkar SG, Singh CI (2004) Prevalence of sleep disordered breathing and sleep apnea in middle aged urban Indian men. Am J Respir Crit Care Medicine 169: 168-173.
5. Bixler EO, Vgontzas AN, TenHave T, Tyson K, Kales A (1998) Effects of age on sleep apnea in men: I. Prevalence and severity. Am J Respir Crit Care Med 157: 144-148.

Resolution of Sleep Bruxism using Biomimetic Oral Appliance Therapy

Felix Liao[1] **and G Dave Singh**[2*]

[1]7115 Leesburg Pike, Suite 310, Falla Church, VA 22043, USA

[2]BioModeling Solutions, Inc., 17933 NW Evergreen Parkway, Suite 280, Beaverton, OR 97006, USA

[*]**Corresponding author:** G Dave Singh, DDSc PhD DMD, BioModeling Solutions, Inc., 17933 NW Evergreen Parkway, Suite 280, Beaverton, OR 97006, USA, E-mail: drsingh@drdavesingh.com

Abstract

Background: Evidence suggests that sleep bruxism is centrally regulated, and that the highest risk factor associated with sleep bruxism is obstructive sleep apnea. Current treatments for sleep bruxism include dental night-guards or occlusal splints, which are often provided without upper airway or sleep assessments. Methods: In this case report, we used biomimetic oral appliance therapy to address sleep bruxism by redeveloping the maxilla and repositioning the mandible in a 17 yr. old, female patient.

Results: The upper airway volume increased by 313% (from 7.7 cm^3 to 24.1 cm^3) and the minimum upper airway cross-sectional area increased by 230% from (120 mm^2 to 276.5 mm^2), which improved both sleep bruxism and orthodontic relapse.

Conclusion: We conclude that dentists and orthodontists can help in the recognition and treatment of both sleep bruxism and malocclusion, thereby preventing systemic co-morbidities associated with obstructive sleep apnea.

Keywords: Sleep bruxism; Nocturnal bruxism; Obstructive sleep apnea; Biomimetic; Oral appliance

Abbreviations:

SB: Sleep Bruxism; OSA: Obstructive Sleep Apnea; AOB: Anterior Open Bite; CPAP: Continuous Positive Airway Pressure

Introduction

Bruxism occurs in over 50% of children aged 3-5 yrs., with significant oral and systemic consequences [1]. In adults, a study that relied on self-reporting found that about 8% of a general sample admitted to sleep bruxism (SB) [2]. More specifically, it is thought that about 25% of patients diagnosed with obstructive sleep apnea (OSA) have SB [3]. Indeed, over 50% of patients with mild OSA and 40% of patients with moderate OSA have concomitant SB [4]. Therefore, it appears that SB is related to OSA.

It is thought that SB is a neural response to stress that is mediated via the jaws [5]. Indeed, resolution of episodes of apnea during sleep is thought to eliminate SB [6]. It has been shown in sleep studies that EEG signals spike 4s before an SB event [5], indicating that SB is a centrally-mediated event, and not simply a local, dental occurrence. In fact, the same study [5] showed tachycardia 10s after the SB event, suggesting that SB is associated with a stressor, possibly oxygen desaturation, during sleep. Interestingly, transient hypertension is also associated with SB, as the blood pressure increases by about 25% after SB events [7], indicating that SB is associated with sympathetic activation. It is also thought that SB is associated with micro-arousals during sleep [5], possibly related to upper airway obstruction.

In addition to the above, rhythmic masticatory muscle activity (RMMA) is thought to be secondary to a sequence of events in relation to micro-arousals [8] and, not surprisingly, nearly 90% of SB events occur during periods of sleep arousal. In an earlier study, RMMA was found to be 3 times higher in patients with SB than in controls. However, not all RMMA episodes are accompanied by tooth grinding, and many patients or family members may not be aware of this para-functional activity [8]. But it is thought that contractions of the masticatory muscles are associated with arousal and/or transient oxygen desaturation in patients with OSA [9]. Therefore, we surmise that SB is a sympathetic-activating event likely in response to hypoxia, and appears to be regulated centrally, not peripherally [10].

This case report describes the clinical management of a young patient with SB and anterior open bite (AOB) 3 yrs. after conventional orthodontic treatment, showing resolution of the former and concomitant improvement of the latter.

Case Report

Aside from continuous positive airway pressure (CPAP), oral appliance therapy helps to maintain the upper airway during sleep. But, some cases can develop unwanted occlusal changes and possibly temporo-mandibular joint dysfunction following long-term oral appliance use [11].

This case report refers to a 17 yr. old female (Figure 1) who gave informed consent and signed a patient release form. She was initially referred by a Chiropractor to our dental office with a chief complaint of bruxism.

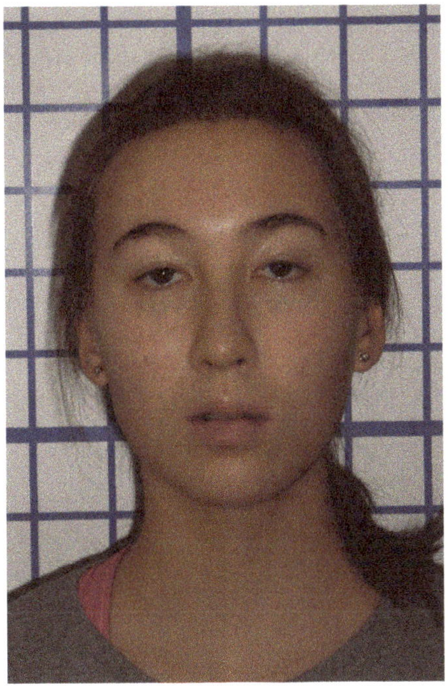

Figure 1: Note the counterclockwise rotation of the head. Sclera is visible below the iris on both sides, suggesting midfacial hypoplasia. The lips apart posture indicates mouth-breathing.

The patient admitted to grinding her teeth and had worn holes through her night-guard (Figure 2). Screening revealed a history of orthodontic treatment at age 14 yrs. Currently, the patient exhibited a significant degree of orthodontic relapse, presenting as AOB. She also admitted to snoring while asleep, as well as having neck and shoulder pain. The patient had a social history of being a tennis player.

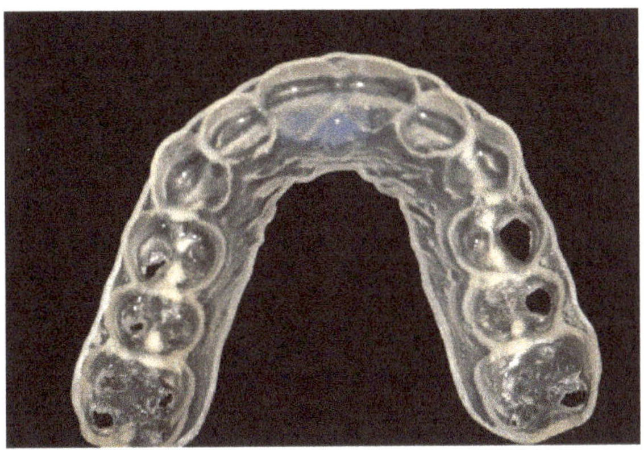

Figure 2: The patient had worn holes through her night-guard, revealing a history sleep bruxism.

Examination and Assessment

After the patient completed a psychometric assessment in the form of an Epworth Sleepiness Scale (ESS) questionnaire, physical and 3D cone-beam CT scan (i-CAT Imaging Sciences International, PA) evaluations were undertaken, including 3D analysis (Invivo5 software, Anatomage Inc., San Jose, CA), which revealed the following findings; An ESS total score of 10. Forward head posture (Figure 3) with counterclockwise rotation of the head (Figure 1), indicating cervical subluxation.

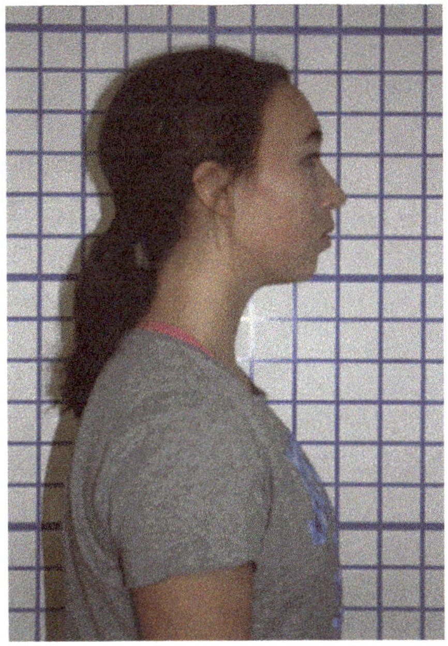

Figure 3: Counterclockwise rotation of the head from lateral aspect, revealing forward head posture and mandibular retrognathia.

Anterior open bite with anterior crowding (Figure 4A and 4B), indicating orthodontic relapse.

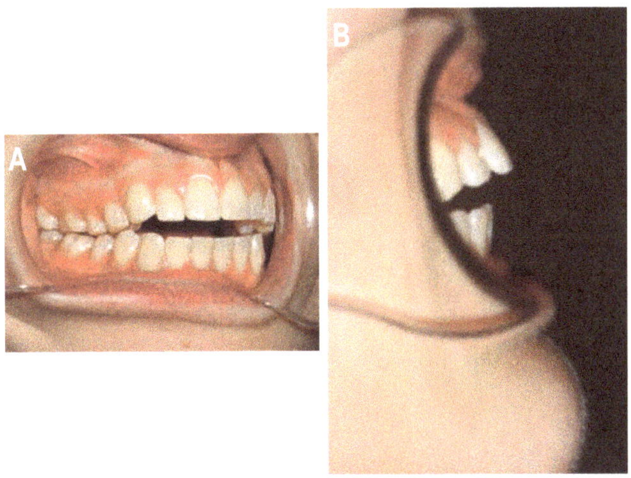

Figure 4: (A) The anterior open bite is evident with minor anterior crowding in the upper arch, indicating orthodontic relapse. (B) The anterior open bite is evident from the lateral aspect, indicating orthodontic relapse.

Flattened cusps of posterior teeth (Figure 5), indicating sleep bruxism.

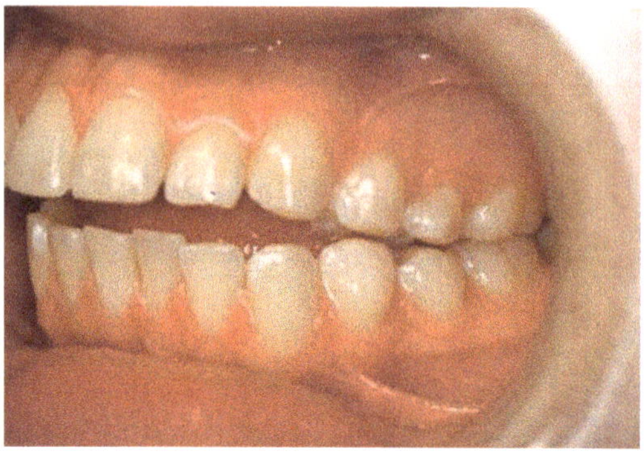

Figure 5: Note the flattened cusps of posterior teeth, indicating sleep bruxism.

Uvula not visible with mouth open (Figure 6) with Mallampati class IV, suggesting upper airway obstruction.

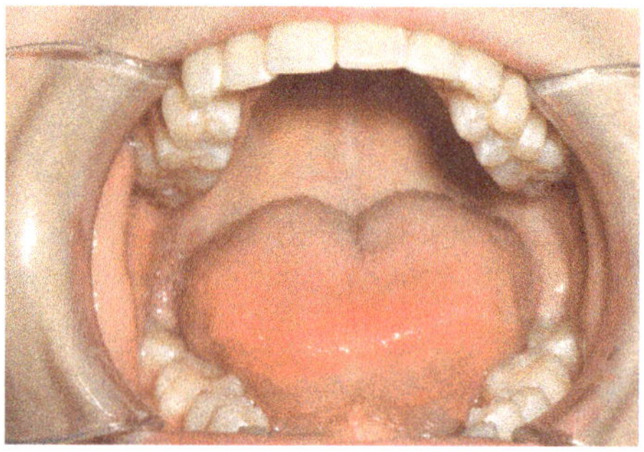

Figure 6: The uvula is not visible with mouth open (Mallampati class IV), suggesting upper airway obstruction.

Nasal and upper airway obstruction with an upper airway volume of 7.7 cm^3 and a minimum cross-sectional area of 120 mm^2 (Figure 7).

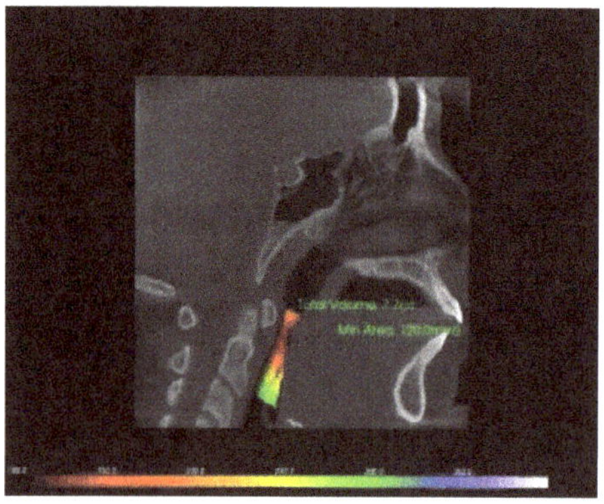

Figure 7: An upper airway volume of 7.7 cm^3 and a minimum cross-sectional area of 120 mm^2 indicates a degree of upper airway obstruction.

Diagnosis

The working and differential diagnoses in this case included; Class I malocclusion with anterior open bite (apertognathia), Maxillary hypoplasia and mandibular retrognathia, Obstructive sleep apnea with hypersomnia, Mandibular dyskinesia, and Cervicalgia.

Therefore, a comprehensive treatment plan was formulated as noted below.

Treatment

The patient was advised to improve her sleep hygiene, including black-out blinds in the bedroom and going to sleep by 11 pm. She was also instructed on keeping her lips closed as much as possible, particularly while at rest. In addition, nutritional counseling [12,13] was implemented. Next, a biomimetic, upper appliance was prescribed (DNA appliance®, Figure 8).

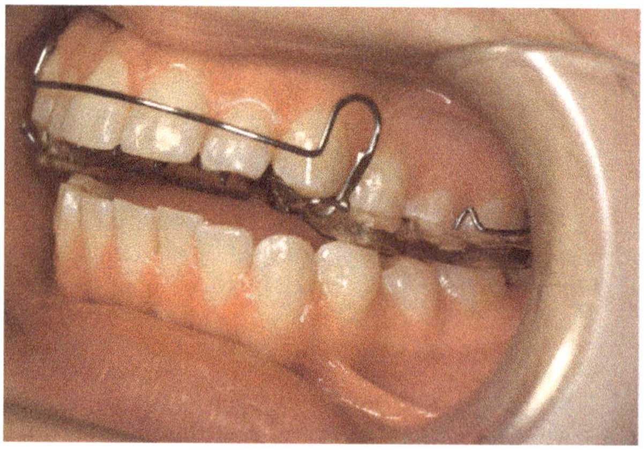

Figure 8: The biomimetic, upper appliance that was prescribed is shown in situ.

The DNA appliance system is designed to correct maxillo-mandibular underdevelopment in both children and adults [14-19]. The patient was instructed to wear the DNA appliance during the late afternoon, early evening and at nighttime during sleep (for approx. 10-12 hrs. in total), but not during the day time and not while eating, partly in line with the circadian rhythm of tooth eruption [20], although this only occurs in children. In addition, a facemask was utilized to protract the maxilla [21]. The patient reported for review and the biomimetic appliance was adjusted every 4 weeks, approximately. At each monthly follow-up, examination for the progress of midfacial development was recorded. Adjustments to the device were performed to optimize its efficacy. Only gentle pressures were transmitted to the teeth, and the functionality of the device was checked with the subject activating a mild force on biting. The patient was encouraged to maintain the sleep, postural and nutritional protocols outlined at the start of treatment.

Results

After 15 months of active treatment, the ESS total score decreased from 10 to 4, the upper airway volume increased from 7.7 cm^3 to 24.1 cm^3 and the minimum cross-sectional area increased from 120 mm^2 to 276.5 mm^2 (Figures 7 and 9).

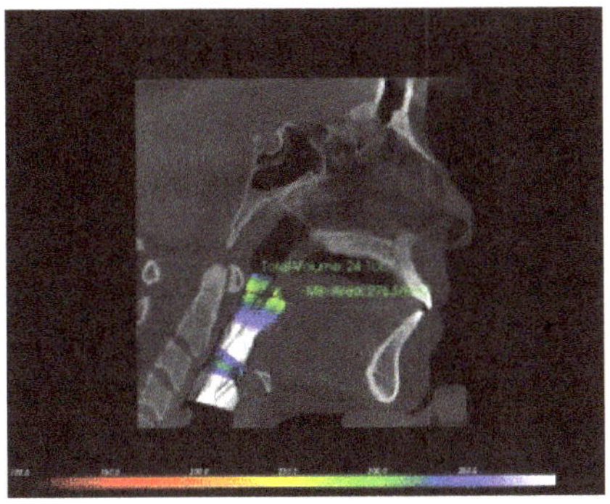

Figure 9: After 15 months of active treatment, the upper airway volume increased to 24.1 cm^3 (from 7.7 cm^3) and the minimum cross-sectional area increased to 276.5 mm^2 from 120 mm^2 (as shown in Figure 7 above).

Thus, the upper airway volume increased by 313% and the minimum upper airway cross-sectional area increased by 230%. Moreover, the patient reported that she was no longer grinding her teeth and was no longer snoring at night. In addition, she noticed an improved facial appearance and smile esthetics (Figure 10A and 10B).

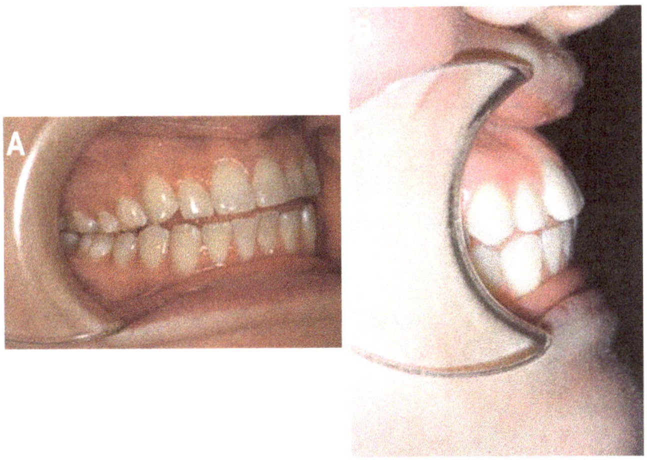

Figure 10: (A) Significant improvement of the anterior open bite, which lays the foundation for final occlusal interdigitation and anterior coupling, using conventional orthodontic techniques. (B) Significant improvement of the anterior open bite from the lateral aspect is evident.

Furthermore, the patient reported that she woke up feeling refreshed and her athletic performance during tennis matches appeared to have improved also.

Discussion

Currently, it is thought that preventive therapy cannot effectively cure sleep bruxism but various treatment protocols for its management are available [22]. This particular case report represents a patient who followed all treatment recommendations conscientiously, and her progress and results appear to reflect her pursuit of health. However, a major limitation of this case report is the lack of a PSG study to document bruxism and OSA at both the baseline and post-treatment phases. However, psychometric measures, such as an Epworth Sleepiness Scale questionnaire were used to confirm the presence of bruxism, its severity and daytime sleepiness. In addition, the patient admitted to grinding her teeth, had worn holes through her night-guard (Figure 2), and the flattened cusps of her posterior teeth (Figure 5) were indicative of sleep bruxism. As a result of biomimetic oral appliance therapy, her upper airway was developed (Figures 7 and 9) so that mouth breathing was corrected and she could revert back to nasal breathing. This change in function appears to have resolved her chief concern of sleep bruxism. In fact, a comparable finding was reported in children that underwent a similar procedure for bruxism [23]. But, in addition, the nasal mode of breathing allowed her lips to contact gently while at rest. This oral posture permitted the tongue to sit in the palate, which is a prerequisite for the resolution of AOB, as noted in this particular case (Figure 10A and 10B).

Currently, the patient is being monitored for long term follow up, and is continuing with atlas-orthogonal chiropractic care as needed. Specifically, an overnight sleep study will be undertaken to assess the patient's sleep architecture and identify any signs of OSA. Indeed, a multi-disciplinary approach will be adopted. For example, it has been shown that both craniofacial [24] and systemic [25] improvements can be achieved using a combination of chiropractic adjustment and biomimetic oral appliance therapy. In addition, oral myofunctional therapy can correct tongue posture and behavior [26,27]. Furthermore, development of the lower arch may be required, using a lower appliance to permit arch re-coordination prior to final occlusal detailing with a finishing phase of orthodontics.

Conclusion

Micro-arousals during sleep are considered to be one of the main factors initiating nocturnal jaw-closing muscles activation or bruxism, which may be related to neurotransmitter and basal ganglia disorders [28]. Therefore, further studies are needed to clarify the pathophysiology of SB and develop new protocols to target therapy for patients with concomitant SB and OSA. A multi-disciplinary approach may be appropriate for patients that present to a dental office with issues relating to SB. The protocol described in this article may also be applicable to cases of posterior open bite associated with mandibular advancement appliance therapy for the management of OSA. That premise remains as the basis for future studies.

Acknowledgement

This work was support by a grant to Dr Felix Liao by The PACE Institute, Oregon, USA, a non-profit entity.

References

1. Hachmann A, Martins EA, Araujo FB, Nunes R (1999) Efficacy of the nocturnal bite plate in the control of bruxism for 3 to 5 year old children. J Clin Pediatr Dent 24: 9-15.
2. Ohayon MM, Li KK, Guilleminault C (2001) Risk factors for sleep bruxism in the general population. Chest 119: 53-61.
3. Subramanian S, Rao S, Majid H, Casturi L, Guntupalli B, et al. (2009) Prevalence and gender and ethnic variance of bruxism and gastroesophageal reflux disease (GERD) in obstructive sleep apnea. Chest 136 (4MeetingAbstracts); 69S.

4. Sjöholm TT, Lowe AA, Miyamoto K, Fleetham JA, Ryan CF (2000) Sleep bruxism in patients with sleep-disordered breathing. Arch Oral Biol 45: 889-896.
5. Bader GG, Kampe T, Tagdae T, Karlsson S, Blomqvist M (1997) Descriptive physiological data on a sleep bruxism population. Sleep 20: 982-990.
6. Oksenberg A, Arons E (2002) Sleep bruxism related to obstructive sleep apnea: the effect of continuous positive airway pressure. Sleep Med 3: 513-515.
7. Nashed A, Lanfranchi P, Rompré P, Carra MC, Mayer P, et al. (2012) Sleep bruxism is associated with a rise in arterial blood pressure. Sleep 35: 529-536.
8. Lavigne GJ, Huynh N, Kato T, Okura K, Adachi K, et al. (2007) Genesis of sleep bruxism: motor and autonomic-cardiac interactions. Arch Oral Biol 52: 381-384.
9. Kato T, Katase T, Yamashita S, Sugita H, Muraki H, et al. (2013) Responsiveness of jaw motor activation to arousals during sleep in patients with obstructive sleep apnea syndrome. J Clin Sleep Med 9: 759-765.
10. Lobbezoo F, Naeije M (2001) Bruxism is mainly regulated centrally, not peripherally. J Oral Rehabil 28: 1085-1091.
11. Pliska BT, Nam H, Chen H, Lowe AA, Almeida FR (2014) Obstructive sleep apnea and mandibular advancement splints: occlusal effects and progression of changes associated with a decade of treatment. J Clin Sleep Med 10: 1285-1291.
12. Price WA (2008) Nutrition and physical degeneration. Price-Pottenger Nutrition Foundation
13. Fallon S (2003) Nourishing Traditions Diet. New Trends Publishing, (2ndedn).
14. Singh GD, Lipka G (2009) Case Report: Introducing the wireframe DNA applianceTM. J Am Acad Gnathol Orthop 26: 8-11.
15. Singh GD, Wendling S, Chandrashekhar R (2011) Midfacial development in adult obstructive sleep apnea. Dent Today 30: 124-127.
16. Singh GD, Utama J (2013) Effect of the DNA Appliance TM on migraine headache: case report. Int J Orthod Milwaukee 24: 45-49.
17. Singh GD, Cress SE (2013) Craniofacial enhancement using a biomimetic oral appliance. Dent Today 32: 92-94.
18. Singh GD, Callister JD (2013) Effect of a maxillary appliance in an adult with obstructive sleep apnea: a case report. Cranio 31: 171-175.
19. Harris WG, Singh GD (2013) Resolution of 'gummy smile' and anterior open bite using the DNA applianceTM: Case Report. J Amer Orthod Soc 30-34.
20. Proffit WR, Frazier-Bowers SA (2009) Mechanism and control of tooth eruption: overview and clinical implications. Orthod Craniofac Res 12: 59-66.
21. Baccetti T, McGill JS, Franchi L, McNamara JA Jr, Tollaro I (1998) Skeletal effects of early treatment of Class III malocclusion with maxillary expansion and face-mask therapy. Am J Orthod Dentofacial Orthop 113: 333-343.
22. Afrashtehfar K, Afrashtehfar CD, Huynh N (2014) Managing a patient with sleep bruxism. J Can Dent Assoc 80: e48.
23. Bellerive A, Montpetit A, El-Khatib H, Carra MC, Remise C, et al. (2015) The effect of rapid palatal expansion on sleep bruxism in children. Sleep Breath.
24. Singh GD and Chapman DC. Craniofacial changes after combined atlas-orthogonal and biomimetic oral appliance therapy. Annals Vert Sub Res. 4, 112-118, 2014.
25. Chapman DC and Singh GD. Combined effect of a biomimetic oral appliance and atlas orthogonist cervical adjustment on leg lengths in adults. Annals Vert Sub Res. 46-50, 2013.
26. Moeller JL, Coceani-Paskay L, Gelb ML (2014) Myofunctional Therapy: A Novel Treatment of Pediatric Sleep-Disordered Breathing. Sleep Med Clin 9: 235–243.
27. Guilleminault C, Huang YS, Monteyrol PJ, Sato R, Quo S, et al. (2013) Critical role of myofascial reeducation in pediatric sleep-disordered breathing. Sleep Med 14: 518-525.
28. Kostrzewa-Janicka J, Jurkowski P, Zycinska K, Przybyłowska D, Mierzwińska-Nastalska E. Sleep-Related Breathing Disorders and Bruxism. Adv Exp Med Biol. 2015 May 29. [Epub ahead of print]

23

Sleep, Pain and Cannabis

Ferguson G and Ware MA

Alan Edwards Pain Management Unit, McGill University Health Centre, Montreal, Quebec, Canada

***Corresponding author:** Dr. Mark A. Ware, A5.140 Montreal General Hospital, 1650 Cedar Avenue, Montreal, Quebec H3G 1A4, Canada, E-mail: mark.ware@mcgill.ca

Abstract

One of the most common reasons that patients report the use of cannabis for medical purposes is to reduce pain and improve sleep. Despite this repeated association, it is not clear whether the effects of cannabis use on pain are mediated by the effect of improved sleep, or vice versa. This distinction may have important therapeutic implications as different cannabis preparations have different pharmacokinetic properties; short acting cannabinoids may therefore initiate sleep but not maintain it, while longer acting cannabinoids may be better at sleep maintenance than initiation. Recent reviews have examined the quantitative outcomes of sleep measures in clinical trials of cannabinoids in a range of disorders but did not focus on pain; others focused exclusively on one cannabinoid preparation. Given the current interest in the potential therapeutic uses of cannabis, we have prepared a general review of sleep, pain and cannabis with a view to identifying gaps in our knowledge that could be addressed in further research.

Keywords: Cannabis; Marijuana; Sleep; Pain

Introduction

One of the most common reasons that patients report the use of cannabis for medical purposes is to reduce pain and improve sleep. Despite this repeated association, it is not clear whether the effects of cannabis use on pain are mediated by the effect of improved sleep, or vice versa. This distinction may have important therapeutic implications as different cannabis preparations have different pharmacokinetic properties; short acting cannabinoids may therefore initiate sleep but not maintain it, while longer acting cannabinoids may be better at sleep maintenance than initiation.

Recent reviews have examined the quantitative outcomes of sleep measures in clinical trials of cannabinoids in a range of disorders [1] but did not focus on pain; others focused exclusively on one cannabinoid preparation [2]. Given the current interest in the potential therapeutic uses of cannabis, we have prepared a general review of sleep, pain and cannabis with a view to identifying gaps in our knowledge that could be addressed in further research.

Cannabinoids: A Primer

Historical evidence suggests that the plant Cannabis sativa has been used for millennia for the treatment of pain and nausea [3]. In cannabis, over 100 cannabinoids (defined as the terpenophenolic compounds found in Cannabis sativa) have been identified, of which the most well-studied are Δ9-tetrahydrocannabinol (THC) and cannabidiol (CBD). The physiological effects of cannabinoids are well described and affect learning and memory, appetite, pain, mood, sleep, movement, reward pathways, as well as effects on the immune system [4,5]. Interestingly, the pharmacological effects of THC appear to be biphasic whereby effects at low doses are different from those at high doses [5].

Two major endogenous cannabinoids have been described: anandamide (AEA) and 2-arachidonoyl glycerol (2-AG). These lipid molecules are synthesized on demand from post-synaptic neurons and bind to G protein-coupled cannabinoid receptors (GPCR) CB1 (located on presynaptic nerve terminals) and CB2 (located on immune cells including microglia and macrophages) [5]. The CB1 receptor is found in the brain regions that have to do with motor control, cognition, emotional responses, motivated behavior, and homeostasis [6]. In humans, the CB1 receptor is found in high density in the central nervous system (CNS) in areas such as the thalamus, hypothalamus, hippocampus, cortex, limbic system, and the basal ganglia [7] (Figure 1).

The role of the CB2 receptor is not as well characterized as the CB1 receptor, but it is believed to have a role in modulation of immune function. CB2 receptors are located in the thymus, lungs, testicles, and spleen and absent from the brain, heart, kidney, and liver [8]. However more recently CB2 receptors were found in the brainstem [9] and their role in neuroinflammation is receiving increased attention [10].

THC acts on CB1 and, to a lesser extent, CB2 receptors and is psychoactive [4]. CBD is non-psychotropic and has a very low affinity for the CB1 and CB2 receptors; CBD has even been found to antagonize CB1 agonists. CBD is currently being examined for suppression of inflammation promoting cytokines in rheumatoid arthritis, and type 1 diabetes, protection against acute and chronic neurodegeneration, anxiety, and cancer. It also has antiemetic and anti-nausea properties [11]. When THC is given to healthy volunteers as a single agent before sleep, overnight memory is impaired in the morning but if equal parts THC: CBD are given there appears to be no memory impairment [12], suggesting that ratios of THC and CBD are important in adverse event profiles.

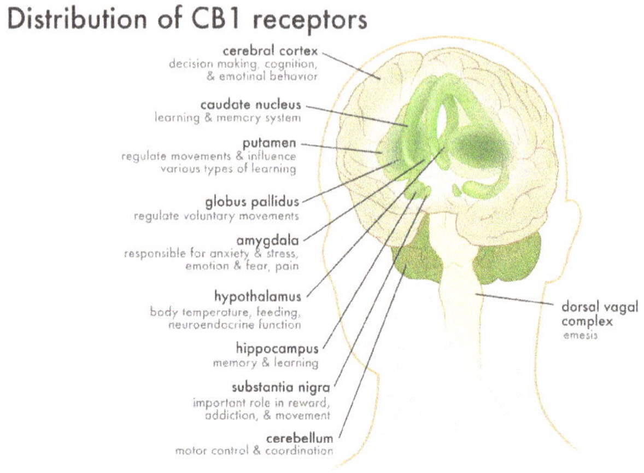

Figure 1: Image courtesy of the Canadian Consortium for the Investigation of Cannabinoids.

Sleep and Pain

Pain is the most common reason for people to seek medical attention, and sleep problems are among the most frequent complaints of acute and chronic pain sufferers. The combined influence of pain and poor sleep can have profound effects on the biological and behavioral state of an individual [13]. Lack of slow wave sleep (SWS) and rapid eye movements (REM) caused by acute or chronic pain has been shown to increase the perception of pain, and recovery from SWS deprivation has a significantly greater analgesic effect than does REM recovery [14].

Pain and sensation are drastically reduced during REM and non-REM sleep [15]. The pathways responsible for this remain poorly understood. Pain is relayed through ascending pathways from the body (spinothalamic tract) and face (trigemino-thalamic tract) to higher cortical areas in the brain [16]. Pain manifests itself in sleep by delaying the onset and fragmenting sleep [17].

Chronic pain patients have a reduction in SWS and poor overall sleep efficiency brought on by microarousals and shifts in sleep stages i.e. sleep fragmentation [18,19]. Ohayon et al. [20] found that 23% of chronic pain sufferers (>= 6 months in duration) had at least one symptom of insomnia and 40.2% of subjects with insomnia symptoms had at least one type of chronic pain. This study however needs to be interpreted cautiously as subjects were not screened for preexisting conditions such as depression which is known to affect sleep. The relationship between pain and sleep may be reciprocal: pain disrupts sleep which in turn exacerbates pain [19].

Monitoring acute pain responses during sleep has shown that noxious intramuscular stimuli force the subject awake regardless of sleep stage, but non-noxious stimuli only causes microarousals [21].

Another study of acute post-operative pain found that total sleep was decreased for 1 to 2 nights and that sleep was fragmented. For the first 2 nights after surgery REM sleep was absent but was made up for on subsequent nights. SWS duration was reduced for up to 4 nights. This study however had many variables as it may not have just been pain that caused the change in sleep but also the hospital environment, stress from surgery and the analgesic medication the patients were administered [13].

Other Conditions Involving Sleep and Pain

There are several well-described conditions which highlight the important interaction between pain and sleep.

Restless leg syndrome

Restless leg syndrome (RLS) is a neurological disorder in which vague painful sensations in the legs occur during periods of muscular inactivity. Pain appears with a circadian rhythm, peaking between midnight and 4:00 am, causing sufferers to be unable to get to sleep [22]. RLS is associated with an increased risk of depression and anxiety [23]; lack of sleep due to RLS contributes to the increase the risk of depressive disorders, and sleep deprivation has been known to exacerbate panic attacks and can even precipitate them in certain individuals [24].

Obstructive sleep apnea

Obstructive sleep apnea (OSA) is defined as a pattern of interrupted breathing during sleep which also causes fractured sleep. Patients with OSA wake up frequently during the night due to lack of oxygen intake caused by the collapse of the upper airway. This causes them to be constantly tired since they are rarely getting to SWS and spend less time in REM sleep [25]. Subjects with major depression are five times more likely to have a sleep related breathing disorder than non-depressive subjects [26]. OSA has been documented in studies of chronic pain patients with disorders such as rheumatoid arthritis and fibromyalgia. Studies of patients with symptoms of fibromyalgia have led some investigators to propose that certain individuals may instead have a sleep apnea syndrome and the medications prescribed for fibromyalgia would actually worsen the sleep apnea symptoms [27]. OSA is more prevalent in chronic pain patients who use opioid-based drugs for pain management compared to the general population [28]. Sleep apnea is also frequently linked to headaches [27].

Cannabinoids and Sleep

Clinical cannabis research is predominantly focused on symptom management using compounds derived from cannabis called cannabinoids, and it has been suggested that one of the additional benefits of cannabinoid use is increasing sleep quality. Indeed one of the main reasons that patients report using herbal cannabis is to improve sleep quality [29]. Given our improved understanding of the endocannabinoid system (ECS), It is worth exploring the underlying rationale for this effect.

Anatomical data suggests that the CB1 receptor may be involved in the modulation of sleep [7]. Research on cannabis and THC extract from the 1970s and 1980s showed that cannabinoids have an effect on sleep by increasing SWS and decreasing REM sleep, but these studies were poorly controlled. The earliest reported studies of the primary psychoactive cannabinoid delta-9-tetrahydrocannabinol (THC) on sleep explored the hypnotic effects of different dose levels of THC [30]; the effect of the isomer delta-8-THC on EEG activity and sleep was explored in cats [31] and rats [32].

In a single dose human study examining cannabinoid effects on sleep, administration of CBD alone increased wakefulness, while THC was found to have no adverse effect on sleep and in some individuals increased the amount of SWS. The effect of equal parts THC and CBD was found to decrease stage 3 sleep, but had no effect on the duration of stage 2 or SWS [12]. This suggests that THC may acts as a sedative whereas CBD as a stimulant.

The physiological role of endocannabinoids on sleep has been explored. Intracerebroventricular injection of AEA enhances SWS and REM sleep through actions at the CB1 receptor [7]. The effect of AEA effect was enhanced when injected into the pedunculopontine tegmental nucleus. It was hypothesized that AEA, acting through CB1, induces an increase in the activity of the cholinergic neurons of the brainstem and basal forebrain that are involved in inducing sleep.

Cannabis and Sleep: Clinical Evidence

It is important to recognize that the effects of cannabis on sleep have been examined in recreational users as well as patients. Among heavy cannabis users, shorter REM latency and a longer sleep onset have been observed compared to controls [33]. Cessation of long-term heavy use of cannabis reduces sleep quality by decreasing total sleep length as well as the amount of SWS [34]. Poor sleep quality was one of the reasons that abstinent heavy cannabis users relapse [35].

Among patients with chronic pain, early experience with the synthetic cannabinoid nabilone found that one of the main reasons nabilone was continuously used was due to improvement in sleep quality [36]. Other observational studies have found that smoked cannabis is used by patients with chronic non-cancer pain to help decrease their pain and improve sleep [37]. Cannabis use in patients with post-traumatic stress disorder has also been reported to increase sleep quality [38].

Clinical trials with synthetic cannabinoids have shown some promise for dealing with sleep and pain. A study by Notcutt et al. [39] on chronic pain found that THC and THC: CBD reduced pain scores in patients but had little to no effect on the duration of sleep, while the perceived quality of sleep increased dramatically. Nabiximols, an oromucosal drug containing a 1:1 ration of THC: CBD drug has been tested for its effectiveness on pain and sleep interactions in several pain conditions including multiple sclerosis (MS) [2]. Nabiximols has been shown to reduce insomnia and daytime fatigue and to improve sleep quality in both MS and neuropathic pain patients. In the patients in whom it was beneficial, no evidence of tolerance or cognitive problems was noted [2]. Rog et al. [40] performed a randomized, control trial on cannabis-based medicine in central pain in MS patients. They found that nabiximols was effective in reducing pain and pain-related sleep disturbances. Nabiximols was also tried on patients with rheumatoid arthritis and was found significantly reduce pain on movement, pain and rest and the quality of sleep [41].

A study done by Ware et al. [42] on fibromyalgia (FM) patients tested the efficacy of another synthetic cannabinoid, nabilone, which mimics the action of THC. FM-related insomnia is usually treated with low-dose tricyclic antidepressants such as amitriptyline. However, nabilone was found to be superior to amitriptyline in improving the sleep quality of FM patients while the effects on pain, mood and quality of life were similar. Drowsiness and dizziness were common adverse events but these were similar to the side effects of amitriptyline.

Dronabinol, a synthetic version of THC, has been found to be useful for nighttime agitation related to severe dementia. Nighttime motor activity was found to decrease in dementia sufferers after the first dose of dronabinol, and while the mechanism of action is not clear, it may be due to sleep induction. Dronabinol was found to have dose dependent side effects and other studies showed effects on the cognition and function of patients but this was not examined in this study [43]. Dronabinol has also demonstrated effectiveness in treating central pain due to MS [44,45]. Intriguingly, THC has been found to stabilize respiratory patterns during all sleep stages and reducing sleep apnea in a dose dependent fashion [46].

A systematic review of cannabinoids and sleep completed in 2013, which addresses many of the articles presented above, points to the fact that many of the studies have bias and were not properly controlled. Despite the poor studies the authors of the review state that cannabinoids may play a role in sleep most specifically when pain is involved but the current evidence was not sufficient enough to say for certain [1].

What Needs to be Studied?

Sleep is a complex and poorly understood phenomenon integral to quality of life. Cannabinoids appear to have a potential role in improving perceived sleep quality, but overall there is very little data on the effects of cannabinoids on sleep architecture. It will be important to demonstrate the long term effects of cannabis and cannabinoid-based medicines, like nabilone and nabiximols, as well as medical cannabis on sleep. They should be validated by further randomized clinical trials and long term surveillance studies [37]. In-depth studies using polysomnography will be needed to understand to a greater extent the effects of cannabinoids on sleep architecture and the relationship of such changes to the patient's perceived quality of sleep [2]. A key question is whether the cannabinoid helps pain and therefore sleep is a secondary effect, or whether they affect sleep primarily and the pain relief is a function of a better rested state and therefore better coping skills.

Cannabinoid medications have typically been used as a last resort for chronic pain patients when other conventional methods have failed. These cases are often very complex and are hard to study since the chronic pain is heterogeneous with variable pathophysiological mechanisms [39]. For many patients with chronic pain, obtaining a good night's sleep can be a huge milestone and an important objective in setting treatment outcomes.

Emerging neurobiological findings show that the ECS system may be involved in areas of the brain associated with depression but further conclusive research is needed [47]. Animal depression studies point to doses of THC 2.5 mg/kg, CBD 200 mg/kg, and cannabichromene (CBC) 20 mg/kg acting as an antidepressant in some animal models. However to date, no clinical trials have been undertaken to test cannabinoids on affective disorders [48]. Due to the link between insomnia and depression, this may give interesting insights into the effect cannabinoids have in depression/insomnia/pain interactions and may help clinicians better understand the potential roles of cannabinoid based medicines, particularly in disorders like fibromyalgia where sleep disturbances, depression, and pain all coexist [42]. Polysomnographic studies of FM patients have shown that sleep architecture is disordered causing a delay in the onset of sleep, poorer sleep efficiency and reduced SWS and REM sleep. Various other non-REM sleep physiology alterations have been found [49]. Studies using polysomnography of FM patients and others using cannabinoid medicines are needed to verify the effect of cannabinoids on sleep architecture in such conditions.

References

1. Gates PJ, Albertella L, Copeland J (2014) The effects of cannabinoid administration on sleep: a systematic review of human studies. Sleep Med Rev 18: 477-487.
2. Russo EB, Guy GW, Robson PJ (2007) Cannabis, pain, and sleep: lessons from therapeutic clinical trials of Sativex, a cannabis-based medicine. Chem Biodivers 4: 1729-1743.
3. Russo E (1998) Cannabis for migraine treatment: the once and future prescription? An historical and scientific review. Pain 76: 3-8.
4. Iversen L (2003) Cannabis and the brain. Brain 126: 1252-1270.
5. Mechoulam R and LA Parker (2012) The Endocannabinoid System and the Brain. Annu Rev Psychol.
6. Rodríguez de Fonseca F, Del Arco I, Bermudez-Silva FJ, Bilbao A, Cippitelli A, et al. (2005) The endocannabinoid system: physiology and pharmacology. Alcohol Alcohol 40: 2-14.
7. Murillo-Rodríguez E (2008) The role of the CB1 receptor in the regulation of sleep. Prog Neuropsychopharmacol Biol Psychiatry 32: 1420-1427.
8. Brown SM, Wager-Miller J, Mackie K (2002) Cloning and molecular characterization of the rat CB2 cannabinoid receptor. Biochim Biophys Acta 1576: 255-264.
9. Van Sickle MD, Duncan M, Kingsley PJ, Mouihate A, Urbani P, et al. (2005) Identification and functional characterization of brainstem cannabinoid CB2 receptors. Science 310: 329-332.
10. Rom S, Persidsky Y (2013) Cannabinoid receptor 2: potential role in immunomodulation and neuroinflammation. J Neuroimmune Pharmacol 8: 608-620.
11. Mechoulam R, Peters M, Murillo-Rodriguez E, Hanus LO (2007) Cannabidiol--recent advances. Chem Biodivers 4: 1678-1692.
12. Nicholson AN, Turner C, Stone BM, Robson PJ (2004) Effect of Delta-9-tetrahydrocannabinol and cannabidiol on nocturnal sleep and early-morning behavior in young adults. J Clin Psychopharmacol 24: 305-313.
13. Roehrs T, Roth T (2005) Sleep and pain: interaction of two vital functions. Semin Neurol 25: 106-116.
14. Onen SH, Alloui A, Gross A, Eschallier A, Dubray C (2001) The effects of total sleep deprivation, selective sleep interruption and sleep recovery on pain tolerance thresholds in healthy subjects. J Sleep Res 10: 35-42.
15. Lavigne G, Zucconi M, Castronovo C, Manzini C, Marchettini P, et al. (2000) Sleep arousal response to experimental thermal stimulation during sleep in human subjects free of pain and sleep problems. Pain 84: 283-290.
16. Willis WD, Westlund KN (1997) Neuroanatomy of the pain system and of the pathways that modulate pain. J Clin Neurophysiol 14: 2-31.
17. Harding SM (1998) Sleep in fibromyalgia patients: subjective and objective findings. Am J Med Sci 315: 367-376.
18. Lavigne McMillan GD, Zucconi M eds. Principles and Practice of Sleep Medicine. Principles and Practice of Sleep Medicine, ed. Kryger M, Roth T, and Demeent W. 2005 Elsevier; Philidelphia: 1246-1255.
19. Smith MT, Haythornthwaite JA (2004) How do sleep disturbance and chronic pain inter-relate? Insights from the longitudinal and cognitive-behavioral clinical trials literature. Sleep Med Rev 8: 119-132.
20. Ohayon MM (2005) Relationship between chronic painful physical condition and insomnia. J Psychiatr Res 39: 151-159.
21. Lavigne G, Brousseau M, Kato T, Mayer P, Manzini C, et al. (2004) Experimental pain perception remains equally active over all sleep stages. Pain 110: 646-655.
22. Michaud M, Dumont M, Selmaoui B, Paquet J, Fantini ML, et al. (2004) Circadian rhythm of restless legs syndrome: relationship with biological markers. Ann Neurol 55: 372-380.
23. Earley CJ (2003) Clinical practice. Restless legs syndrome. N Engl J Med 348: 2103-2109.
24. Winkelmann J, Prager M, Lieb R, Pfister H, Spiegel B, et al. (2005) "Anxietas tibiarum". Depression and anxiety disorders in patients with restless legs syndrome. J Neurol 252: 67-71.
25. Ratnavadivel R, Chau N, Stadler D, Yeo A, McEvoy RD, et al. (2009) Marked reduction in obstructive sleep apnea severity in slow wave sleep. J Clin Sleep Med 5: 519-524.
26. Ohayon MM (2003) The effects of breathing-related sleep disorders on mood disturbances in the general population. J Clin Psychiatry 64: 1195-1200.
27. Menefee LA, Cohen MJ, Anderson WR, Doghramji K, Frank ED, et al. (2000) Sleep disturbance and nonmalignant chronic pain: a comprehensive review of the literature. Pain Med 1: 156-172.
28. Webster LR, Choi Y, Desai H, Webster L, Grant BJ (2008) Sleep-disordered breathing and chronic opioid therapy. Pain Med 9: 425-432.
29. Walsh Z, Callaway R, Belle-Isle L, Capler R, Kay R, et al. (2013) Cannabis for therapeutic purposes: patient characteristics, access, and reasons for use. Int J Drug Policy 24: 511-516.
30. Cousens K, DiMascio A (1973) (-) Delta 9 THC as an hypnotic. An experimental study of three dose levels. Psychopharmacologia 33: 355-364.
31. Wallach MB, Gershon S (1973) The effects of delta8-THC on the EEG, reticular multiple unit activity and sleep of cats. Eur J Pharmacol 24: 172-178.
32. Friedman E, Gershon S (1974) Effect of delta8-THC on alcohol-induced sleeping time in the rat. Psychopharmacologia 39: 193-198.
33. Bolla KI, Lesage SR, Gamaldo CE, Neubauer DN, Funderburk FR, et al. (2008) Sleep disturbance in heavy marijuana users. Sleep 31: 901-908.
34. Vandrey R, Smith MT, McCann UD, Budney AJ, Curran EM (2011) Sleep disturbance and the effects of extended-release zolpidem during cannabis withdrawal. Drug Alcohol Depend 117: 38-44.
35. Babson KA, Boden MT, Harris AH, Stickle TR, Bonn-Miller MO (2013) Poor sleep quality as a risk factor for lapse following a cannabis quit attempt. J Subst Abuse Treat 44: 438-443.
36. Berlach DM, Shir Y, Ware MA (2006) Experience with the synthetic cannabinoid nabilone in chronic noncancer pain. Pain Med 7: 25-29.
37. Ware MA, Doyle CR, Woods R, Lynch ME, Clark AJ (2003) Cannabis use for chronic non-cancer pain: results of a prospective survey. Pain 102: 211-216.
38. Bonn-Miller MO, Babson KA, Vandrey R (2014) Using cannabis to help you sleep: heightened frequency of medical cannabis use among those with PTSD. Drug Alcohol Depend 136: 162-165.
39. Notcutt W, Price M, Miller R, Newport S, Phillips C, et al. (2004) Initial experiences with medicinal extracts of cannabis for chronic pain: results from 34 'N of 1' studies. Anaesthesia 59: 440-452.
40. Rog DJ, Nurmikko TJ, Friede T, Young CA (2005) Randomized, controlled trial of cannabis-based medicine in central pain in multiple sclerosis. Neurology 65: 812-819.
41. Blake DR, Robson P, Ho M, Jubb RW, McCabe CS (2006) Preliminary assessment of the efficacy, tolerability and safety of a cannabis-based medicine (Sativex) in the treatment of pain caused by rheumatoid arthritis. Rheumatology (Oxford) 45: 50-52.
42. Ware MA, Fitzcharles MA, Joseph L, Shir Y (2010) The effects of nabilone on sleep in fibromyalgia: results of a randomized controlled trial. Anesth Analg 110: 604-610.
43. Walther S, Mahlberg R, Eichmann U, Kunz D (2006) Delta-9-tetrahydrocannabinol for nighttime agitation in severe dementia. Psychopharmacology (Berl) 185: 524-528.
44. Svendsen KB, Jensen TS, Bach FW (2004) Does the cannabinoid dronabinol reduce central pain in multiple sclerosis? Randomised double blind placebo controlled crossover trial. BMJ 329: 253.
45. Campbell FA, Tramèr MR, Carroll D, Reynolds DJ, Moore RA, et al. (2001) Are cannabinoids an effective and safe treatment option in the management of pain? A qualitative systematic review. BMJ 323: 13-16.
46. Carley DW, Paviovic S, Janelidze M, Radulovacki M (2002) Functional role for cannabinoids in respiratory stability during sleep. Sleep 25: 391-398.
47. Vinod KY, Hungund BL (2006) Role of the endocannabinoid system in depression and suicide. Trends Pharmacol Sci 27: 539-545.

24

Simultaneous Measurement of Heart Rate Variability and Blinking Duration to Predict Sleep Onset and Drowsiness in Drivers

Akiko Noda[1*], Masahiro Miyaji[2], Yuki Wakuda[3,4], Yuki Hara[5], Fumihiko Yasuma[6], Toshio Fukuda[7], Kunihiro Iwamoto[8] and Norio Ozaki[8]

[1]*Chubu University Graduate School of Life and Health Sciences, Kasugai, Japan*

[2]*Geaduate School of Information Science and Technology, Aichi Prefectural University, Aichi, Japan*

[3]*The University of Tokyo, Tokyo, Japan*

[4]*YRP Ubiquitous Networking Laboratory, Tokyo, Japan*

[5]*Department of Medical Technology, Nagoya University Graduate School of Medicine, Japan*

[6]*Department of Medicine, National Hospital Organization Suzuka National Hospital, Suzuka, Japan*

[7]*Depertment of Micro-Nano Systems Engineering, Graduate School of Engineering, Nagoya University, Nagoya, Japan*

[8]*Department of Psychiatry, Nagoya University Graduate School of Medicine, Nagoya, Japan*

***Corresponding author:** Akiko Noda, PhD, Chubu University Graduate School of Life and Health Sciences, 1200 Matsumoto-cho, Kasugai-shi, Aichi-487-8501, Japan, E-mail: anoda@isc.chubu.ac.jp

Abstract

Excessive sleepiness in drivers greatly increases the risk of traffic accidents. A compact, three-dimensional system for analyzing visual information from a face photograph using an infrared CCD camera was recently designed to monitor drivers. The present study aimed to examine whether temporal changes in autonomic activity as determined by spectral analysis of electrocardiogram heart rate variability (HRV) and blinking duration obtained with this camera system could predict sleep onset in a driving simulation. Ten healthy adults (mean age, 21.8 ± 0.64 years) were enrolled in the study. The subjects sat upright in the driver's seat while we performed standard polysomnography (PSG). HRV was assessed through a spectral analysis of RR intervals of the PSG electrocardiogram. Blinking duration was evaluated by an eyelid movement tracking system within the infrared CCD camera. Blinking duration was significantly prolonged during the 10 seconds before sleep onset compared with that during wakefulness (0.64 ± 0.13 vs. 0.34 ± 0.06 sec, p=0.0004). Subsequently, the high-frequency power of HRV was significantly greater at sleep onset (1201 ± 994.6 vs. 906.9 ± 766.2 ms^2, p=0.001). We conclude that simultaneous measurement of HRV and blinking duration can be utilized to predict sleep onset in an automobile driving simulation.

Keywords: Excessive sleepiness; Blinking duration; Heart rate variability; Sleep onset; Drowsiness; Driver

Abbreviations:

HRV: Heart Rate Variability; LF: Low-Frequency; HF: High-Frequency

Introduction

According to the National Police Agency Traffic Bureau, the numbers of traffic annual fatalities and injuries were approximately 5,000 and 850,000, respectively, in 2012 [1]. Sleepiness and a subsequent sleep onset in drivers are significant risk factors of road traffic fatalities/injuries. In addition, excessive daytime sleepiness was noted among 20-25% of general population in an epidemiologic study [2], and it was particularly prevalent in certain occupations as medical residents, shift workers, and transportation workers [3].

Various safe-driving systems have been developed and installed to prevent traffic accidents, including physiological monitoring for detecting the direction of driver facial movements [4]. As such, development of methodology to predict sleep onset by assessing the adaptive functional state of drivers is urgently needed to reduce the risk of traffic accidents.

Heart rate variability (HRV) is a non-invasive and reliable tool to quantify the autonomic activity in the sympathetic and parasympathetic modulation in humans [5]. The low-frequency (LF) component is a marker of sympathetic and parasympathetic modulation, while the high-frequency (HF) component is solely a marker of vagal modulation.

Sleep onset, typically with subsequent progression to deeper sleep, is associated with a shift to the augmented parasympathetic modulation [6,7]. Hence, circadian and sleep stage-specific effects on HRV are clinically relevant [8].

A compact, in-vehicle camera system was recently designed to monitor driver fatigue and loss of concentration. It is superior to the previous system in its ability to measure head position, gazing direction and eyelid closure through a three-dimentional system for analyzing visual information from a face photograph using an infrared CCD camera.

We investigated this new method, which simultaneously provides a blinking-related index with an infrared CCD camera and HRV parameters, both of which served as predictors of sleep onset in the driving simulation.

Materials and Methods

Ten healthy adults (mean age, 21.8 ± 0.64 years) were enrolled in this study. The study protocol was approved by the appropriate institutional review committee, and all subjects provided written consent of their participation after being informed about the details of the study purpose and methods.

Polysomnography

Standard polysomnography (PSG) [9] (ALICE3, Healthdyne Technologies, PA, USA.) was performed while subjects were in a relaxed sitting position on the driver's seat of a simulated automobile operation. The laboratory environment was dark and quiet during testing, and smoking, caffeinated beverages and physical/mental activities were prohibited during the 30 minutes prior to the PSG study.

Subjects avoided unusual exposure to bright light, noise, and conversation. Measurements were recorded from an electroencephalogram, electrooculogram, electromyogram, and electrocardiogram with a NASA lead. Sleep stage was evaluated by visual analysis according to Rechtshaffen and Kales [9]. Sleep onset was defined as the first three consecutive epochs of sleep stage 1, or the first epoch of sleep stages 2, 3, or 4, and REM sleep.

Heart rate variability

Spectral analysis of HRV (Memcalc/Win, GMS Co., Tokyo, Japan) was performed using RR intervals from the electrocardiogram. Low-frequency (LF; 0.04-0.15 Hz) and high-frequency (HF; 0.15-0.40 Hz) power were calculated by integrating the power spectral density in defined frequency bands. The HF component and LF/HF ratio were used as indices of parasympathetic and sympathetic activity, respectively [5].

Measurement of eyelid movement

An eyelid movement tracking system (Anti Sleep, Smart Eye, Göteborg, Sweden) comprising an infrared CCD camera with a single lens and image processing function was used to obtain facial information, such as head position, gaze direction, and eyelid closure in the driving simulation.

The system required a one-time calibration using special checkerboard at the beginning of the measurement, which enabled measurements in the longitudinal direction. Blinking duration was derived by measuring the time from the time of one eyelid closure to the next eyelid closure.

Data analysis

Data are presented as means ± SD, and were analyzed by the paired t-test. All analyses were performed using the Statview statistical software package (SAS Institute, Inc.; Cary, NC, USA). A P value of <0.05 was considered statistically significant.

Results and Discussion

Blinking duration tended to increase during the transitional period from wakefulness to sleep, with a significantly longer blinking duration during the 10 seconds immediately before sleep onset relative to that during wakefulness (0.64 ± 0.13 vs. 0.34 ± 0.06 sec, p=0.0004; Figure 1a).

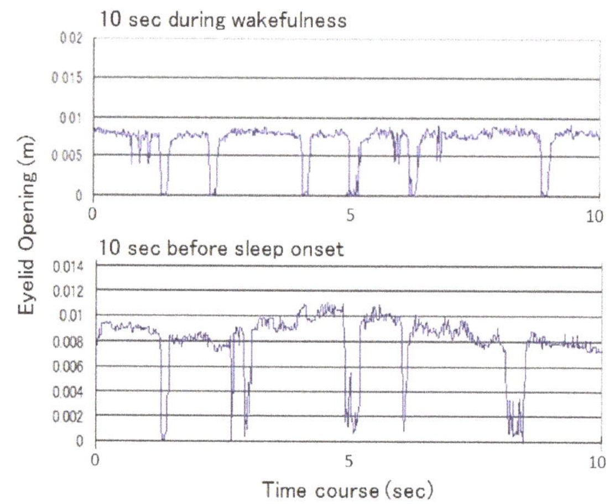

Figure 1a: The time course of blinking duration during wakefulness and during 10 seconds before sleep onset.

We observed no significant differences in eye position, head position, and gazing direction before and after sleep onset. Furthermore, prolonged blinking preceded an increase in HF components in all participants. HF levels increased significantly at sleep onset compared with that during wakefulness (1201 ± 994.6 vs. 906.9 ± 766.2 ms^2, p=0.001; Figure 1b), whereas LF/HF increased during wakefulness.

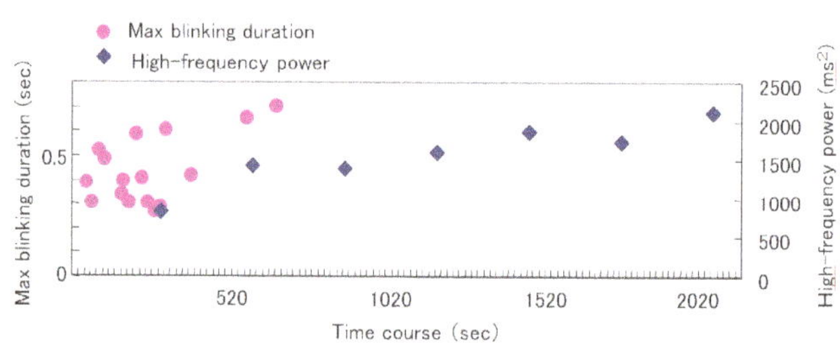

Figure 1b: The time course of blinking duration and high-frequency power associated with sleep onset.

The present study found that changes in HF and blinking duration were significantly associated with sleep onset. Our findings suggest that the combination of prolonged blinking duration and increased HF provides us with the critical information needed to assess the adaptive functional state of drivers (Figure 2).

Autonomic activity can be evaluated by an analysis of HRV, which varies during different sleep stages, showing predominantly parasympathetic activation of the heart during non-REM sleep and increased sympathetic activity during REM sleep [5-8]. Whiletime responsiveness of HRV is not instantaneous enough to detect sleep onset, that of blinking is approximately 1 to 5 seconds, and thus measurement of blinking duration may reliably predict sleepiness in a driver. Electrooculograms have been widely used to measure blinking duration in driving simulations in the past, but this technique requires the subject to have multiple electrodes attached to their face [10]. In addition, simple video cameras which monitor blinking may also lack the accuracy necessary to detect drowsiness [11].

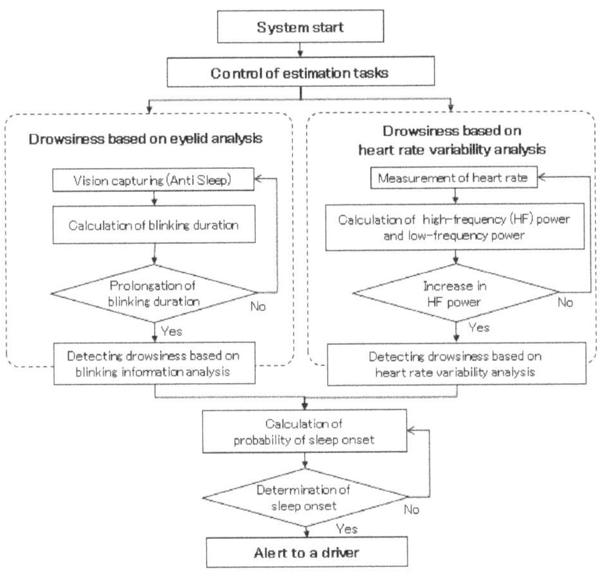

Figure 2: The new system architecture for prediction of sleep onset and drowsiness.

However, an eyelid movement tracking system comprising an infrared CCD camera was recently designed for real-time three-dimensional measurement of eyelid closure in a person sitting in the driver's seat, and demonstrates sufficient accuracy and reliability. Our results suggest that simultaneous recording of both HRV and blinking duration with a CCD camera could help detect sleep onset in young healthy subjects.

Blinking habits vary from person to person, and given the instability in blinking recognition due to head movements before sleep onset and eye size, the device must be improved to allow for optimal image recognition. Diagnostic imaging of blinking in simulator experiments and actual driving experiments, in addition to practical validation of the physiological index, will be important to provide valuable information for increasing the accuracy of sleep detection. In the future, threshold values should be established for the HF components of HRV and blinking time in order to accurately detect sleepiness in a large-sized subject group.

Conclusion

We introduce a new system of estimating sleep onset based on temporal changes in HF components of HRV and blinking duration. Time-series observations of HF components of HRV and blinking duration provide new insight into sleep onset and daytime sleep. Application of this practical approach would help significantly to prevent accidents caused by drivers falling asleep.

Acknowledgements

This study was funded by research grants from the Ministry of Education, Culture, Sports, Science and Technology of Japan.

References

1. National Police Agency Traffic Bureau, Road traffic accidents in 2012.
2. Walsleben JA, Kapur VK, Newman AB, Shahar E, Bootzin RR, et al. (2004) Sleep and reported daytime sleepiness in normal subjects: the Sleep Heart Health Study. Sleep 27: 293-298.
3. Drake C, Roehrs T, Breslau N, Johnson E, Jefferson C, et al. (2010) The 10-year risk of verified motor vehicle crashes in relation to physiologic sleepiness. Sleep 33: 745-752.
4. Hattori A, Tokoro S, Miyashita M, Tanaka I, Ohue K, et al. (2006) Development of Forward Collision Warning System using the Driver Behavioral Information, SAE Technical Paper Series, 2006 SAE World Congress 115: 818-827.
5. Camm AJ, Malik M, Bigger JT, Breithardt G, Cerutti S, et al. (1996) Heart rate variability: standards of measurement, physiological interpretation and clinical use. Task Force of the European Society of Cardiology and the North American Society of Pacing and Electrophysiology. Circulation 93: 1043-1065.
6. Stein PK, Pu Y (2012) Heart rate variability, sleep and sleep disorders. Sleep Med Rev 16: 47-66.
7. Fukuda T, Wakuda Y, Hasegawa Y, Arai F, Kawaguchi M, et al. (2005) Sleep quality estimation based on Chaos analysis for heart rate variability. IEEJ Trans. EIS 125: 43-49.
8. Boudreau P, Yeh WH, Dumont GA, Boivin DB (2013) Circadian variation of heart rate variability across sleep stages. Sleep 36: 1919-1928.
9. Rechtschaffen A, Kales A (1968) A manual of standardized terminology, Techniques and scoring system for sleep stage of human subjects. Public Health Service, United States Government Printing Office, Washington, DC.
10. Caffier PP, Erdmann U, Ullsperger P (2003) Experimental evaluation of eye-blink parameters as a drowsiness measure. Eur J Appl Physiol 89: 319-325.
11. Abe T, Nonomura T, Komada T, Asaoka S, Ueno A, et al. (2011) Detecting deteriorated vigilance using percentage of eyelid closure time during behavioral maintenance of wakefulness tests. Int J Psychophysiol 82: 269-274.

25

Sleep Apnea Symptoms and Cardiovascular Disease Risks among Haitian Medical Students

Diana M Rosenthal[1], Donaldson F Conserve[2], Dodley Severe[3], Michaele A Gedeon[3], Ferdinand Zizi[1], Georges Casimir[4], Samy I McFarlane[5] and Girardin Jean Louis[1*]

[1]*Department of Population Health, Center for Healthful Behavior Change, NYU School of Medicine, NY, USA*

[2]*Department of Health Promotion, Arnold School of Public Health, Education, and Behavior, University of South Carolina, Columbia, SC, USA*

[3]*University of the Aristide Foundation, Haiti, USA*

[4]*Department of Psychiatry, SUNY Downstate Medical Center, Brooklyn, NY, USA*

[5]*Department of Endocrinology, SUNY Downstate Medical Center, Brooklyn, NY, USA*

[*]**Corresponding author:** Girardin Jean Louis, Professor of Population Health and Psychiatry, Department of Population Health, Center for Healthful Behavior Change, New York University School of Medicine, 227 East 30th Street, 6th Floor, NY 10016, USA, E-mail: Girardin.jean-louis@nyumc.org

Abstract

Sleep apnea is a prevalent sleep disorder that disproportionately affects blacks and has been previously studied among Caribbean-born blacks in Brooklyn, New York, but there has been negligible research in the Caribbean, specifically Haiti, and developing countries on this pressing health issue. A total of 373 medical students (mean age=20.6 years ± 2.3 years) from a medical school in Haiti participated in this study. Participants were administered a questionnaire assessing their sleep health and cardiovascular outcomes. The rate of sleep apnea symptoms was: snoring (13.2%), excessive daytime sleepiness (73.7%), and difficulty maintaining sleep (25.3%). Many reported falling asleep while watching television (68.2%) or while driving (7.8%). Based on logistic regression analysis, reported nocturnal breathing pauses was the most important predictor of the likelihood of reporting a history of cardiac disease (14.96; 95% CI=1.27–76.07). Findings suggest that more aggressive effort should be made to increase screening of sleep apnea among Haitians, thereby increasing the likelihood for early detection and treatment to reduce sleep-related risk of cardiovascular disease.

Keywords: Sleep apnea; Cardiovascular disease; Haiti; Medical students

Introduction

Sleep apnea is a prevalent sleep disorder that disproportionately affects blacks [1-4]. OSA has been previously studied in Caribbean-born blacks in New York [4], but there has been negligible research in the Caribbean, specifically Haiti, and developing countries on this pressing health issue. There is significant evidence that quality of nocturnal sleep plays a role in regulating Blood Pressure (BP) levels based on evidence that shows a significant association between poor nocturnal sleep and non-dipping behavior as well as the presence of sleep apnea [5]. Such evidence has concluded that OSA is an indicator of cardio metabolic risk.

In Haiti, there are a number of structural and historical factors that may play role in producing sleep apnea. For instance, Haiti is the poorest country in the Americas and one of the poorest in the world (with a GDP per capita of US $846 in 2014) with significant needs in basic services. According to the World Health Organization (WHO), the total expenditure on health per capita (Intl $, 2014) is 131 and the total expenditure on health as percent of GDP is 7.6% in 2014 [6]. In addition, Haiti was struck by a 7.0 magnitude earthquake that left much devastation and long term psychological effects on the survivors. Although Haiti has been recovering from the earthquake, a number of challenges remain and survivors may still be suffering from post-traumatic stress disorder (PTSD). In a study conducted among 246 Haitian students 2 years after the earthquake, a prevalence of 36% for PTSD and 32% for depression was reported [7] and another study found higher PTSD symptoms among female university students than male [8]. Findings from a recent systematic review suggest that sleep apnea is positively associated with PTSD and major depressive disorder [9]. In 2015, five years after the earthquake, the reported life expectancy at birth in Haiti was 62/66 (m/f) [10]. According to WHO, 48% of total deaths in Haiti are attributed to non-communicable diseases (NCDs); furthermore, the probability of dying from one of the four main NCDs (cardiovascular, respiratory, diabetes, and cancer) is 24% for Haitians between ages 30 and 70 [6].

The probability of death from one of the four main NCDs for Haitians may be influenced by the structural and historical factors associated with the presence of sleep fragmentation and sleep apnea in various communities. Research conducted in a Haitian community without electricity showed that sleep fragmentation differed by age groups; however, this Haitian sample reported a greater average time in bed than reported for developed countries like the United States (9.3 *vs.* 7 hours to 8 hours), but the average sleep duration of this sample was shorter at 7 hours [11]. Further research is needed to determine other co-contributing factors to the presence of sleep apnea including socio-demographic and cultural determinants, and if sleep apnea is associated with the high NCD mortality rate in Haiti. The aim of this study is to examine the presence of sleep fragmentation and sleep apnea in a sample of Haitian medical students, and observe the factors potentially impacting the occurrence of this health phenomenon.

Methods

A total of 373 medical students participated in the study. The average age was 20.6 years ± 2.3 years (range=16 years to 35 years). Of the sample, 67.4% were women and 32.6% were men. The data was collected in two waves among students at the Medical School in Port-au-Prince, Haiti. Eligible participants were approached by a health educator (or medical student) who explained the purpose of the study and provided answers to questions raised by the participants. The health educator assisted all participants in completing the questionnaires. Questionnaires were available in both French and Haitian Creole, requiring approximately 15 minutes to complete.

Study variables

Self-reported data relating to history of hypertension and cardiac disease were collected in the questionnaire. For this study, we asked participants several questions such as: "Do you have a history of cardiac problems?" with a binary (yes/no) response option. Participants were also asked to give yes/no answers based on whether they experienced habitual snoring, excessive daytime sleepiness, and sleep fragmentation. Subjective questions as well as self-rated items on health status, sleep apnea symptoms, insomnia, and daytime functioning were also asked. For example, participants were asked to rate their health status from "excellent" to "poor" and rate their satisfaction with their current sleep status from "very satisfactory" to "very trouble." The questionnaire also assessed the number of hours spent in bed, number of hours actually spent sleeping, and daytime napping.

Statistical analysis

The present analysis examined sleep characteristics and assessed their associations with cardiovascular outcomes. Frequency and measures of central tendency were used to describe the sample. In preliminary analyses, Pearson and Spearman correlations were used to explore relationships between variables of interest. Relationships of sleep characteristics with cardiovascular outcomes (i.e., hypertension and heart disease) were examined with multiple logistic regression analysis. Factors were selected based on their theoretical importance. Demographic and health risks were adjusted in the regression model. SPSS 21.0 was used for the statistical analyses.

Results

The rate of OSA symptoms in this sample was: snoring (13.2%), witnessed apneas (25.7%), and excessive daytime sleepiness (73.7%). Many of the respondents indicated falling asleep while watching television (68.2%) or while driving (7.8%). Overall, 27.8% reported difficulty initiating sleep, 25.3% difficulty maintaining sleep, and 56.6% early morning awakening; 45.5% reported excessive tossing and turning while sleeping; 61.3% indicated daytime napping and 9.8% used sleep medicine. Of the sample, the average time spent in bed at night was 6.48 hours ± 1.9 hours and the average time spent in bed sleeping at night was 5.99 hours ± 1.5 hours. For the cardiovascular outcomes, 25.5% reported a history of hypertension and 10.5% a history of heart disease. More than half (61.5%) reported difficulty concentrating during the day and 68.5% rated their health status as good to excellent and 31.5% as fair to poor. Most of the participants (62.1%) were satisfied with their habitual sleep. The average weight and height of the participants were 69.5 kg ± 27.5 kg, 1.63 m ± 0.17 m, respectively.

In Table 1, we contrast sleep characteristics of participants reporting adverse cardiovascular outcomes (i.e., hypertension or heart disease). Based on logistic regression analysis, difficulty breathing at night was the most important predictor of the likelihood of reporting a history of cardiac problems. The corresponding multivariate-adjusted odds ratio was 14.96 (95% CI=1.27–76.07). Sleep factors were not significantly associated with the presence of hypertension (Table 1).

Variable	N	No (%)	Yes (%)
Snoring	365	317 (86.85)	48 (13.15)
Witnessed Apneas	366	272 (74.3)	94 (25.7)
Excessive Daytime Sleepiness	361	95 (26.3)	266 (73.7)
Falling Asleep Watching TV	368	117 (31.8)	251 (68.2)
Falling Asleep Driving	256	236 (92.2)	20 (7.8)
Difficulty Initiating Sleep	367	265 (72.2)	102 (27.8)
Difficulty Maintaining Sleep	363	271 (74.7)	92 (25.3)
Early Morning Awakening	357	155 (43.4)	202 (56.6)
Excessive Tossing and Turning	365	199 (54.5)	166 (45.5)
Daytime Napping	362	140 (38.7)	222 (61.3)
Use of Sleep Medicine	368	332 (90.2)	36 (9.8)

Adverse cardiovascular outcomes were reported as binary (yes/no) responses. The number and percentage of these self-reported outcomes in our sample of medical students are presented respectively in Table 1.

Table 1: Sleep characteristics of participants reporting adverse cardiovascular outcomes.

Discussion

To our knowledge, this is the first study to examine symptoms of OSA and self-reported cardiovascular outcomes among Caribbean men and women residing in Haiti. The main finding of the study is that a significant number of Haitians reported sleep apnea symptoms (i.e., snoring and excessive daytime sleepiness) and that difficulty breathing at night is a strong predictor of the likelihood of reporting a history of heart disease. Excessive daytime sleepiness, another symptom highly suggestive of greater sleep apnea risk, was also more common among medical students in Haiti. Specifically, 73.7% of the participants reported excessive daytime sleepiness. By contrast, the estimated rate of daytime sleepiness in the 2005 Sleep in America poll was 27% [12]. Comparatively, estimates of daytime sleepiness in Sweden, France, and in the UK were 16%, 20%, and 15%, respectively [13-16]. Furthermore, the rates of daytime sleepiness in our study were similar to the rates among Caribbean-born blacks in Brooklyn, NY (33%). However, these rates are higher than those generally observed for blacks (19%) in the U.S. [17], who typically experience more severe daytime sleepiness than do age-matched whites [18,19]. These findings support the notion that blacks do not constitute a homogenous group regarding snoring and daytime sleepiness, two of the most frequent symptoms of sleep apnea.

Students in our sample reported an average time spent in bed at night of 6.48 hours ± 1.9 hours, and the average time spent in bed sleeping at night was 5.89 hours ± 1.5 hours. This compares to an average sleep time of 9.3 hours ± 1.2 hours and 7.0 hours ± 1.0 hours, respectively with a previous study [11]. This noticeable discrepancy in bed and sleep time is possibly due to the difference in the study samples. It can be expected that medical students sleep less and spend more time studying, while community members in the other may have a more sedentary lifestyle without electricity [11]. In addition, our sample consisted of a younger age group, while the participants in the other study ranged from 18 years to ≥ 65 years of age. In contrast, in a Jamaican lifestyle survey conducted with 2,432 participants, they reported sleeping 8.2 hours ± 1.8 hours [20].

Similar to other studies, we found an association between history of cardiac disease and sleep apnea symptoms, although the confidence interval for the regression model suggests a great deal of variability [21-23]. Furthermore, the Sleep Heart Health Study showed that sleep apnea increases the risk of heart failure by 140%, the risk of stroke by 60%, and the risk of coronary heart disease by 30% [24]. One implication of these findings is that public health efforts should promote adequate screening and timely diagnosis of sleep apnea among Haitians in order to prevent heart disease. Caribbean patients with a history of heart disease should receive a brief screening for sleep apnea while attending regular visits in primary-care facilities. Screening instruments should be made available and can be easily administered by the medical staff. Appropriate referrals for comprehensive sleep assessment should be encouraged.

Conclusion

As expected, sleep apnea risk factors, specifically difficulty breathing at night, was a predictor of heart disease. In addition, the Haitian participants reported high rates of sleep apnea symptoms (i.e., snoring, difficulty breathing at night and excessive daytime sleepiness) similar to Caribbean-born blacks studied in the U.S. Of note, since Haitian medical students in our sample represent a particular age group and occupational setting, estimates from our sample are not generalizable to population-based estimates.

Based on the geographic location, almost all of the medical students were from Port-au-Prince area, so it is not a reflection of the entire country. Likewise, our sample comprised young medical students who were not seeking sleep services. Our data suggests that blacks in developing countries may be at risk of developing sleep apnea. Furthermore, based on these findings, it can be said that Caribbean individuals at-risk for OSA can experience increased risks when they immigrate to the U.S. Our previous study showed that Caribbean-born blacks were at greater risk of developing sleep apnea compared with US-born blacks [4]. This suggests that more aggressive effort should be made to increase screening rates for sleep apnea in the Caribbean, thereby increasing the likelihood for early detection and treatment to prevent cardiovascular complications. Future studies should assess sleep patterns among Haitians using more robust epidemiologic methodologies.

Acknowledgement

This research was supported by funding from the National Institutes of Health R01MD007716.

References

1. Smedley BD, Stith AY, Nelson AR (2002) Unequal treatment: Confronting racial and ethnic disparities in health care. National Academies Press.
2. Williams DR (2003) The health of men: structured inequalities and opportunities. Am J Public Health 93: 724-731.
3. Williams NJ, Jean Louis G, Ravenell J, Seixas A, Islam N, et al. (2016) A community-oriented framework to increase screening and treatment of obstructive sleep apnea among blacks. Sleep Med 18: 82-87.
4. Zizi F, Jean Louis G, Fernandez S, von Gizycki H, Lazar JM, et al. (2008) Symptoms of obstructive sleep apnea in a Caribbean sample. Sleep Breath 12: 317-322.
5. Silva A, Moreira C, Bicho M, Paiva T, Clara J (2000) Nocturnal sleep quality and circadian blood pressure variation. Rev Port Cardiol 19: 991-1005.
6. WHO (2014) Noncommunicable diseases (NCD) country profiles. Haiti.
7. Silvestre G, Anacréon P, Théodore M, Silvestre E, Garcia Dubus E (2014) Risk Factors for Posttraumatic Stress Disorder in Haitian Students. Psychology 5: 849.
8. Burnett HJ, Helm H (2013) Relationship between posttraumatic stress disorder, resilience, and religious orientation and practices among university student earthquake survivors in Haiti. Int J Emerg Ment Health 15: 97-104.
9. Gupta MA, Simpson FC (2015) Obstructive sleep apnea and psychiatric disorders: a systematic review. J Clin Sleep Med 11: 165-175.
10. World Health Organization (WHO) (2015) Haiti: Statistics.
11. Knutson KL (2014) Sleep duration, quality, and timing and their associations with age in a community without electricity in Haiti. Am J Hum Bio 26: 80-86.
12. Friedman M, Bliznikas D, Klein M, Duggal P, Somenek M, et al. (2006) Comparison of the incidences of obstructive sleep apnea-hypopnea syndrome in African-Americans versus Caucasian-Americans. Otolaryngol Head Neck Surg 134: 545-550.
13. Ohayon MM, Caulet M, Philip P, Guilleminault C, Priest RG (1997) How sleep and mental disorders are related to complaints of daytime sleepiness. Arch Intern Med 157: 2645-2652.
14. Ohayon MM, Guilleminault C, Priest RG, Caulet M (1997) Snoring and breathing pauses during sleep: telephone interview survey of a United Kingdom population sample. BMJ 314: 860.

15. Cumberbatch CG, Younger NO, Ferguson TS, McFarlane SR, Francis DK, et al. (2011) Reported hours of sleep, diabetes prevalence and glucose control in jamaican adults: analysis from the Jamaica lifestyle survey 2007-2008. Int J Endocrinol.

16. Soldatos CR, Allaert FA, Ohta T, Dikeos DG (2005) How do individuals sleep around the world? Results from a single-day survey in ten countries. Sleep Med 6: 5-13.

17. Qureshi AI, Giles WH, Croft JB, Bliwise DL (1997) Habitual sleep patterns and risk for stroke and coronary heart disease A 10-year follow-up from NHANES I. Neurology 48: 904-910.

18. Ancoli Israel S, Klauber MR, Stepnowsky C, Estline E, Chinn A, et al. (1995) Sleep-disordered breathing in African-American elderly. Am J Respir Crit Care Med 152: 1946-1949.

19. Durrence HH, Lichstein KL (2006) The sleep of African Americans: a comparative review. Behav Sleep Med 4: 29-44.

20. Findley LJ, Weiss JW, Jabour ER (1991) Drivers with untreated sleep apnea: a cause of death and serious injury. Arch Intern Med 151: 1451-1452.

21. USDHHS (1993) Wake Up America National Sleep Alert.

22. Kiely J, McNicholas W (2000) Cardiovascular risk factors in patients with obstructive sleep apnoea syndrome. Eur Respir J 16: 128-133.

23. Mehra R, Benjamin EJ, Shahar E, Gottlieb DJ, Nawabit R, et al. (2006) Association of nocturnal arrhythmias with sleep-disordered breathing: The Sleep Heart Health Study. Am J Respir Crit Care Med 173: 910-916.

24. Wright J, Johns R, Watt I, Melville A, Sheldon T (1997) Health effects of obstructive sleep apnoea and the effectiveness of continuous positive airways pressure: a systematic review of the research evidence. BMJ 314: 851.

Sleep Patterns in a Carbon Monoxide (CO) Poisoning Patient

Fructuoso Ayala-Guerrero[1*], Indira J Arreguín-González[2] and Carlos Raúl Castillo-Montoya[3]

[1]*School of Psychology, National Autonomous University of Mexico, Mexico*

[2]*Unit of Physical Medicine and Rehabilitation Centre Region, UMAE Lomas Verdes, Mexican Social Security Institute, Mexico*

[3]*Autonomous Metropolitan University (UAM) Iztapalapa, Mexico*

[*]**Corresponding author:** Fructuoso Ayala-Guerrero, 1School of Psychology, National Autonomous University of Mexico, 3004 University Avenue Col. Copilco-University, CP 04510, Mexico, E-mail: fayala@unam.mx

Abstract

Importance: The functional anatomy of the brain, especially of the subcortical structures, is one of the least understood areas in neurophysiology. A great deal of the understanding of the functional neuroanatomy is derived from the study of patients whose brain has been damaged under different circumstances. Carbon monoxide (CO) poisoning affects particularly the basal ganglia and subcortical white matter, providing insight into the functional neuroanatomy of this complex region of the central nervous system. Since the regulating mechanisms of the sleep-wake cycle depend on multiple brain regions, damage of any of these regions may result in states of vigilance disturbances.

Methods: Sleep was recorded and scored using 30-s epochs according to standard methods, including central and occipital EEG (C3-A1, C4-A2, O1-A1 and O2-A2), submental EMG and periorbital EOG. Oronasal airflow and thoracic and abdominal respiratory effort were also monitored throughout the night.

Results: In addition to disruption of continuity and alterations in the sleep architecture, total sleep time was significantly reduced in the patient under study; consequently, sleep efficiency was severely affected. Reduction in total time spent in REM sleep was related to the mean duration but not to the number of REM sleep episodes displayed across the recording of sleep. Cardiac and respiratory activities exhibited a tendency across the sleep-wake cycle different to that observed in healthy subjects.

Conclusions: This report suggests that cortical and subcortical brain damage caused by CO poisoning induces sleep disturbances and functional modification of the autonomic nervous system. Therapies to improve the sleep quality of patients exposed to CO poisoning should be implemented.

Keywords: CO poisoning; Insomnia; Fragmented sleep; Sleep efficiency

Introduction

The functional anatomy of the brain, especially of the subcortical structures, is one of the least understood areas in neurophysiology. A great deal of the understanding of the functional neuroanatomy is derived from the study of patients whose brains have been damaged under different circumstances.

Carbon monoxide (CO) poisoning affects particularly the basal ganglia and subcortical white matter, providing insight into the functional neuroanatomy of this complex region of the central nervous system [1].

Initial symptoms displayed by individuals under CO poisoning usually include severe headache, nausea, weakness, confusion, heart arrhythmias, myocardial infarction, coma, or death [2,3]. If the patient survives, he or she will develop diverse neuropsychological sequelae [4-7].

Recent studies using detailed neuropsychological evaluations show that significant decrements in cognitive performance may be common, even years after recovery from the main symptoms [6,8,9].

Some reports integrate several cases to assess different kinds of brain damage during the first week after CO poisoning [10,11]. In these reports, it was described that about two-thirds of the patients under study had abnormal imaging studies, the globus pallidus was the most frequently injured area (39-63%), followed by the deep subcortical white matter (28-32%). Cortical, mesial temporal lobe and other subcortical lesions were occasionally detected.

It has been suggested that there may be a significant correlation between the regions that are hypoperfused during the acute stage and the neuropsychiatric disorders that develop later [12]. Some studies have described more lesions in the white matter than in the globus pallidus, whereas others have observed a similar incidence [13]. The Precise identification of brain lesions and neuropsychological deficits that may benefit from therapy is important for patient recovery.

On the other hand, the sleep wake cycle may be affected by different factors. Since the regulating mechanisms of this cycle depend on multiple brain regions, any damage of some of these regions may result in states of vigilance disturbances.

Sleep is a reversible behavioral state [14], which consists of rapid eye movement (REM) sleep and non-REM (NREM) sleep. NREM sleep is further divided into stages N1, N2, and N3 based on electroencephalographic (EEG) patterns. N3 is also termed slow-wave sleep (SWS) or delta sleep and comprises stages 3 and 4 of older nomenclature [15]. In adult humans, sleep consists of about 5% wake, 5% N1, 50% N2, 15% N3, and 25% of REM sleep.

There are multiple hypotheses about the primary function of sleep. Among these hypotheses, restorative and cognitive effects are the most accepted. There is increasing evidence that sleep is necessary for neural plasticity and memory consolidation [16]. NREM sleep is important for declarative memory consolidation, whereas REM sleep helps non declarative and emotional memory. NREM spindle density is positively linked to verbal memory and slow-wave density is positively linked to retention of same day memory.

The lower brain stem is an essential area to generate waking, NREM, and REM sleep states; however when other several brain regions are injured, such as the medulla, mesencephalon, preóptic area of the hypothalamus, thalamus, and neocortex, the amount of NREM and REM sleep is reduced. Similarly, waking state is regulated by several neuronal groups localized in the midbrain, the posterior and lateral hypothalamus, and the basal forebrain. These arousal systems are characterized by long axons and extensive projections to widespread brain regions, involving the diencephalon, the limbic system, and neocortex. Arousal systems also control the thalamocortical neurons, which in turn, regulate the oscillatory mechanisms intrinsic to thalamocortical networks that underlie NREM or synchronized EEG patterns.

On the other hand, sleep is characterized by rapid fluctuations in autonomic activity controlling systemic blood pressure, and heart rate. In normal subjects non-REM sleep is related to a very high vagal activity while REM sleep is associated with a significant withdrawal of vagal activity and an increased influence of sympathetic control of heart rate [17].

Therefore sleep represents a physiological state for a better understanding of the variability of heart rate since autonomic activity can be studied in the absence of factors such as physical activity and cortical functions which modulate heart rate variability

As previously described, brain damage induced by CO poisoning involves different areas related to regulating mechanisms of states of vigilance. Consequently, patients suffering from this damage have a high risk of presenting sleep-wake disturbances.

The aim of this study is to analyze the sleep characteristics of a patient that was exposed to CO inhalation and as consequence, suffers extensive brain damage.

Material and Methods

The study was approved by the institutional Research Ethics Committee. It was carried out in a 30-year-old female found unconscious after 36 hours of CO inhalation and brought to the hospital for medical attention. After intubation, she was transferred to the intensive care unit, where she remained for two weeks after which; she was transferred to the Department of Neurology Services. Her vital signs at admission were as follows: blood pressure: 110/70; pulse rate: 82 beats/min; respiratory rate: 20/min; temperature: 36.6°C. After assessing her clinical history, the diagnosis of CO poisoning was suggested and oxygen therapy via face mask (15 lit/min) was immediately started. Hyperbaric O2 therapy was not available.

Personal history showed that prior CO poisoning, the patient was healthy without antecedents of tabaquism or alcoholism. Additionally, she has not had any sleep or depressive problems before the accident.

Her brain computed tomography scan demonstrated generalized mild cerebral cortex damage. Differentiation between grey and white matter on the left frontal and parietal regions became confuse.

MRI showed multiple cerebral lesions affecting the cortical grey matter and the subcortical white matter from the frontal, parietal, and temporal lobes, as well as on the left occipital lobes, left hippocampal gyrus, both cerebellar hemispheres and both globus pallidus.

Central nervous system damage coincided with cognitive and neurologic disturbances [9]. These observations lead to the diagnosis of syndrome of upper motoneurone, secondary right hemiparesis, ischemic encephalopathy, sensory aphasia, anomies, confabulations, amnesic syndrome, and left hemineglect. The patient's intellectual coefficient was severely deteriorated.

Brain stem evoked potentials

Auditory evoked potentials were normal; in contrast, visual evoked potentials showed bilateral long lasting latencies for P100 components suggesting a slowing conduction of bilateral optic nerves.

Sleep studies

Previous to polysomnographic recording, the patient's sleep habits were integrated by means of a sleep questionnaire. Then, a Grass Comet Model 25 Acquisition System was used to obtain a polysomnographic recording throughout the night from 23:00 to 8:00 hr.

Sleep was recorded and scored using 30-s epochs according to standard methods, including central and occipital EEG (C3-A1, C4-A2, O1-A1 and O2-A2), submental EMG and periorbital EOG with a high-pass filter at 0.5 Hz and a low-pass filter at 45 Hz [18].

Oronasal airflow and thoracic-abdominal respiratory effort were also monitored throughout the night.

Total sleep time was obtained and the sleep efficiency was calculated. The total time spent in each sleep stage during the recording period was assessed and the percentage within the period was calculated. Mean duration of each sleep state as well as of the sleep cycles were obtained. Sleep and REM sleep latencies were also obtained. Scoring reliability was 91%, when comparing the independent judgment of two scorers.

Results

EEG

EEG recordings across the sleep-wake cycle were similar to those of normal subjects.

At the beginning of the recording, the patient was awake. During this period, brain activity consisted of a low voltage mixed frequency wave pattern and alpha rhythm (Figure 1).

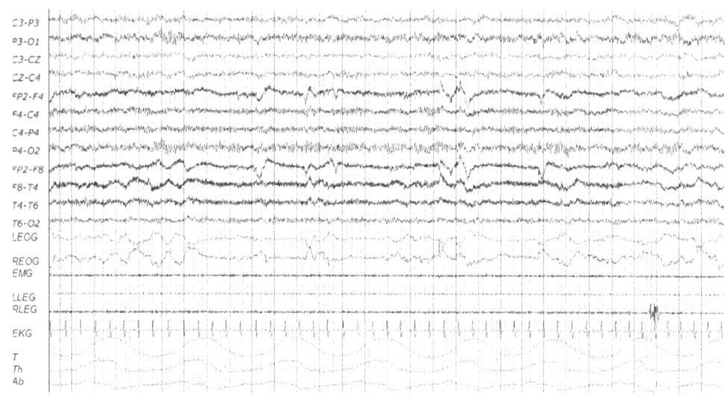

Figure 1: Polysomnographic recording during Wakefulness. EEG is characterized by low voltage mixed frequency waves and alpha rhythm recorded particularly on occipital leads.

After a variable period of relaxed wakefulness, the patient entered stage N1 of sleep, a transitional phase between full wakefulness and light sleep. During this stage, the EEG patterns were similar to those in normal individuals (Figure 2).

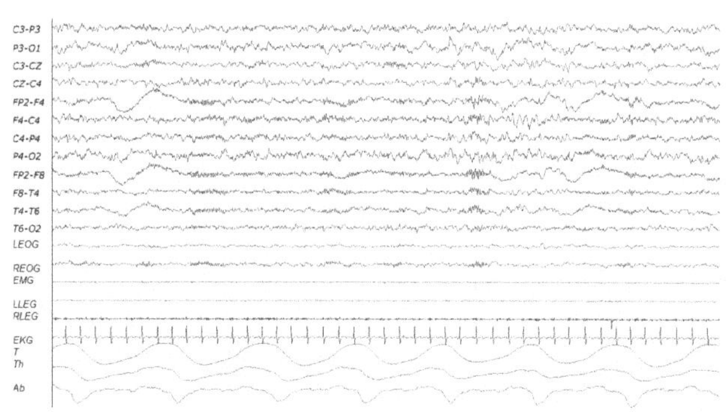

Figure 2: Stage N1 of sleep. Mixed frequency and theta waves are observed. Some vertex waves are observed on central recordings.

Stage N1 of sleep was usually followed by stage N2, where sleep spindles sometimes presented interhemispheric asynchrony (Figure 3).

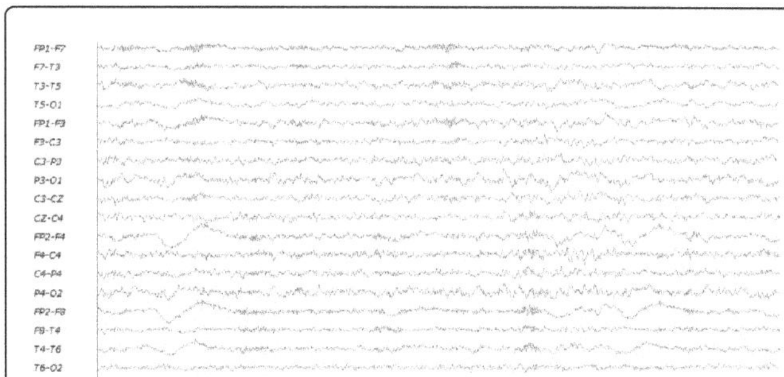

Figure 3: Stage N2 of sleep. Interhemispheric asymmetry of sleep spindles distribution is observed.

As stage N2 of sleep developed, sporadic high voltage slow waves appeared gradually, until meet the criteria for stage N3 of sleep (Figure 4). After a variable period of sleeping time, the patient went into REM sleep displaying the characteristic EEG patterns (Figure 5).

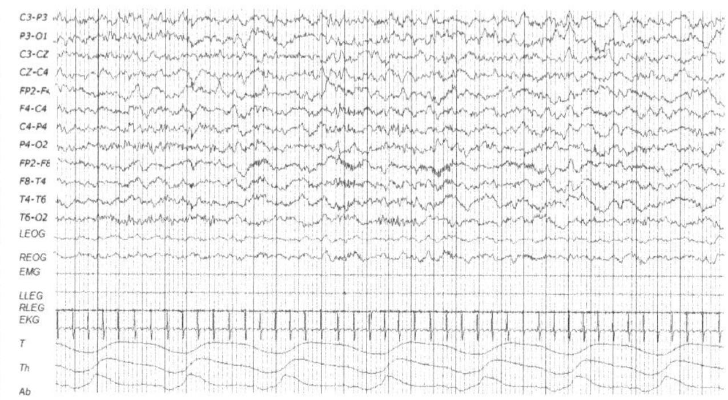

Figure 4: Stage N3 of sleep. Delta waves on EEG recordings are observed.

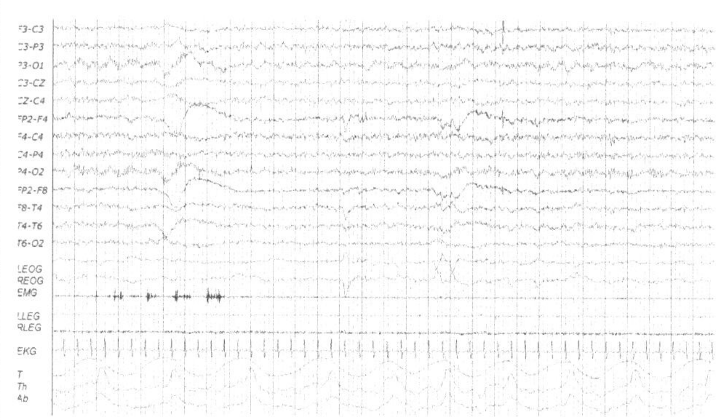

Figure 5: REM sleep. An EEG pattern of mixed frequency and theta waves is observed. Rapid eye movements are also present on EOG recordings.

When present, saw tooth waves sometimes preceded or coincided with eye movements.

Quantitative data

Sleep recordings revealed that in comparison with normative data14 this patient show lower sleep efficiency, more nocturnal wake time, and more awakenings lasting longer than 3 minutes. These disturbances were related to an important sleep fragmentation. The patient also showed altered sleep architecture, with higher percentage of nonrapid eye movement (NREM) stage 1 and lower percentage of rapid eye movement (REM) sleep compared to those in normative data. Quantitative sleep data are integrated in Table 1.

Latency to stage N2	**25 min**
Wake after sleep onset	128 min
Sleep efficiency	58%
Total sleep time	280 min
Total recording time	483 min

Time awake (%)	42
Stage N1 (%)	17
Stage N2 (%)	59
Stage N3 (%)	13
REM sleep (%)	11
Latency of REM sleep	91 min
Number of REM periods	4
Total number of stage changes	114
Stage changes index	24.4

Table 1: Quantitative data.

EMG

In contrast to waking state, low amplitude EMG activity was present throughout all NREM sleep stages. A discrete change in EMG amplitude in the waking to sleeping transition was generally observed. The EMG during stage 2 sleep was usually present at low amplitude. When passing to delta sleep, it was still present although its tracing occasionally fell to very low levels, similar to those of REM sleep. At this stage, muscle tone was extremely low or absent, though some twitches were present.

Heart rate

Patient showed across the sleep-waking cycle a mean heart rate of 90.10 ± 10.20 (Mean ± SD). The extremes between minimal (32 bpm) and maximal (145 bpm) values were greater during wakefulness followed by those in SWS (68 against 111 bpm), whereas during REM sleep the shortest extremes were displayed (81against 106 bpm). Heart variability expressed as bradycardia and tachycardia were present during wakefulness, but not during both SWS and REM sleep.

Respiratory activity

During steady NREM sleep, breathing was remarkably regular in both amplitude and frequency showing the lowest index of variability of all vigilance states. During quiet wakefulness and throughout N1, N2, and N3 sleep phases breathing frequency averaged 16.0 breaths/min, it slightly decreased to 14.0 breaths/min when passing to the first episode of REM sleep and it oscillated from 15 to 21 breaths/min during the second REM sleep episode. Breathing irregularity during REM sleep consisted of sudden changes involving both amplitude and frequency of respiratory movements, which were at times interrupted by central apneas lasting 10 to 30 sec. The breathing irregularities did not occur at random but were linked to bursts of REMs.

Oximetry

Oximetry values were periodically checked throughout sleep. The patient displayed high oxygen saturation levels reaching a total average of 95.53% distributed as follows: wakefulness, 96.01%; NREM sleep, 94.86; and REM sleep, 94.98%. Any event of oxygen desaturation was not observed.

Discussion

People suffering brain damage usually develop sleep disturbances [19-22], as confirmed in this study. These disturbances can lead to mood disorders, anxiety, irritability, and a general feeling of physical and mental fatigue. It can also originate poor work performance and occupational accidents.

Sleep disturbances have been observed in people having different levels of brain damage from mild to severe. Since sleep is a complex process involving several parts of the brain, a variety of sleep disturbances can develop after brain injury.

Some studies show that sleep abnormalities may persist months and even years following brain damage [23,24].

In addition to disruption of sleep continuity, alterations in its architecture were observed in the patient under study. Total sleep time was significantly reduced; consequently, sleep efficiency was severely affected. These findings are similar to those of other authors who observed sleep fragmentation after traumatic brain injury (TBI) [23-25]. Light sleep (stages N1 and N2) showed percentage proportions higher than those in normative data, while time percentage spent in REM sleep showed an important reduction. This reduction was related to the mean duration but not to the number of REM sleep episodes displayed across the recording of sleep.

Longer time spent awake after sleep onset and more frequent awakenings observed in this patient affected total sleep time and sleep efficiency. These results are in line with previous studies which have found mainly an increment of wakefulness and number of awakenings into the sleeping period after TBI [23-26].

Apart from the increasing in sleep stages N1 and N2, no other differences were noted in the distribution of sleep stages in TBI patients. Poor sleep exhibited by our patient may be a result of brain lesions affecting sleep-regulating mechanisms, as well as psychological factors such as anxiety and depression.

The complex interactions between depression, anxiety or post-traumatic stress disorder symptoms and sleep disturbances deserve further attention since these psychiatric conditions affect sleep architecture. Prospective studies should, therefore, include thorough evaluations for such conditions.

Autonomic variables

It has been reported that there is a fall in heart rate and respiratory activity when passing from relaxed wakefulness to light sleep. These physiological variations are a reflex of parasympathetic activation. The increase in parasympathetic activity remains across NREM sleep [27-32]. During REM sleep, HR returns to waking levels or it remains below waking, but above NREM sleep levels [33-35], while respiratory activity becomes irregular.

These sleep related changes in heart and respiratory rates appear to be mediated mainly by changes in autonomic circulatory control [36].

Studies that have investigated the effect of sleep and sleep stages on autonomic control have made the assumption that stage effects are independent of time during the sleep period. A number of studies have described that cardiac activity shows systematic changes over the sleep period [27,34,37,38]. The present results indicate that HR does not change significantly over time within both NREM and REM sleep. It appears that regulation of the autonomous nervous systems on the cardiac activity was absent across the sleep period.

In contrast, an important increase of heart rate was observed in the early morning coinciding with patient's arousal. This HR acceleration may reflect an activation of the sympathetic tone.

The present results contrast with normative findings related to autonomic control of cardiac activity during sleep [39]. The data indicate that parasympathetic nervous system activity remains at a low level throughout both NREM sleep and REM sleep. In contrast, sympathetic nervous system activity, as indicated by the high heart rate average, remains elevated throughout the sleep period showing an additional increase during the early morning that coincides with the awaking period. These findings may reflect a damage of cerebral regions that regulate the heart rate variability induced by carbon monoxide poisoning.

Usually, respiratory activity undergoes important modifications becoming deeper and more regular with NREM sleep, while it turns shallower, irregular, and more frequent during REM sleep.

However, average respiratory rate of the studied patient shows regular levels across the vigilance states from waking state to NREM sleep and a slight non-significant decrement in the first REM sleep episode. This activity became faster and irregular during the second REM sleep episode. Our findings about sleep stage-dependent variations in the heart rate Variability signal and respiratory rate contrast with previous reports.

Conflict of Interest

The authors declare that there is no conflict of interest in this study.

References

1. Hurley RA, Hopkins RO, Bigler ED, Taber KH (2001) Applications of functional imaging to carbon monoxide poisoning. J Neuropsychiatry Clin Neurosci 13: 157-160.
2. Henry JA (1999) Carbon monoxide: not gone, not to be forgotten. J Accid Emerg Med 16: 91-92.
3. Turner M, Hamilton-Farrell MR, Clark RJ (1999) Carbon monoxide poisoning: an update. J Accid Emerg Med 16: 92-96.
4. Pavese N, Napolitano A, De Iaco G, Canapicchi R, Collavoli PL, et al. (1999) Clinical outcome and magnetic resonance imaging of carbon monoxide intoxication. A long-term follow-up study. Ital J Neurol Sci 20: 171-178.
5. Hopkins RO, Weaver LK, Bigler ED (2000) Longitudinal outcome following carbon monoxide poisoning. J Int Neuropsychol Soc 6: 393.
6. Dunham MD, Johnstone B (1999) Variability of neuropsychological deficits associated with carbon monoxide poisoning: four case reports. Brain Inj 13: 917-925.
7. Choi IS, Cheon HY (1999) Delayed movement disorders after carbon monoxide poisoning. Eur Neurol 42: 141-144.
8. Gale SD, Hopkins RO, Weaver LK, Bigler ED, Booth EJ, et al. (1999) MRI, quantitative MRI, SPECT, and neuropsychological findings following carbon monoxide poisoning. Brain Inj 13: 229-243.
9. Arreguín-González IJ, Ayala-Guerrero F, Gasca-Zamudio PD, Melo-Balderas MA (2014) Funciones neurocognitivas alteradas en paciente intoxicada por monóxido de carbono. Neurología (Barcelona).
10. Tom T, Abedon S, Clark RI, Wong W (1996) Neuroimaging characteristics in carbon monoxide toxicity. J Neuroimaging 6: 161-166.
11. O'Donnell P, Buxton PJ, Pitkin A, Jarvis LJ (2000) The magnetic resonance imaging appearances of the brain in acute carbon monoxide poisoning. Clin Radiol 55: 273-280.
12. Kao CH, Hung DZ, ChangLai SP, Liao KK, Chieng PU (1998) HMPAO brain SPECT in acute carbon monoxide poisoning. J Nucl Med 39: 769-772.
13. Lee MS, Marsden CD (1994) Neurological sequelae following carbon monoxide poisoning clinical course and outcome according to the clinical types and brain computed tomography scan findings. Mov Disord 9: 550-558.
14. Carskadon MA, Dement WC (2011) Normal human sleep: an overview. In: Kryger M, Roth T, and Dement W (eds.) Principles and practice of sleep medicine. (2ndedn). Saunders; Philadelphia: 16-26.
15. Schulz H (2007) Phasic or transient? Comment on the terminology of the AASM manual for the scoring of sleep and associated events. J Clin Sleep Med 3: 752.
16. Wang G, Grone B, Colas D, Appelbaum L, Mourrain P (2011) Synaptic plasticity in sleep: learning, homeostasis and disease. Trends Neurosci 34: 452-463.
17. Otzenberger H, Gronfier C, Simon Ch, Charloux A, Ehrhart J, et al. (1998) Dynamic heart rate variability: a tool for exploring sympathovagal balance continuously during sleep in men. Am J Physiol 275: H946–H950.
18. Retschaffen A, Kales A (1968) A manual of standardized terminology, techniques, and scoring system for sleep stages of human subjects. U.S. Public Health Service, U.S. Government Printing Office: Washington, D.C.
19. Beetar JT, Guilmette TJ, Sparadeo FR (1996) Sleep and pain complaints in symptomatic traumatic brain injury and neurologic populations. Arch Phys Med Rehabil 77: 1298-1302.
20. Cohen M, Oksenberg A, Snir D, Stern MJ, Groswasser Z (1992) Temporally related changes of sleep complaints in traumatic brain injured patients. J Neurol Neurosurg Psychiatry 55: 313-315.
21. Clinchot DM, Bogner J, Mysiw WJ, Fugate L, Corrigan J (1998) Defining sleep disturbance after brain injury. Am J Phys Med Rehabil 77: 291-295.
22. Perlis ML, Artiola L, Giles DE (1997) Sleep complaints in chronic postconcussion syndrome. Percept Mot Skills 84: 595-599.
23. Prigatano GP, Stahl ML, Orr WC, Zeiner HK (1982) Sleep and dreaming disturbances in closed head injury patients. J Neurol Neurosurg Psychiatry 45: 78-80.
24. George B, Landau-Ferey J (1986) Twelve months' follow-up by night sleep EEG after recovery from severe head trauma. Neurochirurgia (Stuttg) 29: 45-47.
25. Kaufman Y, Tzischinsky O, Epstein R, Etzioni A, Lavie P, et al. (2001) Long-term sleep disturbances in adolescents after minor head injury. Pediatr Neurol 24: 129-134.
26. Lenard HG, Pennigstorff H (1970) Alterations in the sleep patterns of infants and young children following acute head injuries. Acta Paediatr Scand 59: 565-571.
27. Furlan R, Guzzetti S, Crivellaro W, Dassi S, Tinelli M et al. (1990) Continuous 24-hours assessment of the neural regulation of systemic arterial pressure and R-R variabilities in ambulant subjects. Circulation 81: 537–547
28. Berlad II, Shlitner A, Ben-Haim S. Lavie P (1993) Power spectrum analysis and heart rate variability in Stage 4 and REM sleep: evidence for state-specific changes in autonomic dominance. J Sleep Res 2: 88–90.
29. Orr W, Lin B, Adamson P, Vanoli E (1993) Autonomic control of heart rate variability during sleep. Sleep Res 22: 26.
30. Vanoli E, Adamson PB, Ba-Lin P, Pinna GD, Lazzara R, Orr WC (1995) Heart rate variability during specific sleep stages. A comparison of healthy subjects with patients after myocardial infarction. Circulation 91: 1918–1922.
31. Bonnet MH, Arand DL (1998) Heart rate variability in insomniacs and matched normal sleepers. Psychosom Med 60: 610-615.
32. Burgess HJ, Trinder J, Kim Y (1996) Cardiac parasympathetic nervous system activity does not increase in anticipation of sleep. J Sleep Res 5: 83-89.

33. Zemaityte D, Varoneckas G, Sokolov E (1984) Heart rhythm control during sleep. Psychophysiology 21: 279-289.
34. Van de Borne P, Nguyen H, Biston P, Linkowski P, Degaute JP (1994) Effects of wake and sleep stages on the 24-h autonomic control of blood pressure and heart rate in recumbent men. Am J Physiol 266: H548-554.
35. Morgan BJ, Crabtree DC, Puleo DS, Badr MS, Toiber F, et al. (1996) Neurocirculatory consequences of abrupt change in sleep state in humans. J Appl Physiol 80: 1627-1636.
36. Narkiewicz K, Phillips B, Somers VK (2000) Influence of sleep and sleep apnea on autonomic control of the cardiovascular system: Sleep Apnea: Implications in Cardiovascular and Cerebrovascular Disease. Bradley TD, Floras JS (eds.) Marcel Dekker: New York: 135–158.
37. Degaute JP, van de Borne P, Linkowski P, Van Cauter E (1991) Quantitative analysis of the 24-hour blood pressure and heart rate patterns in young men. Hypertension 18: 199-210.
38. Parati G, Castiglioni P, Di Rienzo M, Omboni S, Pedotti A, et al. (1990) Sequential spectral analysis of 24-hour blood pressure and pulse interval in humans. Hypertension 16: 414-421.
39. Tobaldini E, Nobili L, Strada S, Casali KR, Braghiroli A, et al. (2013) Heart rate variability in normal and pathological sleep. Front Physiol 4: 294.

Sleep Quality in Adolescents: What's Discriminates Good from Poor Sleepers?

Sílvia HM Pucci* **and M Graça Pereira**

School of Psychology, University of Minho, Braga, Portugal

***Corresponding author:** Sílvia HM Pucci, School of Psychology, University of Minho, Braga, Portugal, E-mail: shmpucci@gmail.com

Abstract

Background: The study focused on discriminating adolescents with good versus poor sleep quality.

Method: The sample consisted of 272 adolescents and a transversal design was used. The instruments assessed socio-demographic data, psychological morbidity, sleep quality, family sleep behavior, excessive daytime sleepiness, sleep habits and social skills.

Results: The results revealed that age, caffeine intake, psychological morbidity, excessive daytime sleepiness, and family sleep behavior were variables that discriminated good from poorer sleepers in terms of adolescents' sleep quality.

Conclusions: The results emphasize the role of family on sleep quality and the need to include family members in intervention programs. Programs should be sensitive to adolescents' age and gender.

Keywords: Adolescent; Sleep; Psychological morbidity; Caffeine

Introduction

The phase of adolescence is marked by changes that occur on many different aspects of the individual's life, including changes in sleep patterns [1]. Sleep plays an active role in the brain during an individual's overall development, especially regarding restorative functions [2]. Several studies have reported a trend of insufficient and poor sleep, in adolescents [3,4]. A study that analyzed 5226 adolescents classified 20% as poor sleepers.

The study showed that the prevalence of poor sleep, increased with age, grade level, and older adolescents showed worse sleep efficiency, problems in falling asleep, and more sleep disturbances [5]. At the same time, a research that focused on disturbed sleep and associated factors, in 1221 adolescents, found that almost 35% of adolescents showed poor sleep that increased with age [4].

Psychological factors may affect sleep patterns in adolescents, interacting with biological regulatory processes, like autonomy to decide the right time to go to bed, use of technology/electronic equipment, social activities, and parental-set-bedtime [6]. It is possible to extend adolescents' sleep with parent's intervention on set-bedtime; and with the combination of "extended sleep" and "early bedtime"; positive outcomes may be achieved regarding depression, fatigue and sleepiness [6].

There is a range of possible causes and consequences of sleep quality in adolescents, and psychological morbidity seems to be one important and relevant factor. Some studies have linked psychological morbidity, i.e., depression/anxiety, with adolescents' sleep.

In fact, a study that estimated the relationship between anxiety/depression and sleep, in a non-clinical child sample aged 6 to 11 years old found, through mothers' reports, that children with troubled sleep had higher odds of developing depression and anxiety [7]. Other interesting research [8] found an association between childhood sleep problems and anxiety and depression, later on, in adulthood. The authors found that adulthood's anxiety was predicted by the persistence of sleep problems in adolescence.

Another psychological variable with great relevance to sleep quality in adolescents is family functioning, although there is a lack of studies that focused on the association between these two variables [9]. A study that focused on the perceived sleep quality, health habits, and psychological factors revealed that having a good environment at home was essential for sleep quality and quantity, among adolescents [10].

As indicators of poor sleep quality, are the problems of initiating and maintaining sleep among children and adolescents that are common with varying prevalence's estimations, probably due to the methodology and design of the studies [11]. Excessive daytime sleepiness (EDS) is one of the most common clinical consequences of inadequate sleep, having a big prevalence among teenagers [12].

In fact, daytime sleepiness is closely associated with sleep habits that youngsters develop and follow during adolescence [13] and is related to mood disorders and psychological morbidity [14-16].

Several studies have shown that sleep habits and sleep quality, in adolescents, are related. In fact, sleep habits change according to age, and adjustments in sleep schedules and time spent in bed, need to be done [17]. The use of electronic equipment is an important factor that influences adolescents' sleep. Studies have shown that among the most important impairments for good sleep quality are adolescents' habits, such as watching television [18]. Adolescents with less hours of sleep, who watched television at night, also have a higher consumption of caffeine intake [19].

In fact, psychoactive substances are also related to sleep quality, in adolescents. Caffeine is one of the most consumed substance worldwide, by adults and adolescents. Caffeine is quickly absorbed, reaching a plasmatic high in about 30 to 75 minutes when consumed orally [20]. A literature review focusing on caffeine and sleep concluded that in children and adolescents, poor sleep quality and caffeine intake is related [21].

Taking in consideration the literature reviewed, the present study focused on the variables that discriminate adolescents with good versus poor sleep quality [22]. According to the literature, we expect that psychological morbidity, daytime sleepiness and more problems with family sleep behaviors will discriminate poor from good sleepers [23]. Knowing which variables are the most important and discriminating adolescents' sleep quality will help health care professionals to plan interventions, in this population [24].

Method and Material

Participants

Participants were 272 adolescents from two public schools, aged between 12 and 18 years old (M = 15.48, SD = 1.61). The majority of students were female (58%), with married parents (79%), with mothers (51%) and fathers (73%) consuming alcohol. Of the total sample, 31% had a daily intake of caffeine, 47% consumed beverages with caffeine and 23% consumed energetic drinks.

Design and settings

The study used a transversal design. The research was approved by the General Education Committee. The data were collected in two secondary public schools in the Northern region of Portugal. The participation was voluntary, and the parents signed an informed consent regarding their adolescent's participation. The instruments were completed by adolescents, at school, during class.

The inclusion criteria were 1) age between 12 and 18; 2) being a student in the class the day of the assessment; 3) parent's approval to be part of the study. Exclusion criteria included parent's non-approval of the adolescent's inclusion in the study.

Assessments

Pittsburgh sleep quality index (PSQI): This instrument assesses sleep quality during the previous month and has 19 items [25]. PSQI is composed of seven components that evaluate daytime dysfunction, sleep medication, sleep disturbances, sleep efficiency, sleep duration, sleep latency and sleep quality. In the present study only the total scale was used and the Cronbach's alpha was 0.60.

Modified excessive sleepiness scale (MESSA): The instrument assesses the propensity of adolescents to fall asleep in different situations and is composed of 13 items [26]. In this study, only the total scale was used and the Cronbach's alpha for the total scale was .78.

Hospital anxiety and depression scales (HADS): The instrument assesses the levels of depression and anxiety [27]. It has 14 items that give a psychological morbidity global score. There are two subscales (anxiety and depression). The cutoff score for clinical depression and anxiety is 8. In this study, only the total scale was used and the Cronbach's alpha was 0.76.

Howard family sleep questionnaire (HFSQ): This scale assesses the cumulative impact of family dynamics on sleep behavior and is composed of 52 items that assess physical and cultural aspects of the family environment that influence sleep (e.g. "we eat dinner together", "we respect each other's needs for quiet once one of us goes to bed", "on weekends, we have no set bedtime [28]. In this study, Cronbach's alpha was 0.70.

Sleep habits questionnaire (SHQ): This 12 item questionnaire assesses the impact of behaviors that may influence sleep in adolescents (e.g. how many times a week do you play video-games after bedtime, how many times a week do you read, study or, do homework after bedtime) [29]. In the present study, Cronbach's alpha was 0.70.

Data extraction/scoring

Data was abstracted from the instruments that were scored regarding the original instructions of their authors i.e., summing the items according to the Likert scale. In the Pittsburgh Sleep Quality Index, Howard Family Sleep Questionnaire, and the Sleep Habits Questionnaire, a higher score indicates poor sleep quality, poor family sleep behaviors, and poor sleep habits, respectively.

Regarding the Modified Excessive Sleepiness Scale, Hospital Anxiety and Depression Scales, a higher score indicates respectively the presence of excessive daytime sleepiness, and more anxiety and depression. Information regarding age, gender, the consumption of caffeine and energetic beverages was abstracted from a sociodemographic questionnaire.

Data analysis

A discriminant analysis was used to determine which variables differentiated adolescents with good versus poor sleep quality based on the sample median (stepwise method).

This statistical procedure determines which variables differentiate the two groups allowing to know the best predictors of sleep quality. The stepwise procedure in particular allows seeing which variables are included in the prediction of group membership (good versus poorer sleepers).

Results

The results showed that age, caffeine intake, psychological morbidity, daytime sleepiness and family sleep behaviors discriminated adolescents who had good versus poor sleep quality (Table 1). Low function values indicate good sleep quality (mean = -0.354) and higher function values indicate poor sleep quality (mean = 0.519). Therefore, lower values of the discriminant function belong to the good sleep quality group.

The variables that present the highest coefficient in absolute value are the most important. Therefore, adolescents with psychological morbidity (-0.619) and family sleep behavior (-0.455), i.e., less depression/anxiety and less problems with family sleep behaviors belong to the good sleepers group. Adolescents with more excessive daytime sleepiness (0.435), being older (0.370) and drinking more caffeine beverages (0.335; 0.328) belong to the poorer sleepers.

Based on the results, groups were significantly different and the discriminant function was significant (Wilk's Lambda = 0.844; Qi2 = 44.83; $p<0.000$) (Table 2). The classification matrix identified 66.5% of cases as correctly classified, i.e., in group 0, 79.6% are good sleepers and in group 1, 45.5% are poor sleepers.

Variables	Good sleepers		Poor sleepers		Wilks' Lambda	F	P
	Mean	SD	Mean	SD			
Age	15.26	1.7	15.77	1.3	0.975	6.776	0.01
Caffeine Intake	1.25	0.46	1.40	0.57	0.98	5.319	0.022
Use of Energy Drinks	1.22	0.59	1.41	0.7	0.98	5.537	0.019
HADS (Depression/Anxiety)	20.06	3.29	18.23	3.5	0.934	18.92	0
MESSA (Daytime Sleepiness)	11.63	6.1	13.95	6.0	0.966	9.336	0.002
HFSQ (Family Sleep)	99.95	10.9	95.75	10.1	0.963	10.222	0.002

Table 1: Significant psychosocial variables that discriminate poor from good sleep quality in adolescents.

Sleep Quality	Function
HADS	-0.619
HFSQ	-0.455
MESSA	0.435
Age	0.37
Energy Drinks	0.335
Caffeine Intake	0.328

Table 2: Matrix of the factorial structure factors that discriminate sleep quality.

Discussion

This study analyzed the differences between adolescents with good versus poor sleep quality in terms of their social demographic and psychological characteristics. The results showed that age was a discriminant variable between adolescents with good versus poor sleep quality. A meta-analysis, reviewing 41 studies about adolescent's sleep patterns concluded that as age increased there was a trend for later sleep patterns [27]. Another study focusing on age and sleep patterns showed that older students had more depression and daytime sleepiness [28]. Older adolescents reported a few hours of sleep, when compared with two different aged groups (older teenagers and pre-teens) [29]. The results found in this study concerning age are in accordance with the majority of studies, showing that age is a determinant for adolescent's sleep quality.

Daytime sleepiness was also an important variable for the discrimination of adolescent sleep quality. A literature review showed, through laboratory experiments, that poor sleep quality and insufficient sleep hours were related to daytime sleepiness [12]. Age and poor sleep quality were also predictors of sleepiness in children and teenagers in a recent German study [30].

The intake of caffeine and energetic beverages discriminated adolescents in terms of sleep quality. Literature has suggested that youngster's sleep quality may also be related to the consumption of psychoactive substances. Adolescents with poor sleep quality had twice as much intake of stimulant substances to decrease daytime sleepiness and drank more alcoholic drinks per day than good sleepers. However, there were no differences on caffeine and energy drink consumption between the two groups [31].

On the other hand, a more recent study with 225 adolescents concluded that 79% drank caffeine and that higher intake of caffeine was negatively associated with sleep quality [32], which was corroborated by other studies [19].

Family variables were an important discriminant factor between good and poor sleep quality. In line with our results, a recent study analyzed the relationship between parents and adolescent sleep patterns and psychological functioning, finding a relationship between parents and children sleep patterns; and a relationship between stress perception, depression symptoms, family environment and subjective sleep disturbances in adolescents. Adolescents' sleep disturbances were independently predicted by stress, perceived negative parental styles and mother's poorer sleep [33]. Another study found a significant association for parents and adolescents regarding sleep patterns sleep disturbances, depression and family environment. In the face of these results, the authors concluded that there might be a bidirectional association between family function, family environment, well-being and adolescent's sleep, and that mothers and children sleep and well-being are related [34]. Our results are in accordance with this literature, emphasizing the important role of parents in promoting sleep quality with adolescents.

This study found that psychological morbidity was a very important variable discriminating adolescents' sleep quality. In fact, several studies have shown the association between sleep problems and psychological symptoms, in adolescents [2,35]. A study analyzed the relationship between sleep and suicidal behaviors in students and concluded that sleep disturbances were associated with suicidal ideation [36]. Interestingly, after adjusting for the statistical effect of depression, this relationship ceased to exist, leading the authors to hypothesize that it was mediated by depression.

Another study that assessed sleep quality as a predictor of sleep patterns found that lower sleep quality was related to depressions self-reports [31]. An association between sleep problems and anxiety and depression was also found in another study, showing that emotional problems could be predicted by sleep problems [37]. This relationship between sleep quality and psychological morbidity seems to be bidirectional. In any case, psychological morbidity either a cause or a consequence of poor sleep quality, is an important variable to be addressed in future interventions.

This study emphasizes how important variables such as caffeine intake and family sleep behaviors, that are less researched, need to be addressed and incorporated in health promotion interventions regarding sleep quality, in adolescents.

Limitation

The Cronbach alpha of the Pittsburgh Sleep Questionnaire Index was acceptable but low 0.60 (total scale). Finally, the use of only self-reported instruments and the cross-sectional design are also limitations.

Conclusion/Clinical Implications

This study concluded that age, caffeine intake, psychological morbidity, daytime sleepiness and the influence of family on sleep behaviors were discriminant factors for sleep quality among adolescents. It is crucial to take these variables into consideration in health promotion programs with this population.

Psychological morbidity and family factors were important discriminating variables in adolescent sleep quality. Intervention with teenagers should, therefore, pay attention to depression and anxiety symptoms and should include the family, in order to promote better sleep quality.

Systemic intervention is crucial to promote healthy habits in the family, addressing in particular, the consumption of caffeine and other psychoactive substances, and family sleep behaviors that impacts adolescents sleep quality.

Future studies should focus on detecting poor sleep quality causes, in order to understand possible bidirectional relationships and comorbidities and use longitudinal designs to understand the influence of these variables, over time.

Acknowledgement

The present research had a support of Erasmus Mundus 15.

Disclosure

No author indicated any conflicts of interest.

References

1. Carskadon MA, Vieira C, Acebo C (1993) Association between puberty and delayed phase preference. Sleep 16: 258-262.
2. Dahl RE, Lewin DS (2002) Pathways to adolescent health sleep regulation and behavior. J Adolesc Health 31: 175-184.
3. Wolfson AR, Carskadon MA (1998) Sleep schedules and daytime functioning in adolescents. Child Dev 69: 875-887.
4. Zhou HQ, Shi WB, Wang XF, Yao M, Cheng GY, et al. (2012) An epidemiological study of sleep quality in adolescents in South China: a school-based study. Child Care Health Dev 38: 581-587.
5. Xu Z, Su H, Zou Y, Chen J, Wu J, et al. (2012) Sleep quality of Chinese adolescents: distribution and its associated factors. J Paediatr Child Health 48: 138-145.
6. Carskadon MA (2011) Sleep in adolescents: the perfect storm. Pediatr Clin North Am 58: 637-647.
7. Johnson EO, Chilcoat HD, Breslau N (2000) Trouble sleeping and anxiety/depression in childhood. Psychiatry Res 94: 93-102.
8. Gregory AM, Caspi A, Eley TC, Moffitt TE, O'Connor TG, et al. (2005) Prospective Longitudinal Associations Between Persistent Sleep Problems in Childhood and Anxiety and Depression Disorders in Adulthood. J Abnorm Child Psych 33: 157-163.
9. Adam EK, Snell EK, Pendry P (2007) Sleep timing and quantity in ecological and family context: a nationally representative time-diary study. J Fam Psychol 21: 4-19.
10. Tynjälä J, Kannas L, Levälahti E, Välimaa R (1999) Perceived sleep quality and its precursors in adolescents. Health Promot Int 14: 155-166.
11. Dewald JF, Meijer AM, Oort FJ, Kerkhof GA, Bögels SM (2010) The influence of sleep quality, sleep duration and sleepiness on school performance in children and adolescents: A meta-analytic review. Sleep Med Rev 14: 179-189.
12. Millman RP; Working Group on Sleepiness in Adolescents/Young Adults; AAP Committee on Adolescence (2005) Excessive sleepiness in adolescents and young adults: causes, consequences, and treatment strategies. Pediatrics 115: 1774-1786.
13. Cain N, Gradisar M (2010) Electronic media use and sleep in school-aged children and adolescents: A review. Sleep Med 11: 735-742.
14. Carskadon MA (1990) Patterns of sleep and sleepiness in adolescents. Pediatrician 17: 5-12.
15. Carskadon MA, Wolfson AR, Acebo C, Tzischinsky O, Seifer R (1998) Adolescent sleep patterns, circadian timing, and sleepiness at a transition to early school days. Sleep 21: 871-881.
16. Leotta C, Carskadon M, Acebo C, Seifer R, Quinn B (1997) Effects of acute sleep restriction on affective response in adolescents: Preliminary results. Sleep Res 26: 201.
17. Colrain IM, Baker FC (2011) Changes in sleep as a function of adolescent development. Neuropsychol Rev 21: 5-21.
18. Noland H, Price JH, Dake J, Telljohann SK (2009) Adolescents' sleep behaviors and perceptions of sleep. J Sch Health 79: 224-230.
19. Lodato F, Araújo J, Barros H, Lopes C, Agodi A, et al. (2013) Caffeine intake reduces sleep duration in adolescents. Nutr Res 33: 726-732.
20. Mandel HG (2002) Update on caffeine consumption, disposition and action. Food Chem Toxicol 40: 1231-1234.
21. Roehrs T, Roth T (2008) Caffeine: sleep and daytime sleepiness. Sleep Med Rev 12: 153-162.
22. Buysse DJ, Reynolds CF 3rd, Monk TH, Berman SR, Kupfer DJ (1989) The Pittsburgh Sleep Quality Index: a new instrument for psychiatric practice and research. Psychiatry Res 28: 193-213.
23. Billings T, Berg-Cross L (2010a) The Modified Epworth Sleepiness Scale for Adolescents: A Brief Measure of Daytime Sleepiness in Adolescents. Howard University, Washington, DC.
24. Zigmond AS, Snaith RP (1983) The hospital anxiety and depression scale. Acta Psychiatr Scand 67: 361-370.
25. Billings T, Bangash O, Berg-Cross L (2010) Predicting Sleep Problems in Adolescents: Validation of the Family Sleep Questionnaire. Howard University, Washington.
26. Billings T, Berg-Cross L (2010b) Sleep Competing Activities and Sleep Problems. Howard University, Washington, DC.
27. Gradisar M, Gardner G, Dohnt H (2011) Recent worldwide sleep patterns and problems during adolescence: a review and meta-analysis of age, region, and sleep. Sleep Med 12: 110-118.
28. Yang CK, Kim JK, Patel SR, Lee JH (2005) Age-related changes in sleep/wake patterns among Korean teenagers. Pediatrics 115: 250-256.
29. Taylor DJ, Jenni OG, Acebo C, Carskadon MA (2005) Sleep tendency during extended wakefulness: insights into adolescent sleep regulation and behavior. J Sleep Res 14: 239-244.
30. Urschitz MS, Heine K, Brockmann PE, Peters T, Durst W, et al. (2013) Subjective and objective daytime sleepiness in schoolchildren and adolescents: results of a community-based study. Sleep Med 14: 1005-1012.
31. Lund HG, Reider BD, Whiting AB, Prichard JR (2010) Sleep patterns and predictors of disturbed sleep in a large population of college students. J Adolesc Health 46: 124-132.
32. Anderson BL, Juliano LM (2012) Behavior, sleep, and problematic caffeine consumption in a college-aged sample. J Caffeine Res 2: 38-44.

33. Bajoghli H, Alipouri A, Holsboer-Trachsler E, Brand S (2013) Sleep patterns and psychological functioning in families in northeastern Iran; evidence for similarities between adolescent children and their parents. J Adolescence 36: 1103-1113.

34. Kalak N, Gerber M, Kirov R, Mikoteit T, Pühse U, et al. (2012) The relation of objective sleep patterns, depressive symptoms, and sleep disturbances in adolescent children and their parents: A sleep-EEG study with 47 families. J Psychiat Res 46: 1374-1382.

35. Johnson EO, Roth T, Breslau N (2006) The association of insomnia with anxiety disorders and depression: exploration of the direction of risk. J Psychiatr Res 40: 700-708.

36. Liu X (2004) Sleep and adolescent suicidal behavior. Sleep 27: 1351-1358.

37. Gregory AM, O'Connor TG (2002) Sleep problems in childhood: a longitudinal study of developmental change and association with behavioral problems. J Am Acad Child Adolesc Psychiatry 41: 964-971.

The Role of Race/Ethnicity and Gender in the Association between Inadequate Sleep and Hypercholesterolemia

Alethea N Hill[1], Natasha J Williams[2], Idoko Salifu[2], Chimene Castor[3], Jenna Gibilaro[3], Samy I McFarlane[4] and Girardin Jean-Louis[2,*]

[1]College of Nursing, Adult Health Nursing Department, University of South Alabama, USA

[2]Center for Healthful Behavior Change, Division of Health and Behavior, Department of Population Health, NYU Langone Medical Center, USA

[3]Department of Nutritional Sciences, Howard University, USA

[4]Department of Medicine, Division of Endocrinology, SUNY Downstate Medical Center, USA

[*]**Corresponding author:** Girardin Jean-Louis, Ph.D., Professor of Population Health, Center for Healthful Behavior Change, Department of Population Health, New York University School of Medicine, 227 East 30th St, 6th Floor, New York, NY 10016, USA, E-mail: girardin.jean-louis@nyumc.org

Abstract

Background: Evidence links aberrant sleep durations with elevated serum cholesterol levels or, hypercholesterolemia (HC), an established risk factor for coronary heart disease (CHD). Few studies have assessed the relationship between key sociodemographic indicators including gender and race/ethnicity and HC.

Methods: A total of 40,679 Americans who participated in the 2008-2009 National Health Interview Survey (NHIS) provided data for this cross-sectional analysis. Participants were recruited using a nationally representative cross-sectional household interview survey, which uses a multi-stage area probability design. Participants provided sociodemographic information, physician-diagnosed chronic conditions, and habitual sleep duration, categorized as <6 hours, or >8 hours, referenced to 7 hours. We used NHIS-provided weights to adjust for use of complex design.

Results: Of the total sample (n=40,679), 85% reported their race/ethnicity as non-Hispanic white and 15% as non-Hispanic black; 56% of the participants were female. Adjusted logistic regression analyses showed significant association between sleep duration and presence of HC among blacks, but not among whites. Blacks reporting short (<6 hours) or long sleep durations (>8 hours) had a greater risk of HC relative to blacks sleeping 7 hours habitually [OR=1.12, 95% CI: 1.11-1.13; OR=1.13, 95% CI: 1.12-1.14; p<0.001, respectively]. Black females reporting short or long sleep duration had greater risk of reporting HC compared with black males sleeping 7 hours [OR=1.11, 95% CI: 1.10-1.11; OR=1.10, 95% CI: 1.10-1.10; p<0.001, respectively].

Conclusion: Our study supports the relationship between inadequate sleep and traditional risk factors for CHD, namely, HC. Future lifestyle interventions should consider the role of sleep in addressing CHD risk and CHD morbidity.

Keywords: Inadequate sleep; Sleep duration; Hypercholesterolemia; Coronary heart disease; Race; Gender

Introduction

Sleep duration is an important risk factor to assess as clinicians strive to improve the health-related quality of life and management of chronic diseases in their patient population [1,2]. The effect of inadequate sleep duration on physiological mechanisms and body systems often manifest as disease processes including depression [3,4], obesity [5-7], diabetes mellitus [8-13], and hypertension [6,14,15]. In addition, several studies have evidenced associations, often preceded by aberrant lipid metabolism, between sleep duration and atherosclerosis [16-19].

Hypercholesterolemia (HC), an established risk factor of atherosclerosis and coronary heart disease, is highly prevalent in the U.S. In 2010, approximately 26% of adults reported high cholesterol placing them at risk for cardiovascular morbidity and mortality [20]. HC has been associated with inadequate sleep duration [18,21-23]; however, there are inconsistencies in the literature with some reporting no association [24], and others reporting an association for short or long duration. In addition, most studies have been devoted to specific subgroups including adolescents [21] individuals with bipolar disorders [25] and longer time in bed/fragmented sleep among older individuals [22,26].

Studies exploring associations between HC and sleep duration have examined the role of gender and have shown that women reporting short sleep duration are at greater risk of developing HC. For example, Sabanayagam and Shankar [18] found that sleep duration <5 hours among women had positive associations. Gangwisch et al. [21] showed that each additional hour of sleep in women was associated with a significant decreased odds of being diagnosed with HC in young adulthood (OR=0.83, 95% CI: 0.73-0.95). But inconsistencies in the literature remain. In the Coronary Artery Risk Development in Young Adults (CARDIA) study, sleep duration was positively associated with total cholesterol, however, when reproductive-related factors were controlled for, the results were attenuated and no longer significant [23]. Williams et al. [13] found increased HDL in normotensive women, but not hypertensive women reporting short sleep duration.

Only a few studies have examined racial/ethnic differences. Sabanayagam et al. [18] reported a positive association between sleep duration and hypercholesterolemia was stronger in other ethnic groups, and did not observe a significant race/ethnicity interaction. However, the data did not characterize "other racial/ethnic groups" and it is unclear if these results are applicable to non-Hispanic blacks (hereafter referred to as blacks), Hispanics, or Asians. Similarly, the CARDIA study using a sample of 503 black and white adults did not find significant race interactions [23].

There is growing evidence that sleep duration varies across racial/ethnic groups [27,28]. Cross-sectional studies demonstrate that blacks [27] and other ethnic groups report shorter and longer sleep duration relative to whites. Of note, very few studies have explored race/ethnic interactions on the association between sleep duration and HC. This is particularly important given the disproportionate burden of cardiovascular disease morbidity and mortality among blacks [29]. Given the role of HC as a prominent risk factor for coronary heart disease and the high prevalence of inadequate habitual sleep duration in the U.S., we investigated the role of gender and race/ethnicity on the association between sleep duration and HC.

Methods

The National Health Interview Survey (NHIS) is an ongoing, cross-sectional, in-person household interview survey conducted annually by the Centers for Disease Control's National Center for Health Statistics. NHIS uses a multistage area probability design, sampling non-institutionalized representatives of the civilian population of the U.S. Probability samples of the adult population of all 50 states and District of Columbia were obtained. Details on sample design are provided elsewhere [30].

We used data from 40,679 adults ≥18 who participated in the 2008-2009 NHIS for this cross-sectional analysis. Participants were recruited using a nationally representative cross-sectional household interview survey, which uses a multistage area probability design. Participants provided sociodemographic, physician-diagnosed chronic conditions and data on habitual sleep time. We used NHIS-provided weights to adjust for use of complex design.

Measures

HC was based on self-report of whether a physician had ever diagnosed the participant as having high cholesterol. Self-reported body mass index (BMI) was assessed as weight in kilograms/height in meters squared. A BMI in the range of 18.5 and 24.9 was considered normal; BMI ≥ 25-29 was considered overweight, while a BMI ≥ 30 was considered obese. BMI was dichotomized as normal/underweight vs. overweight/obese. Age was measured as a continuous variable. Education was measured as 1) less than high school, 2) completed high school, or 3) greater than high school. Self-reported race/ethnicity was measured as non-Hispanic white, non-Hispanic black, Asian, and Hispanic. Sleep duration was measured with the question, "On average, how many hours of sleep do you get in a 24-hour period?" coded as <6 hours, or >8 hours referenced to 7-8 hours. Socioeconomic status was based on reported annual individual income (<\$35,000; \$35-\$55,000; >\$55,000).

Analysis

Descriptive analysis was used to ascertain prevalence of variables of interest. In order to test the first hypothesis, we used multivariable regression models. We also assessed if the associations varied by race and race-sex groups by adding interaction terms into separate fully adjusted models. A p<0.05 value was considered as a significant. Analysis was conducted using SPSS, version 20.0 (SPSS Inc., Chicago, IL).

Results

Of the total sample of 40,679, 85% reported their race/ethnicity as white and 15% as black; 56% of the participants were female. Table 1 compares sociodemographic and health characteristics of participants who reported HC compared to those who did not. In unadjusted regression analysis showed that overall participants who reported long sleep duration (>8 hours) were more likely to have reported HC than individuals reporting habitual sleep duration of 7-8 hours [OR=1.28, 95% CI: 1.22-1.31 p<0.001].

Variables	Reported HC (28.5%)	Reported No HC (71.5%)
Age (± SD)	58.2 ± 14.9	45.2 ± 17.4
Blacks	14.1	16.7
Female sex	56.1	56.7
Income >\$35,000	57	58.3
Married	80.8	61.9
Education, ≥HS	80.8	83.6
Smoking history	48.9	38.3
Current drinking	78.3	75.1
Cancer	13.7	6.5
Coronary heart disease	11.5	2.3
Diabetes	37.7	6.4
Heart Attack	8.8	2
Hypertension	58.1	22.4
Stroke	6.5	2
Obese	43	34.6
Arthritis	82.7	80.8
Vision Problems	16.7	9.2
Emotional distress	3.9	2.2
Walk ¼ mile	60.8	16.6
Healthy sleep 7 h	28.6	31.8
Short sleep <6 h	25.2	18.7
Long sleep >8 h	26.7	20

Table 1: Sociodemographic and health characteristics for HC.

However, no significant associations were observed for short sleep in the entire sample. Adjusted logistic regression analyses showed significant association between sleep duration and presence of HC among blacks, but not among whites. Blacks reporting short (<6 hours) or long sleep durations (>8 hours) had a greater risk of HC relative to blacks sleeping 7 hours habitually [OR=1.12, 95% CI: 1.11-1.13; OR=1.13, 95% CI: 1.12-1.14; p<0.001, respectively]. Black females reporting short or long sleep duration had greater risk of reporting HC compared with black males sleeping 7 hours [OR=1.11, 95% CI: 1.10-1.11; OR=1.10, 95% CI: 1.10-1.10; p<0.001, respectively].

Discussion

Traditionally, most studies have focused on comparing whites to all other racial/ethnic groups, or controlling for race/ethnicity in regression models. Given, the increasing racial/ethnic disparities in health outcomes, and sleep duration, it is important to ascertain these differences, as policy makers and clinicians could develop and disseminate appropriate interventions, making such efforts a public health priority. Our results corroborate previous findings that short sleep duration in women is positively associated with HC, and this study went a step further in examining this association in black women. We focused on this population, as national prevalence rates indicate that blacks have two or more risk factors for cardiovascular disease [31] as compared to whites. The fact that black women reporting short or long sleep duration were more likely to report HC is quite alarming and should be a public health priority. Black women report several traditional risk factors for cardiovascular disease; yet, prevention efforts to reduce morbidity and early mortality have proven inadequate [32]. None of the previous studies on HC and sleep duration have reported these findings, and it is likely due to variations in methodological and statistical techniques.

These findings are consistent with other studies that have shown a pattern of association between sleep duration and HC. However, the association for the total sample was significant only for long sleep duration. Sabanayagam et al. [18] found a positive association among women reporting short sleep duration and the inverse among men. Gangwisch et al. [21] found an association in short sleep duration and adolescent females, but not among males. Notably, in our study, short and long sleep may increase risk of HC in black women. The reasons for the observed differences in studies are not clear, but are likely due to variations across studies, including older and young adults, and individuals with comorobdities. Sabanayagam et al. [18] also used the NHIS dataset, and finding that the observed differences in the results are likely due to approaches used in categorizing short and long sleep duration, and adjusting for different covariates. This raises the importance of establishing covariates and the need for large-scale investigations with large multi-ethnic groups.

Findings also highlight the need to address potential mechanism. Some evidence suggests that short sleep duration is associated with increased inflammation [33]. The inflammatory process is related to an in increased in low density lipoprotein [23] molecules that accumulate in the blood stream, but the contribution of sleep to this development is not entirely clear. Conceivably, the relationship could be mediated by other social, lifestyle and environmental factors. The participants in this study with high cholesterol also reported several comorbidities including history of hypertension, current drinker, current smoker, and diabetes. These findings indicate that multilevel interventions for CHD that address sleep, is of growing importance in addressing racial/ethnic health disparities.

While the study does suggest the role of gender, particularly comparing black females with short or long sleep duration with black males with 7 hours of sleep, unlike the CARDIA study [23] we could not control for factors related to reproduction, which could account for these findings. Other limitations of this study are that sleep duration are self-reported, which increases the likelihood of over- or underreporting of the actual hours slept. In addition, we could not assess other sleep disorders including sleep apnea and insomnia, both of which have been linked to CHD [34-37]. Despite these limitations, these findings are robust because we used a large nationally representative sample of the U.S. population and controlled for several covariates to explore this association.

Conclusions

This study represents a significant addition to the literature on the role of race and gender in HC. Our study supports the relationship between inadequate sleep and traditional risk factors for CHD, namely, HC. Future lifestyle interventions should consider the role of sleep in addressing CHD risk and CHD morbidity. It underlines the need for further research that could bring to light not just associations but possible mechanistic factors.

References

1. Knutson KL, Van Cauter E, Rathouz PJ, DeLeire T, Lauderdale DS (2010) Trends in the prevalence of short sleepers in the USA: 1975-2006. Sleep 33: 37-45.
2. Knutson KL, Spiegel K, Penev P, Van Cauter E (2007) The metabolic consequences of sleep deprivation. Sleep Med Rev 11: 163-178.
3. Watson NF, Harden KP, Buchwald D, Vitiello MV, Pack AI, et al. (2014) Sleep duration and depressive symptoms: a gene-environment interaction. Sleep 37: 351-358.
4. Roberts RE, Duong HT (2014) The prospective association between sleep deprivation and depression among adolescents. Sleep 37: 239-244.
5. Donat M, Brown C, Williams N, Pandey A, Racine C, et al. (2013) Linking sleep duration and obesity among black and white US adults. Clin Pract (Lond) 10.
6. Buxton OM, Marcelli E, Short and long sleep are positively associated with obesity, diabetes, hypertension, and cardiovascular disease among adults in the United States. Social science & medicine 2010; 71: 1027-36.
7. Al Lawati NM, Patel SR, Ayas NT (2009) Epidemiology, risk factors, and consequences of obstructive sleep apnea and short sleep duration. Prog Cardiovasc Dis 51: 285-293.
8. Zizi F, Pandey A, Murrray-Bachmann R, Vincent M, McFarlane S, et al. (2012) Race/ethnicity, sleep duration, and diabetes mellitus: analysis of the National Health Interview Survey. Am J Med 125: 162-167.
9. Gangwisch JE, Heymsfield SB, Boden-Albala B, Buijs RM, Kreier F, et al. (2007) Sleep duration as a risk factor for diabetes incidence in a large U.S. sample. Sleep 30: 1667-1673.
10. Kim MJ, Lee GH, Kim CS, Kim WS, Chung YS, et al. (2013) Comparison of three actigraphic algorithms used to evaluate sleep in patients with obstructive sleep apnea. Sleep Breath 17: 297-304.
11. Yaggi HK, Araujo AB, McKinlay JB (2006) Sleep duration as a risk factor for the development of type 2 diabetes. Diabetes Care 29: 657-661.
12. Buxton RB (2010) Interpreting oxygenation-based neuroimaging signals: the importance and the challenge of understanding brain oxygen metabolism. Front Neuroenergetics 2: 8.
13. Williams CJ, Hu FB, Patel SR, Mantzoros CS (2007) Sleep duration and snoring in relation to biomarkers of cardiovascular disease risk among women with type 2 diabetes. Diabetes Care 30: 1233-1240.
14. Pandey A, Williams N, Donat M, Ceide M, Brimah P, et al. (2013) Linking sleep to hypertension: greater risk for blacks. Int J Hypertens 2013: 436502.
15. Cappuccio F, Short sleep duration and obesity: Evidence from population-based studies in children, adolescents and adults across the world. Sleep, 2007. 30: p. A129-A129.

16. Abe T, et al. Sleep duration is significantly associated with carotid artery atherosclerosis incidence in a Japanese population. Atherosclerosis 2011; 217: 509-513.
17. Nagai M, Hoshide S, Nishikawa M, Shimada K, Kario K (2013) Sleep duration and insomnia in the elderly: associations with blood pressure variability and carotid artery remodeling. Am J Hypertens 26: 981-989.
18. Sabanayagam C, Shankar A (2012) Sleep duration and hypercholesterolaemia: Results from the National Health Interview Survey 2008. Sleep Med 13: 145-150.
19. Altman NG, Izci-Balserak B, Schopfer E, Jackson N, Rattanaumpawan P, et al. (2012) Sleep duration versus sleep insufficiency as predictors of cardiometabolic health outcomes. Sleep Med 13: 1261-1270.
20. Services, U.D.o.H.a.H., National Center for Health Statistics. Health, United States, 2012: With Special Feature on Emergency Care. 2013: Hyattsville, MD.
21. Gangwisch JE, Malaspina D, Babiss LA, Opler MG, Posner K, et al. (2010) Short sleep duration as a risk factor for hypercholesterolemia: analyses of the National Longitudinal Study of Adolescent Health. Sleep 33: 956-961.
22. van den Berg JF, Miedema HM, Tulen JH, Neven AK, Hofman A, et al. (2008) Long sleep duration is associated with serum cholesterol in the elderly: the Rotterdam Study. Psychosom Med 70: 1005-1011.
23. Petrov ME, Kim Y, Lauderdale D, Lewis CE, Reis JP, et al. (2013) Longitudinal associations between objective sleep and lipids: the CARDIA study. Sleep 36: 1587-1595.
24. Bjorvatn B, Sagen IM, Øyane N, Waage S, Fetveit A, et al. (2007) The association between sleep duration, body mass index and metabolic measures in the Hordaland Health Study. J Sleep Res 16: 66-76.
25. Soreca I, Wallace ML, Frank E, Hasler BP, Levenson JC, et al. (2012) Sleep duration is associated with dyslipidemia in patients with bipolar disorder in clinical remission. J Affect Disord 141: 484-487.
26. Mezick EJ, Matthews KA, Hall M, Kamarck TW, Buysse DJ, et al. (2009) Intra-individual variability in sleep duration and fragmentation: associations with stress. Psychoneuroendocrinology 34: 1346-1354.
27. Nunes J, Jean-Louis G, Zizi F, Casimir GJ, von Gizycki H, et al. (2008) Sleep duration among black and white Americans: results of the National Health Interview Survey. J Natl Med Assoc 100: 317-322.
28. Grandner MA, Patel NP, Jean-Louis G, Jackson N, Gehrman PR, et al. (2013) Sleep-related behaviors and beliefs associated with race/ethnicity in women. J Natl Med Assoc 105: 4-15.
29. Mensah GA (2005) Eliminating disparities in cardiovascular health: six strategic imperatives and a framework for action. Circulation 111: 1332-1336.
30. [No authors listed] (2000) Design and estimation for the National Health Interview Survey, 1995-2004. Vital Health Stat 2: 1-31.
31. Clark LT, Ferdinand KC, Flack JM, Gavin JR 3rd, Hall WD, et al. (2001) Coronary heart disease in African Americans. Heart Dis 3: 97-108.
32. Ford ES (2013) Trends in predicted 10-year risk of coronary heart disease and cardiovascular disease among U.S. adults from 1999 to 2010. J Am Coll Cardiol 61: 2249-2252.
33. Motivala SJ (2011) Sleep and inflammation: psychoneuroimmunology in the context of cardiovascular disease. Ann Behav Med 42: 141-152.
34. Somers VK (2008) Sleep apnea and cardiovascular disease-An American Heart Association/American College of Cardiology Foundation Scientific Statement from the American Heart Association Council for High Blood Pressure Research Professional Education Committee, Council on Clinical Cardiology, Stroke Council, and Council on Cardiovascular Nursing. Journal of the American College of Cardiology 52: 686-717.
35. Gottlieb DJ, Yenokyan G, Newman AB, O'Connor GT, Punjabi NM, et al. (2010) Prospective study of obstructive sleep apnea and incident coronary heart disease and heart failure: the sleep heart health study. Circulation 122: 352-360.
36. Adedayo AM, Olafiranye O, Smith D, Hill A, Zizi F, et al. (2014) Obstructive sleep apnea and dyslipidemia: evidence and underlying mechanism. Sleep Breath 18: 13-18.
37. Sands-Lincoln M (2013) Sleep Duration, Insomnia, and Coronary Heart Disease Among Postmenopausal Women in the Women's Health Initiative. Journal of Womens Health 22: 477-486.

Timing of Activities and their Effects on Circadian Rhythm in the Elderly with Dementia

Albert J Safi and Nancy A Hodgson*

The Johns Hopkins University School of Nursing, Maryland, USA

***Corresponding author:** Nancy A. Hodgson, The Johns Hopkins University School of Nursing, 525 North Wolfe Street, Room 422, Baltimore, Maryland, 21205, USA, E-mail: nhodgso1@jhu.edu

Abstract

Study Background: Circadian rhythm disorders (CRDs) occur in over 60 percent of patients with dementia and are associated with increased morbidity and mortality and poor quality of life. Regulating the circadian system through the use of light and activity has been shown to alter core clock processes and suggests that activities delivered at strategic times may be an effective mechanism through which to entrain (or reset) disrupted circadian rhythms in persons with dementia. However, the nature and optimal timing of daily activities remains relatively unknown.

Methods: The object of this review is to examine the role of timed activities in regulating circadian activity in older adults living with dementia. A rapid review process was used to identify relevant research with the search terms circadian rhythm, timed activity, sleep, dementia, and other relevant combinations.

Results and Conclusions: Symptoms of CRD in older adults with dementia may be alleviated by participating in activities at their corresponding optimal time window. Future research needs to evaluate single and multiple activity interventions with emphasis on optimal timing to treat or mediate disrupted circadian patterns in older adults with dementia.

Keywords: Circadian; Dementia; Activity

Introduction

The time of day at which we decide to do daily activities and tasks can determine our likelihood of having better health and resiliency in response to the effects of aging, especially dementia [1]. Synching daily activities with the proper brain state leads to efficiency, production, protective health benefits, and properly entrained circadian rhythms, which can lead to a predictable sleep-wake cycle [2]. Circadian rhythms refer to the cyclical changes and fluctuations of biological processes occurring over about a 24-hour period (1 day). These biological processes are entrainable and endogenous and are mainly driven by the brain's biological "clock" [3]. A human's intrinsic clock is slightly longer than 24 hours, but environmental cues—the solar-dark cycle being the most important and profound—impinge on the individual to entrain their circadian rhythm to a 24-hour period [4,5]. These environmental and external cues are referred to as zeitgebers [5]. There is a growing interest in forging a link between the effects of aging on circadian rhythms and the effects of aging on sleep [6-8]. Sleep provides neurological and physiological benefits that are crucial to promoting health and bodily function [9]. No other timed activity synchrony is more important to brain plasticity and resilience than the one between sleep and the sleep/wake cycle [10].

Circadian rhythm disorders (CRDs) occur in over 60 percent of patients with Alzheimer's disease and related dementias and are associated with increased morbidity and mortality and poor quality of life [10,11]. CRD symptoms include late afternoon/evening agitation (e.g., "sundowning") and irregular sleep-wake rhythms such as daytime hypersomnia, frequent night wakenings, and poor sleep efficiency [12-14]. CRDs pose the greatest burden to family caregivers of persons with dementia, and are the principal causes of distress, poor quality of life (QoL), and institutionalization in this growing population [8,15].

CRD symptoms are at their peak during moderate stages of dementia due to the combined effects of poor physical and cognitive health on one's response to zeitbegers such as light (photic stimuli) and structured social and physical activity (nonphotic stimuli) that regulate, or entrain, the circadian clock. Figure 1 below depicts cyclical events that may lead to disrupted circadian rhythms in older adults with dementia.

Regulating the circadian system through the use of light and activity has been shown to alter core clock processes and suggests that activities delivered at strategic times may be an effective mechanism through which to entrain (or reset) disrupted circadian rhythms. However, the nature and optimal timing of these activities remains relatively unknown [16-18].

The purpose of this paper is to provide a systematic review of the research on the role of timed activities in regulating circadian activity in older adults living with dementia. Our intent is to evaluate both the nature or type of activities and the optimal timing of activities that align with the optimal daily circadian cycle. Of particular emphasis was to identify activities that could be useful in entraining disrupted circadian cycles in individuals with dementia. This review is the first to our knowledge to examine the key features and ideal scheduling of daily activities to reduce symptoms of CRDs.

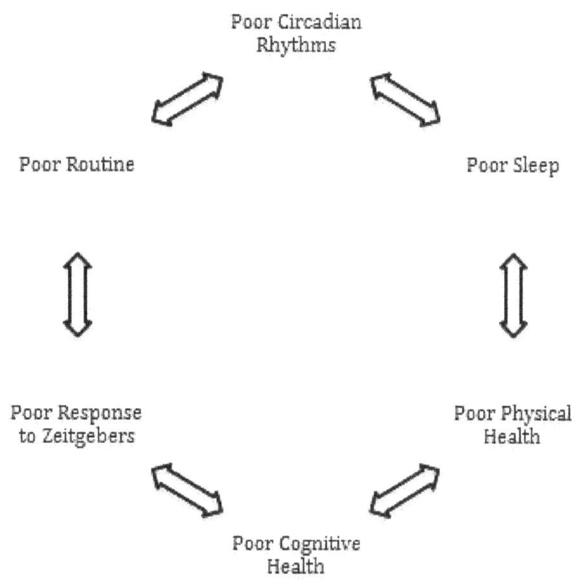

Figure 1: Cycle of influence on circadian rhythm disorders in older adults with dementia.

Methods

A rapid review process was used to identify relevant articles [19]. Six electronic databases, MEDLINE (PubMed), CINAHL, Embase, PsycINFO (OVID), Scopus, and Cochrane Database, were searched to identify relevant studies published in the last 10 years, from January 2004 through October 2014. Search terms and their combinations included: condition (dementia, cognitive impairment, or cognitively impaired), activity (physical, cognitive, social), circadian (sundowning, sleep-wake rhythm), timing (timed, scheduled, routine) and older adult. Both authors assessed all titles and abstracts identified by the literature search for relevance.

Potentially relevant articles were then retrieved for full-text review. Each retrieved study was examined along the following criteria to determine eligibility for inclusion in this review: 1) published in a peer-reviewed journal and in English; 2) testing of an activity intervention; 3) inclusion of individuals over age 65 years with a physician diagnosis or caregiver report of any type of dementia; and 4) at least one outcome related to a factor affecting circadian rhythm (Figure 1). Using these criteria, the search yielded an initial set of 2,952 articles. The titles and abstracts were reviewed for relevance, which excluded 2,910 non-relevant studies. Articles were excluded if they had no activity component to the intervention, if the primary outcomes did not include factors related to circadian disruption in persons with dementia (Figure 1), if the activity interventions also included pharmacological treatment (melatonin), drug trials, or were conducted in lab or clinic setting. Forty two studies were retained for full review; this in turn yielded nine studies [20-28] that met full review criteria (Table 1).

Author	Study Population	Intervention	Timing Addressed	Circadian Related Factors	Circadian related findings
Forbes et al. [20]	Aging population with dementia	Systematic Review of physical activity interventions	No	Cognitive function	Exercise interventions have promising effects on cognitive function
Andrade et al. [21]	Aging population with Alzheimer's	Multi-disciplinary exercise program	No	Physical & Cognitive function	The intervention group displayed increased frontal cognitive function, less body sway, and greater functional capacity
Yoon et al. [22]	Aging population with dementia	Cognitive and physical activity program	No	Cognitive function	A cognitive and physical activity program had significant beneficial effects compared to only a cognitive program
Vreugdenhil et al. [23]	Community dwelling patients diagnosed with Alzheimer's	Physical activity	No	Physical & Cognitive function	Physical activity improved physical and cognitive health compared to a control
Schmidt et al. [24]	Older morning chronotypes & young evening chronotypes	Cognitive activity	Yes	Physical & Cognitive function, Routine	Older individuals performed cognitive tasks better in the morning
Kemoun et al. [25]	Aging population with dementia	Physical activity	No	Physical & Cognitive function	The intervention group had improved cognitive test scores and improved walking efficiency
Christofoletti et al. [26]	Aging population with dementia	Multi-disciplinary exercise program	No	Physical & Cognitive function	Observed attenuation in decline of global cognition after multidisciplinary intervention compared to a single exercise

Kramer et al. [27]	Aging population, animal models	Systematic Review of physical activity interventions	No	Cognitive function	Physical activity moderated age related declines in cognition, brain function, and brain structure
Richards et al. [28]	Aging population with dementia living in nursing homes	Individualized Social Activity Intervention (ISAI)	Yes	Sleep & Routine	In individuals with sleep efficiency worse than 50%, ISAI group had less daytime sleep, a lower day/night sleep ratio, fell asleep faster, and were awake less at night

Table 1: Studies of Activity Influence on Circadian Related Factors in Persons with Dementia

Characteristics of Studies

Table 1 summarizes the essential components of the nine studies. Although there is no recognized classification system for activity based interventions, those reviewed here can be grouped into physical, social or cognitive activities. Two studies were reviews of physical activity interventions and seven studies tested cognitive, physical or social activity interventions (or combinations) in samples of older adults with dementia. While the studies discussed implications for reducing behavioral symptoms of circadian rhythm disorders, most studies included outcomes measures of physical and cognitive function as precursors to circadian disruption in this population. Two studies in the review included measures of sleep quality or sleep routine but no study in the review directly measured circadian rhythm (via actigraphy, behavioral or observational measures) as an outcome. Taken as a whole, there appears to be a very small body of evidence supporting the role of physical, cognitive and social activity in improving factors influencing circadian patterns. Only two of the studies discussed timing for delivery of activities in general terms (e.g., delivered between 9 am and 5 pm) [24,28].

Consideration of timing

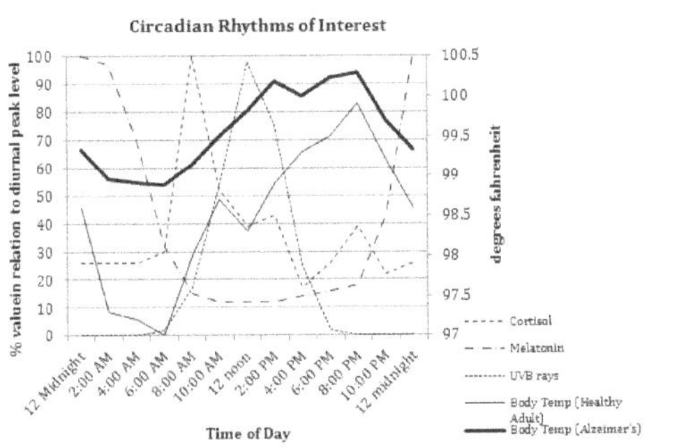

Figure 2: Endogenous Factors Affecting Circadian Rhythm in Older Adults with Dementia

Many factors may contribute to the optimal time window for cognitive, physical, and social activities. Exogenous factors such as light (UVB rays), and endogenous factors such body temperature, cortisol, and melatonin are the largest drivers of circadian patterning [29]. As depicted in Figure 2, the circadian rhythms of hormones in the body adjust to sync with the dynamic light-dark cycles of the sun. For example, melatonin, the hormone involved in sleep onset, is inversely related to UVB rays suggesting sun fall induces sleep and sunrise induces waking.

In all humans, circadian rhythms are adapted to optimize the daily rhythm of environmental engagement [30]. Thus, engaging in activities at times when biological circadian processes are conducive to the specific activity can create optimal efficiency and output [31]. As aging occurs, circadian rhythms begin to become asynchronous. Studies have shown that enhancement of zeitgebers in elderly nursing home residents can have beneficial effects on their sleep [32]. By adopting a highly regular lifestyle, behavioral circadian rhythms become synchronous, and can accommodate for age-related declines in endogenous circadian entrainment mechanisms. In the following section we describe the optimal activities to complete at the specific time of day based on the factors depicted in Figure 2.

Morning (6 am to 10 am)

The sun is beginning to rise signaling humans to wake. Sensory recovery gradually happens as an individual wakes up and becomes alert. Body temperature progressively rises upon waking and plays a major role in alertness and function [33]. Blood levels of the hormone cortisol begin to increase as the sun begins to rise, and melatonin is sharply dropping. The majority of adulthood is spent waking between these hours.

As mid morning approaches, about two to three hours after wake, body temperature and cortisol create an optimum environment for cognitive based activities [34]. Elderly populations exhibit a phenomena where circadian rhythms of body temperature and motor activity are phase delayed [35], but their sleep/wake cycle is not delayed or delayed to the same degree. This phenomena creates extra time upon waking before optimal cognitive performance is reached compared to a healthy adult without CRD [22]. For persons with dementia, performing activities tailored to an individual based on their functional and mental status during the day are important in maintaining a consistent sleep-wake cycle and suggest that late morning is the optimal time for engaging in cognitive activities [22,36].

Afternoon (12 pm to 3pm)

Some mental alertness carries over after noon, but cortisol is sharply dropping causing a dip in performance of nearly any type during the afternoon hours. Improved reaction time, cognitive function, and energy levels are observed after short naps after a relatively short waking period [37]. In the elderly with dementia, naps can elicit negative results if too much time is spent sleeping or napping during the day [38].

Napping and sleeping during the day is an extremely common occurrence among older adults with dementia and has been attributed to a lack of structured routine and no meaningful engagement in activities. Ohayon and Zulley [38] exhibited a linearly increasing trend of napping with age. Tanaka and colleagues [39] found that a combination of a structured 30-minute afternoon nap followed by moderate intensity exercise in the evening improved sleep quality, reduced subjective daytime sleepiness, and improved mental health.

Late Afternoon (3 pm to 6 pm)

Body temperature will reach its peak, which make blood flow, dexterity, grip strength, and limb control optimal during this time [40]. Other factors play a role in making this window ideal for physical activity. By this time, the brain is fatigued and cortisol levels are relatively low. Some sort of physical activity whereby the individual is actively engaged can help entrain circadian rhythms for later relaxation. Physical activity too late in the evening will delay melatonin onset and sleep onset. Therefore, performing an engaging physical activity in the late afternoon is optimal for healthy circadian rhythms. While the evidence supporting physical interventions aiding in sleep and circadian issues is promising and made up the majority of studies in the review [23,25,27], no study addressed optimal timing of physical activity for elderly populations with dementia.

Evening (6 pm to 10pm)

As the evening progresses, melatonin levels begin to rise quickly, cortisol levels drop, and the sun sets. This period should be for relaxing and winding down in preparation for sleep. Interventions to induce sleep for persons with dementia include the use of massage and touch to stimulate blood flow, reduce stress hormone production, induce relaxation, and can ease individuals into a calm relaxed state [41].

Sleep (~10 pm to ~6 am)

The synchrony of sleep timing with endogenous biological processes, solar-dark cycle, and conscious activities further promote healthy circadian patterning [6,9]. Morgenthaler et al (2006) graded the evidence regarding non-pharmacological treatments of sleep disturbance in older adults. The authors list stimulus control therapy, relaxation training, cognitive behavior therapy, sleep restriction therapy, multicomponent therapy, biofeedback, and paradoxical intention as, individually, effective therapies in the treatment of chronic insomnia. The evidence was lacking when it came to sleep hygiene education, imagery training, and cognitive therapy—as single therapies or when added to other approaches—being effective [42]. In addition, the review did not investigate having a steady "routine" of timed activities as a treatment, and individuals with dementia were excluded from the review. Nonetheless, based on the evidence presented in this review, having an organized daily routine—especially one that is in sync with the sun's oscillation—in theory, should provide the basis for improving circadian patterns and therefore improved sleep. The reduced rate of insomnia in the elderly from maintenance of a daily routines study warrants further examination of timed activity protocols for aging populations, especially those with dementia [43].

Conclusion

Based on the collective literature examined in this literature review, when older adults with dementia engage in cognitive, physical, social, and relaxation activities at their optimal times, their circadian rhythms may have a higher likelihood of becoming properly entrained to environmental cues leading to improved sleep quality and reduced circadian rhythm disruption. Future research needs to be done to determine the mechanisms underlying the optimal timing of activities, which activities are most effective, which combinations are effective, and how these activities actually aid in resetting circadian rhythm in those with dementia.

Acknowledgement

Dr. Hodgson has been supported in part by funds from the National Institute on Nursing Research (Grant P30 NR014131-01).

References

1. Figueiro MG, Hamner R, Higgins P, Hornick T, Rea MS (2012) Field measurements of light exposures and circadian disruption in two populations of older adults. J Alzheimers Dis 31: 711-715.
2. Shirani A, St Louis EK (2009) Illuminating rationale and uses for light therapy. J Clin Sleep Med 5: 155-163.
3. Sack RL, Auckley D, Auger RR, Carskadon MA, Wright KP Jr, et al. (2007) Circadian rhythm sleep disorders: part II, advanced sleep phase disorder, delayed sleep phase disorder, free-running disorder, and irregular sleep-wake rhythm. An American Academy of Sleep Medicine review. Sleep 30: 1484-1501.
4. Thome J, Coogan AN, Woods AG, Darie CC, Häßler F (2011) CLOCK Genes and Circadian Rhythmicity in Alzheimer Disease. J Aging Res 2011: 383091.
5. Monk TH (2010) Enhancing circadian zeitgebers. Sleep 33: 421-422.
6. Dang-Vu TT, Desseilles M, Peigneux P, Maquet P (2006) A role for sleep in brain plasticity. Pediatr Rehabil 9: 98-118.
7. Wu YH, Swaab DF (2007) Disturbance and strategies for reactivation of the circadian rhythm system in aging and Alzheimer's disease. Sleep Med 8: 623-636.
8. Alessi CA, Martin JL, Webber AP, Kim E, Harker O, et al. (2005). Randomized, controlled trial of a nonpharmacological intervention to improve abnormal sleep/wake patterns in nursing home residents. Journal of the American Geriatrics Society, 53: 803–810.
9. Zelinski EL, Deibel SH, McDonald RJ (2014). The trouble with circadian clock dysfunction: Multiple deleterious effects on the brain and body.Neuroscience & Biobehavioral Reviews, 40, 80-101.
10. Pollak CP, Perlick D, Linsner JP, Wenston J, Hsieh F (1990) Sleep problems in the community elderly as predictors of death and nursing home placement. J Community Health 15: 123-135.
11. Zee PC, Vitiello MV (2009) Circadian Rhythm Sleep Disorder: Irregular Sleep Wake Rhythm Type. Sleep Med Clin 4: 213-218.
12. Kim P, Louis C, Muralee S, et al. 2005. Sundowning syndrome in the older patient. Clin Geriatr 13(4): 32–36
13. Yesavage JA, Friedman L, Ancoli-Israel S, Bliwise D, Singer C, et al. (2003) Development of diagnostic criteria for defining sleep disturbance in Alzheimer's disease. J Geriatr Psychiatry Neurol 16: 131-139.
14. Volicer L, Harper DG, Manning BC, Goldstein R, Satlin A (2001) Sundowning and circadian rhythms in Alzheimer's disease. Am J Psychiatry 158: 704-711.
15. Bachman D, Rabins P (2006) "Sundowning" and other temporally associated agitation states in dementia patients. Annu Rev Med 57: 499-511.
16. Forbes D, Morgan DG, Bangma J, Peacock S, Pelletier N, et al. (2004) Light therapy for managing sleep, behaviour, and mood disturbances in dementia. Cochrane Database Syst Rev : CD003946.
17. Moghekar A, O'Brien RJ (2012) Con: Alzheimer's disease and circadian dysfunction: chicken or egg? Alzheimers Res Ther 4: 26.
18. Bedrosian TA, Nelson RJ (2012) Pro: Alzheimer's disease and circadian dysfunction: chicken or egg? Alzheimers Res Ther 4: 25.
19. Harker J, Kleijnen J (2012) What is a rapid review? A methodological exploration of rapid reviews in Health Technology Assessments. Int J Evid Based Healthc 10: 397-410.

20. Forbes D, Thiessen EJ, Blake CM, Forbes SC, Forbes S (2013) Exercise programs for people with dementia. Cochrane Database Syst Rev 12: CD006489.
21. Andrade LP, Gobbi LT, Coelho FG, Christofoletti G, Riani Costa JL, Stella F (2013). Benefits of Multimodal Exercise Intervention for Postural Control and Frontal Cognitive Functions in Individuals with Alzheimer's Disease: A Controlled Trial. Journal of the American Geriatrics Society, 61(11), 1919-1926.
22. Yoon JE, Lee SM, Lim HS, Kim TH, Jeon JK, et al. (2013). The effects of cognitive activity combined with active extremity exercise on balance, walking activity, memory level and quality of life of an older adult sample with dementia. Journal of physical therapy science, 25(12), 1601.
23. Vreugdenhil, A, Cannell J, Davies A, Razay G (2012). A community-based exercise programme to improve functional ability in people with Alzheimer's disease: a randomized controlled trial. Scandinavian journal of caring sciences, 26(1), 12-19.
24. Schmidt C, Peigneux P, Cajochen C, Collette F (2012). Adapting test timing to the sleep-wake schedule: effects on diurnal neurobehavioral performance changes in young evening and older morning chronotypes. Chronobiology international 29(4): 482-490.
25. Kemoun G, Thibaud M, Roumagne N, Carette P, Albinet C, et al. (2010) Effects of a physical training programme on cognitive function and walking efficiency in elderly persons with dementia. Dement Geriatr Cogn Disord 29: 109-114.
26. Christofoletti G, Oliani MM, Gobbi S, Stella F, Bucken Gobbi LT, et al. (2008) A controlled clinical trial on the effects of motor intervention on balance and cognition in institutionalized elderly patients with dementia. Clin Rehabil 22: 618-626.
27. Kramer AF, Erickson KI, Colcombe SJ (2006) Exercise, cognition, and the aging brain. J Appl Physiol (1985) 101: 1237-1242.
28. Richards KC, Beck C, O'Sullivan PS, Shue VM (2005) Effect of individualized social activity on sleep in nursing home residents with dementia. J Am Geriatr Soc 53: 1510-1517.
29. McEachron DL (2012) Timing is everything: a chronobiologist's perspective on health, illness, and circadian rhythms. Interview by Gloria F. Donnelly. Holist Nurs Pract 26: 188-193.
30. Murray G, Nicholas CL, Kleiman J, Dwyer R, Carrington MJ, et al. (2009) Nature's clocks and human mood: the circadian system modulates reward motivation. Emotion 9: 705-716.
31. Cardinali DP, Furio AM, Reyes MP, Brusco LI (2006) The use of chronobiotics in the resynchronization of the sleep-wake cycle. Cancer Causes Control 17: 601-609.
32. Ancoli-Israel S, Klauber MR, Jones DW, Kripke DF, Martin J, et al. (1997) Variations in circadian rhythms of activity, sleep, and light exposure related to dementia in nursing-home patients. Sleep 20: 18-23.
33. Waterhouse J, Drust B, Weinert D, Edwards B, Gregson W, et al. (2005) The circadian rhythm of core temperature: origin and some implications for exercise performance. Chronobiol Int 22: 207-225.
34. Valdez P, Ramírez C, García A (2012). Circadian rhythms in cognitive performance: implications for neuropsychological assessment.ChronoPhysiology and Therapy, 2012, 2-81.
35. Satlin A, Volicer L, Stopa EG, Harper D (1995) Circadian locomotor activity and core-body temperature rhythms in Alzheimer's disease. Neurobiol Aging 16: 765-771.
36. Judge, KS., Camp, CJ Orsulic-Jeras S. (2000) Use of Montessori-based activities for clients with dementia in adult day care: Effects on engagement. American Journal of Alzheimer's Disease and Other Dementias 15.1 (2000): 42-46.
37. Milner CE, Cote KA (2009) Benefits of napping in healthy adults: impact of nap length, time of day, age, and experience with napping. J Sleep Res 18: 272-281.
38. Ohayon MM, Zulley J (1999). Prevalence of naps in the general population. Sleep and Hypnosis.
39. Tanaka H, Taira K, Arakawa M, Urasaki C, Yamamoto Y, et al. (2002) Short naps and exercise improve sleep quality and mental health in the elderly. Psychiatry Clin Neurosci 56: 233-234.
40. Wolff G, Esser KA (2012) Scheduled exercise phase shifts the circadian clock in skeletal muscle. Med Sci Sports Exerc 44: 1663-1670.
41. Staedt J, Stoppe G (2005) Treatment of rest-activity disorders in dementia and special focus on sundowning. Int J Geriatr Psychiatry 20: 507-511.
42. Morgenthaler T, Kramer M, Alessi C, Friedman L, Boehlecke B, et al. (2006) Practice parameters for the psychological and behavioral treatment of insomnia: an update. An american academy of sleep medicine report. Sleep 29: 1415-1419.
43. Zisberg A, Gur-Yaish N, Shochat T (2010) Contribution of routine to sleep quality in community elderly. Sleep 33: 509-514.

Titration and Technology - A Single or Multidimensional Perspective?

Khem Ballaho*

Freelance Clinical & Business Consultant, USA

***Corresponding author:** Khem Ballaho, Freelance Clinical & Business Consultant, USA, E-mail: khemarb@yahoo.com

Abstract

Oftentimes we look at titration as a one-way street where the techs increase pressure until the patients exhibit acceptable or normal range AHI (<5/hour). Depending on the diagnosis, CPAP is usually the first line of defense to address obstructive sleep apnea (OSA). While this the gold standard for OSA, advancement in technology continually evolve and offer more dynamic modes that can further increase adherence to therapy due to comfort and varying pressure requirements. The other related hurdle to optimized therapy is the transfer of settings from in-lab titrations to home-care devices. Settings are sometimes changed or modified per physicians' approval in order to fulfill prescription orders even if the complete settings and sub-settings that optimized the titrations in-lab (and experience of the patients) are not fully transcribed due to manufacture differences and/or the limitations of the DME inventory.

This article is of two-folds, one-to look at titration in and outside of the lab for long-term therapy adherence; and two-utilizing technology as additional standard of practice.

Keywords: Titration; Obstructive sleep apnea; CPAP devices; APAP; Adherence to therapy; Multi-dimensional approach to PAP therapy; OSA

Introduction

Is it time to consider automatic titration devices into our standards of practice? According to a study published in 2008 on Reliability of Home CPAP Titration with Different Automatic CPAP Devices "Pressure behaviour and pressure recommendation significantly differ between Auto CPAP (APAP) machines both after one night and one week of home titration" (Series, Plante & Lacasse) [1]. This study points out that pressure requirements vary either nightly, weekly, and so on. Thus, APAP should provide a more appropriate therapy for OSA patients in the long run due to varying pressure needs.

On the contrary, another study published in 2009 in Sleep Med concluded that "patients with moderate sleepiness treated with CPAP, we found no difference in effectiveness between an algorithm-based pressure and an auto-titrated pressure" (Noseda, Andre, Portmans, Kentos, de Maertelaer & Hoffman) [2]. This study seems as a contrast to the former, and therefore begs the question as to which perspective is correct or better?

Furthermore, "Home self-titration of CPAP is as effective as in-laboratory manual titration in the management of patients with OSA" (Fitzpatrick, Alloway, Wakeford, Macl ean, Munt & Day, 2003) [3]. With this study performed two decades ago and with more recent development in automatic CPAP titration algorithms-the premise of automatic CPAP or APAP being as effective as in-lab titration should also not be ignored. Newer APAP algorithms offer more precise and highly-sensitive algorithms in detecting flow limitations, snoring and apneas. Other algorithms even offer central apnea detection where if central sleep apnea (CSA) events are identified, no additional increase in pressure will happen in order to avoid exacerbating CSA events.

On the regulatory side, the American Association of Sleep Medicine (AASM) guidelines are based on clinical studies and evidence-based medicine along with many years of experienced clinicians' input on how titrations should progress [4]. However, even with this said, we must also be reminded of each patient's physiological uniqueness and that the goal of titration should not be a one-night solution; rather, an opening experience for patients that will depend on the therapeutic settings obtained in titration on a nightly basis for the rest of their lives (for the most patients) [5].

Optimal pressure for many techs that have years of experience is typically achieved within the first 2 hours and followed by a few minor adjustments after 4 am or during the last cycles of rapid eye movement (REM) stage of sleep (4th or 5th) within a 6-7 hour titration period [6]. More challenging patients may present co-morbidity or co-morbidities (with cardiovascular disease, obesity hypoventilation syndrome, chronic obstructive pulmonary disorder or restrictive lung disease) and will be more than likely be titrated with bi-level modes eventually. Among these are spontaneous, SV (servo ventilation), volume assured with iVAPS (intelligent volume assured pressure support) or AVAPS (automatic volume assured pressure support), or with back-up rate modalities such as spontaneous-timed (S/T)-either within the first night of titration or the following scheduled titration. Most sleep labs follow this protocol if the initial titration is deemed to be a failed or unsuccessful titration where optimal pressures or settings were not achieved with the reduction of AHI to normal levels and/or arousal index as well (with REM-supine recording while on determined pressure settings and without further abnormal apneic or oxygen desaturation index) [7].

Moreover, looking deeper into the titration night-what really happens with patients during the titrations? What physiological and chemical changes occur as patients go through titrations? For one, there are various changes in hemodynamics (O_2, CO_2, bicarbonates, pH, leptin, grehlin, cortisol, etc.) when patients experience changes in their breathing patterns as well as alterations in their sleep architectures (appropriate levels of varying sleep stages). Along these lines, there are also simpler factors such as positional or behavioral changes that are affecting the patients during titration nights. These changes are considerably important not only for the clinicians' perspectives but also the patients'. Therefore, transcribing these factors into simple prescriptions may or may not fully serve both perspectives. There should be added emphasis on how to fully translate optimal titrations into fewer settings written on prescription pads. Another option is to take all these factors in consideration and allocate future assessments and reassessments of these factors to fully obtain optimal titration-even after the fact. We also have to remember that the physiological changes experienced by the patients continue long after the one-night titration.

After understanding the standards in obtaining the optimal pressure settings for OSA patients, other factors that are affecting how OSA is managed have emerged recently. In less than a decade, two things have evolved tremendously in the sleep industry–the roles of insurance companies and technology. Strategic changes in reimbursements (insurance systems) to increase standards of practice and access to care due to the improvements and acceptance of sleep disorders have been implemented. On the other hand, manufacturers have spent enormous resources in advancing their algorithms on their PAP, bi-level and other non-invasive devices (modalities).

These two additional factors have become advantageous to clinicians and patients on the clinical and management side of patients, particularly on the home care setting where the Durable Medical Equipment (DME) clinicians who are typically respiratory therapists (RT) by training, set up patients with their devices, perform their follow up meetings with patients by downloading data from their devices and troubleshooting therapy issues from mask troubles, pressure setting changes, and many other issues with collaboration with the patients' physicians.

These changes have positive effects on patient care after the in-lab titration

The drop-off rates-the estimated number of patients that either stop their therapy completely or have become sporadic users of their devices-were once between 50-55% within the last decade. Other Durable Medical Equipment (DME) companies have claimed higher compliance rates. However, as an industry, we still have varying figures at this point and there is still no absolute numbers to figure out more accurate compliance levels due to a decentralized system of sleep patient management. Needless to say, we have plenty of room for improvement, given the technological advancements we have and the existing pressure from insurance companies as well as the government (Center for Medicare and Medicaid System) to provide better long-term services to our patients [8].

There is a possible way to obtain an accurate rate of patients who fall out of therapy, adhere to long-term compliance, and many other useful data in gauging the effects of more recent improvements in technology (PAP devices, masks, humidifiers, and accessories) by means of collecting usage from devices; however, not all devices are capable of giving the same data among manufacturers. We can only refer to the bulk of patients who are placed on data-capable devices to justify the premise on the advantages of utilizing APAP devices versus single-pressure CPAP devices in optimizing patient therapies.

Going back to titration, by looking into the existing gap between the optimal settings obtained from the in-lab experience and the devices set in the patients' homes, we can presume that objectives vary among DMEs who set up patient devices. DMEs' PAP settings are transcribed directly from the sleep titration settings (written off as prescriptions by the sleep physicians) or slightly modified depending on what devices are available on-hand that has comparable features, settings and sub-settings with the physicians' approval [9].

Pressures (cmH_2O) are typically the main settings considered when preparing devices for home care. Whereas other settings or sub-settings are sometimes ignored that potentially have added to the optimized settings experienced by the patients during the titration in the sleep labs. This possible dilemma-actual mirroring of optimal titration to translate into prescribed device settings that will be utilized for patients at home every night should further be discussed and enforced in order to possibly increase successful adherence of OSA patients with their therapies. Pressure settings are important; however, if there are other settings/sub-settings that helped with optimizing the overall therapy for patients, then these factors must also be included and transferred over to the patients' home devices.

On a relative note, why do some patients complain of experiencing plateaus in their therapies whereas they don't feel the same way as how they did during their first time with PAP (positive airway pressure) therapy? Some complain after a month or a few months later after successful initial nights or weeks on PAP therapy. If we consider that therapy and titration is straight-forward, nevertheless, a multi-dimensional endeavor at the same time, we could conclude that these later complaints by patients are brought about by so many other factors that we have not localized yet [10].

Similarly, patients attend their titration nights with a straight-forward frame of mind that they will be exposed to air pressures until the best pressure eliminates their apneas and they sleep undisturbed. However, there are so many other variables that come to play-their discomfort and preference with masks, sleeping positions that they are used to, height and texture of pillows or blankets, the hissing sounds of mask intentional and unintentional leaks-at times called mask farts, etc. In short, the entire process and experience are again-multi-dimensional.

On this note, Automatic PAP devices (APAPs) have come a long way and established legitimacy in its performance, particularly with "patients with moderate sleepiness treated with CPAP, we found no difference in effectiveness between an algorithm-based pressure and an auto-titrated pressure" (Noseda, André, Potmans, Kentos, de Maertelaer, & Hoffmann, 2009) [2] as published in Sleep Med.

So, the question begs-can we implement this approach and standardize APAP as the gold standard to optimally treat OSA for the long-term perspective–possibly increasing patient adherence to therapy while reducing drop-off rates and lessen troubleshooting work for clinicians in DMEs who manage these patients with physicians?

Bridging the gap between optimal titrations and device settings set for homecare with APAP configurations have been practiced by Kaiser Permanente and the VA (Veterans Admin.) hospitals by focusing on performing home sleep testing (HSTs with 3-4-channel devices) and APAPs for many years now. The other factor that the two big organizations (VA and Kaiser Permanente) add to the mix is a regimented follow up schedule with patients. In the VA, patients are usually seen 2 weeks after the initial device setup, followed by another follow at 30 days, then 6 months, and eventually yearly scheduled meetings (if adherence to therapy has been established with the patient). This method is also considered as titration–but outside of a sleep lab–allowing for the APAP algorithm to take over and to find varying optimal pressures on a nightly basis. Some more complicated than OSA patients (with co-morbidities such as obesity hypoventilation and COPD) are treated with mechanical (non-invasive) ventilation, thus, requiring more robust follow up schedules.

In summary, titration should not only be seen as a sleep lab experience. It should not be a one-time-deal. Multi-dimensional therapeutic perspectives might prove to be more efficient (with particular patient segments) in addressing multi-dimensional patients, especially since we do have current advanced technologies to support the industry (such as APAP technology and more advanced modalities) and the need of many patients in addressing their nightly-changing optimal pressure requirements. In the meantime, there can also be reduced troubleshooting times with DME clinicians and increased adherence to therapy with properly transcribed titration settings and sub-settings.

We should think about the present and future experience of each patient. Therefore, from screening, diagnosis, treatment, and long-term management–all should be a part of the titration. The goal is to successfully make the patient experience the therapy while keeping in mind a long-term titration of the patient months and years to come otherwise, we miss out on the goal and definition of therapy. The disease we are addressing is a chronic one–not a one-night-disorder. Thus, titration can be optimized inside or outside the sleep labs and that technology as well as data can add values towards increased compliance to therapy.

References

1. Sériès F, Plante J, Lacasse Y (2008) Reliability of home CPAP titration with different automatic CPAP devices. Respir Res 9: 56.
2. Noseda A, André S, Potmans V, Kentos M, de Maertelaer V, et al. (2009) CPAP with algorithm-based versus titrated pressure: A randomized study. Sleep Med 10: 988-992.
3. Fitzpatrick MF, Alloway CE, Wakeford TM, MacLean AW, Munt PW, et al. (2003) Can patients with obstructive sleep apnea titrate their own continuous positive airway pressure? Am J Respir Crit Care Med 167: 716-722.
4. Kushida CA, Chediak A, Berry RB, Brown LK, Gozal D, et al. (2008) Clinical guidelines for the manual titration of positive airway pressure in patients with obstructive sleep apnea. J Clin Sleep Med 4: 157-171.
5. Yamashiro Y, Kryger MH (1995) CPAP titration for sleep apnea using a split-night protocol. Chest 107: 62-66.
6. Mulgrew A, Fleetham JA (2006) How best to determine optimal nasal CPAP in patients with OSAH? Thorax 61: 186-187.
7. Ai-Ping C, Aboussouan LS, Minai OA, Paschke K, Laskowski D, et al. (2013) Long-Term Continuous Positive Airway Pressure Therapy Normalizes High Exhaled Nitric Oxide Levels in Obstructive Sleep Apnea. J Clin Sleep Med 9: 529-535.
8. Rowley JA, Tarbichi AG, Badr MS (2005) The use of a predicted CPAP equation improves CPAP titration success. Sleep Breath 9: 26-32.
9. Montesi SB, Bakker JP, Macdonald M, Hueser L, Pittman S, et al. (2013) Air leak during CPAP titration as a risk factor for central apnea. J Clin Sleep Med 9: 1187-1191.
10. Collen J, Holley A, Lettieri C, Shah A, Roop S (2010) The impact of split-night versus traditional sleep studies on CPAP compliance. Sleep Breath 14: 93-99.

31

Towards a Novel Measure to Determine Improvement of Cognitive Functioning Following Cognitive Behavioral Therapy for Insomnia

Gosselin D[1], Campbell K[1], Grenier J[1,2] and De Koninck J[1*]

[1]*School of Psychology, University of Ottawa, Canada*

[2]*Montfort Hospital, Ottawa, Canada*

[*]**Corresponding author:** Joseph De Koninck, School of Psychology, University of Ottawa, 136, Jean-Jacques Lussier, Ottawa, Ontario, Canada, E-mail: jdekonin@uottawa.ca

Abstract

Background: Cognitive impairments are often reported by individuals with insomnia. Yet, objective performance-based measures of cognitive functioning have yielded inconsistent results. The present study aims to investigate sustained attention and vigilance in individuals with insomnia by employing a novel task based on the Schröger and Wolff paradigm. This innovative auditory distraction task measures two different cognitive processes: 1) the ability to sustain attention in order to detect the duration of auditory stimuli; and 2) the ability to detect auditory stimulus change, which requires a switch of attention. A standard psychomotor vigilance test (PVT) was also employed for comparison purposes.

Methods: Cognitive behavioral therapy for insomnia was delivered to 5 participants. Performance on the psychomotor vigilance test and the novel auditory distraction task were examined prior to and following treatment.

Results: Accuracy of detection in the psychomotor vigilance test significantly improved following treatment. Similarly, the novel distraction task led to a significant improvement of accuracy of detection of auditory stimulus duration following treatment. However, processes related to the switching of attention upon presentation of auditory stimulus change were not altered following treatment.

Conclusion: Insomnia seems to affect sustained attention and vigilance. Such processes do appear to be responsive to therapy, unlike the ability to switch attention when relevant. The novel auditory distraction task examined in this study seems to be a promising clinical outcome measure of sustained attention and vigilance for insomnia, as it was observed to have the benefit of being devoid of a ceiling effect, which was found with the psychomotor vigilance test. Further investigation of this novel application is warranted.

Keywords: Insomnia; Cognitive behavioral therapy for insomnia; Cognitive impairment; Sustained attention; Vigilance

Introduction

Insomnia is the most prevalent sleep disorder, affecting an estimated 6% to 15% of the general population [1,2]. Insomnia is characterized by persistent difficulties in initiating or maintaining sleep with significant distress or impairment in daytime functioning that occur despite adequate opportunities for sleep [3,4]. Substantial societal and personal costs are associated with insomnia. High rates of motor-vehicle accidents, increased health care use, and economic burden linked to work absenteeism or reduced productivity have been documented [5-8]. At an individual level, fatigue, reduced motivation and initiative, as well as mood disturbance are frequently reported by individuals with insomnia [9]. Cognitive impairments typically involving attention, memory, and/or executive functions also represent a significant number of the complaints shared by individuals with insomnia. These subjective complaints have not however always been found to be correlated with objective performance-based measures. Indeed, different meta-analyses have highlighted a lack of consistency in the performance data. Riedel and Lichstein [10] reviewed 13 different studies using various cognitive measures and concluded that only a few of them confirmed the presence of significant cognitive impairments, and these were mainly related to psychomotor functions. Fulda and Schulz [11] arrived at a similar conclusion. In their review of 18 studies, they also noted a lack of consistent evidence of objective cognitive deficits associated with insomnia. Fulda and Schulz [11] however indicated that cognitive tasks that required vigilance were the most likely to be compromised by insomnia. More recently, Shekleton et al. [12] evaluated 18 other studies and suggested that the effect of insomnia on cognitive functions was small and subtle. In addition, the results from the various studies were inconsistent: some studies reported an effect, while others did not using essentially identical tasks. The authors did however note that tasks having a high cognitive load, presumably involving complex, higher cognitive processes, appeared to be the most sensitive to insomnia. Fortier-Brochu et al. [13] reviewed 24 studies and also indicated that insomnia had only small or moderate effects on cognitive functions, in particular on cognitively demanding tasks involving processes such as working and episodic memory, and problem solving. However, no significant differences were observed for less-demanding, simpler tasks. In brief, the findings from the different meta-analyses highlight that studies to date have failed to find a consistent effect of insomnia on various cognitive functions. These reviews do point out a failure to employ identical methodological procedures. Small changes in the methodology of very similar tasks can have a large effect, thus perhaps accounting for some of the inconsistency of results. Moreover, many studies employ standardized neuropsychological measures and these may not be optimal for revealing the small and subtle cognitive deficits identified by the above-mentioned studies. Buysse et al. [14] and Shekleton et al. [12] also point to another limitation of the use of neuropsychological batteries: they are clinical tools used for the screening of individuals likely to meet the criteria of a specific population on basis of a comparison to normative sample data.

Because of the inconsistencies in the insomnia literature, the extensive sleep deprivation body of research might be used as a starting point for the study of cognitive impairments induced by insomnia. Indeed, although the mechanisms responsible for cognitive deficits in insomnia remain to be elucidated, sleep loss can be considered as a factor contributing to performance decrements. Multiple studies have confirmed the deleterious effect of sleep deprivation on cognitive functioning [15]. These impairments have been hypothesized to be the result of either a frontal central executive dysfunction [16], or a more general inability to sustain attention and maintain vigilance [17]. The cognitive correlates resulting from insomnia and their underlying mechanisms could of course differ from those generated by experimental sleep deprivation [10]. Nevertheless, this is the approach used in the present study because the effects of sleep deprivation could at least point to certain aspects of cognition that might be consistent with insomnia [12]. The present study thus employs a novel task that our lab has found to have strong effects obtained in both total and partial sleep deprivation studies.

Many studies have now found that sleep deprivation mainly affects cognitive tasks that are dependent on the maintenance of active, sustained attention, particularly for monotonous tasks [15,18]. A task that is frequently used in sleep deprivation studies is the psychomotor vigilance test (PVT) [19]. In this task, participants are asked to detect a visual stimulus, presented at random intervals ranging from 2 s to 10 s. As it names implies, the PVT requires the participant to remain vigilant and sustain attention for the entire testing period. Accuracy of detection and speed of responding have repeatedly been shown to be affected by sleep loss [20]. Another advantage to the use of the PVT is that it shows little effects of practice or learning, apart from a slight improvement after the first few trials [21]. It can thus be used in pre-post designs. Unfortunately, in the insomnia field, numerous and different tasks requiring sustained attention and vigilance have been used, making comparisons difficult, and thus possibly contributing to the inconsistency of the results. The PVT has not often been used. This might be because of the relative ease of the PVT. Most individuals with insomnia will rarely fail to detect the target stimulus and as a result, the rate of detection will be very high.

Our lab has carried out an initial sleep deprivation study testing a task developed by Schröger and Wolff [22]. It was designed to examine the automatic switching of attention from an ongoing task and towards a potentially more relevant novel stimulus. However, part of the interest of this task to the study of sleep deprivation and insomnia is that the "primary" task, like the PVT, does require sustained attention and vigilance for its successful completion and thus might be susceptible to the effects of insomnia. However, unlike the PVT, it also measures the extent to which individuals can detect acoustic change and subsequently take action, when appropriate. In the classic paradigm, participants are presented with a sequence of equally probable short and long duration auditory tones and asked to discriminate the duration of the stimuli. As mentioned, this does require sustained attention. An advantage of this task is that the difficulty of the task and thus, the accuracy of detection, can be manipulated by varying the difference in the duration of the two stimuli. In pilot studies carried out in our lab on the effects of sleep deprivation, we have found that tones having duration of 190 ms and 310 ms resulted in detection rates varying from 0.70 to 0.85. Decreasing the difference in duration between the tones produced a task that was too difficult, resulting in participants "giving up". Increasing the difference in duration between the tones produced a task that was too easy, resulting in participants no longer needing to be vigilant to successfully carry out the task. Another feature of the Schröger and Wolff [22] task is that it also examines another cognitive function, the switching of attention to a potentially more relevant event. Thus, at rare and unpredictable times, a feature of the auditory stimulus (for example, its pitch) changes. This deviant feature is however irrelevant to the duration detection task, participants still needing to determine whether its duration is short or long. Evidence of the switch of attention away from the processing of the relevant feature of the stimulus, its duration, and towards the processing of the irrelevant feature is provided by performance on the task. Accuracy of detection of the duration of the deviant deteriorates and speed of responding slows. Such switching of attention has both advantages and disadvantages. On the positive side, detection of change (or novelty) in the environment is crucial for survival. While the driving of a car requires sustained attention and vigilance, it is also critical that the driver is made aware of an environmental event occurring outside of the focus of attention, the honking of a horn. On the negative side, the large majority of potentially highly relevant input turns out to be irrelevant. Thus the switching of attention to these events results in distraction and deterioration in performance. Our initial study indicated that total sleep deprivation was associated with an overall decrease in performance compared to normal sleep, probably because of an inability to sustain attention. After normal sleep, when the deviant stimulus was presented, performance did deteriorate. However, after sleep deprivation, deterioration in performance was less marked. Thus, the sleep-deprived seem to be less able to switch attention to potentially highly relevant stimulus input. Partial sleep deprivation also resulted in an overall deterioration in performance. Its effects on the processing of the deviant stimulus were not however significant. Thus, while partial sleep deprivation does affect the ability to sustain attention, there was little evidence that the ability to switch attention to novel input was compromised.

The present study will examine the use of this Schröger and Wolff [22] distraction task to determine the effects of insomnia on cognitive processing. This task will be used to provide an objective measure of cognitive processing prior to and following cognitive behavioral therapy for insomnia (CBT-I). The PVT was also administered because it is considered to be the gold standard for the assessment of the effects of sleep loss on cognition. Performance on these tasks was thus examined prior to and following CBT-I. Various sleep questionnaires and inventories were also used to determine if treatment altered the subjective reports of the quantity and quality of sleep.

Method

Participants

Five participants (4 women, 1 man) aged between 22 and 59 (M=39.8, SD=16.7) volunteered to participate in this exploratory study. It is recognized that this sample is small but it was reasoned that for any task to be useful in a clinical setting, effects need to be highly consistent across most individuals and therefore be evident even in small samples.

All participants met the inclusion and exclusion criteria described in the Procedure section. For diagnostic purposes, 4 of the participants had mixed insomnia (combination of 2 or 3 of sleep onset, middle and late insomnia). The fifth one had middle insomnia only. Additional sociodemographic and clinical characteristics of the sample are shown in Table 1.

	Sociodemographic characteristics				Clinical characteristics		
Participant	Age (years)	Marital status	Education completed	Occupation	Type of insomnia	Insomnia duration (years)	Sleep medication, type (daily dosage)
1	29	Living with partner	University	Employed	Mixed	4	---
2	56	Married	University	Retired	Mixed	3	---
3	22	Living with partner	University	Employed	Mixed	8	Trazodone (50 mg)
4	33	Married	High-School	Employed	Mixed	23	---
5	59	Divorced	University	Retired	Middle	8	Zopiclone (10 mg)
Mean (SD)	39.8 (16.7)	---	---	---	---	9.2 (8.0)	---

Table 1: Sociodemographic and clinical characteristics of participants.

This study was approved by University of Ottawa and Montfort Hospital (Ottawa, Canada) research ethics boards following the guidelines of the Canadian Tri-Council (Medical, Natural and Social sciences) on ethical conduct involving human subjects. In accordance with these guidelines, all participants provided a written informed consent prior to beginning pre-treatment assessment procedures. Data collection was part of a larger study assessing the efficacy of CBT-I delivered by videoconference.

Procedure

Recruitment: Participants were recruited through referrals from general practitioners in Eastern Ontario (Canada). Twenty individuals indicated they were interested in participating in this study. All potential participants were contacted by telephone and given a brief screening interview to determine eligibility. The inclusion criteria included: 1) between 18 and 65 years of age; and 2) having a diagnosis of persistent insomnia as defined by a combination of criteria deriving from the diagnostic and statistical manual of mental disorders (DSM-5) [3], the international classification of sleep disorders (ICSD-3) [4], and those recommended to be used in insomnia research [9,23]. More precisely, the combination of the insomnia criteria included: a) difficulties initiating and/or maintaining sleep. This was defined as a sleep onset latency and/or wake after sleep onset greater than 30 min; b) poor sleep efficiency. This was defined as a percentage of time asleep while in bed lower than 85%; c) sleep difficulties occurring at least 3 nights a week, for at least 6 months; and d) sleep difficulties causing significant distress or deterioration in daytime functioning. Exclusion criteria were: 1) presence of a sleep disorder other than insomnia (e.g. sleep apnea, narcolepsy, periodic limb movement); 2) presence of a severe psychiatric disorder (e.g. major depression, psychosis, neurocognitive disorders); 3) presence of a medical illness potentially related to disturbances in sleep (e.g. anemia, thyroid disorder); 4) use of medication having a proven impact on sleep (e.g. beta blockers); 5) shift work; and 6) currently participating in or having received a psychological treatment for insomnia within the past 2 years. Current use of sleep medication (stable for at least 2 months) was not an exclusion criterion.

Individual clinical interview: Of the 20 individuals who were interviewed, 5 were deemed to be eligible for the study and were invited to complete a second-stage screening consisting of an individual clinical interview. This interview aimed to confirm the diagnosis of insomnia and to assure the absence of exclusion criteria determined for this study. Three diagnostic tools were administrated to prospective participants: 1) insomnia interview schedule (IIS) [24] to confirm the presence of persistent insomnia; 2) the mini international neuropsychiatric interview (MINI) [25] to rule out any psychiatric disorders; and 3) the montreal cognitive assessment (MoCA) [26] to rule out any cognitive impairment. All 5 individuals were considered eligible to participate in the study. They were then asked to complete the insomnia severity index (ISI) [24], the PVT and the distraction task. An appointment for the first treatment session was then scheduled. Participants were asked to complete a daily sleep diary over 2-weeks prior to treatment initiation.

Treatment: Each participant individually underwent CBT-I. CBT-I has long been established as a first-line treatment of insomnia and its efficacy is supported by strong empirical evidence [27,28]. Protocol used in the present study was based on Morin's [24] clinical procedures; an exhaustive description can be found in Morin's [24] book. In brief, CBT-I combines three main components: educational, behavioral, and cognitive. The educational component involves basic education about insomnia including sleep architecture, circadian rhythms, sleep hygiene, and its cognitive behavioral conceptualization. The behavioral intervention includes stimulus control and sleep restriction, which respectively aim to: 1) reinforce the association between the bed and bedroom with sleep, and establish a regular sleep-wake schedule; and 2) restrict time spent in bed as close as possible to the actual sleep time in order to induce a more consolidated and efficient sleep. The third component, the cognitive intervention, involves reframing faulty beliefs and attitudes that interfere with sleep. All sessions were delivered by a clinical psychologist (JG) with extensive training and experience in CBT-I. Structured guidelines were followed during treatment sessions in order to enhance treatment fidelity. Treatment consisted of 6 weekly sessions lasting 60 min and was delivered by videoconference within Montfort Hospital (Ottawa, Canada). Throughout treatment, participants were again instructed to complete a daily sleep diary. Following treatment, participants were also asked to continue to complete the daily sleep diary for an additional 2-week period.

All 5 participants completed all 6 CBT-I sessions. They also fully complied with treatment protocol and sleep diary procedures at all stages.

Individual post-treatment session: Two weeks following the end of treatment, participants completed the ISI, the PVT and the distraction task. The pre and post-treatment outcome measures were administered by an independent researcher who had no role in the provision of treatment.

Measures

Diagnostic measures

Insomnia interview schedule (IIS): The IIS is a semi-structured interview that includes several questions designed to clarify the nature, characteristics, history, and impact of sleep disturbances [24]. It provides a functional analysis and allows establishing an insomnia diagnosis.

Mini international neuropsychiatric interview (MINI): The MINI is a brief structured diagnostic interview that covers all major axis I psychiatric disorders of the DSM-IV. The MINI has a high reliability with other structured interviews [25,29], and has shown good inter-rater and test-retest reliabilities [30].

Montreal cognitive assessment (MoCA): The MoCA is an instrument aiming to screen mild cognitive impairment, by assessing the following eight cognitive domains: attention and concentration, executive functions, memory, language, visuospatial skills, abstraction, calculation, and orientation. The MoCA has a total possible score of 30; a score equivalent to or greater than 26 indicates the absence of cognitive deficit. This measure of global cognitive function has excellent psychometric proprieties as evidenced by high internal consistency and test-retest reliability, and demonstrates strong sensitivity and specificity to neurocognitive impairment [26].

Subjective outcome measures

Sleep diary: The sleep diary is completed daily upon arising. This diary provides a subjective measure of sleep parameters such as bedtime hour, number and duration of awakenings during the night, and time of arising from bed [24]. The daily sleep diary data is then used to calculate sleep variables useful for clinical and treatment outcome analysis. In the present study, the following sleep measures were derived from the diary: sleep onset latency (SOL: min between lights off and first sleep episode), wake after sleep onset (WASO: min awake between sleep onset and wake time), and sleep efficiency (SE: percentage of time asleep while in bed). These variables were selected because they represent outcome indicators commonly used in insomnia research [31,32]. They also have specific normative thresholds - directly drawn from the diagnostic criteria defining insomnia that allow measuring the clinical significance of participant's outcomes. The sleep diary is the gold standard of subjective sleep measures, and data derived from it have proven to be reliable and valid [31].

Insomnia severity index (ISI): The ISI is a 7-item self-report questionnaire inquiring about insomnia symptoms and related distress over the last 2 weeks [24]. The following dimensions are assessed: 1) perceived severity of problems with sleep onset, sleep maintenance, and early morning awakenings; 2) current satisfaction with sleep; 3) degree of interference of sleep difficulties with daytime functioning; 4) noticeability of quality of life impairments due to sleep disturbances; and 5) degree of distress caused by sleep difficulties. A 5-point likert scale (0=no problem; 4=very severe problem) is used for each item and their sum yields a total score ranging from 0 to 28. Four categories of symptom severity based on total score have been defined: scores 0 to 7=no clinically significant insomnia; 8-14=sub threshold insomnia; 15-21=clinical insomnia of moderate severity; 21-28=severe clinical insomnia. For clinical trials, a minimum threshold score of 11 is recommended [33]. The ISI has strong psychometric proprieties and has been validated as an outcome measure in treatment research [34]. It also permits the measurement of the success of treatment using well-defined parameters: a 7-point reduction in baseline score is considered to be minimal evidence of moderate improvement, while a 9-point or larger reduction corresponds to a marked improvement [33]. A post-treatment reduction to a score equal or lower than 7 has also been used as an index of remission [35]. These indicators were thus selected as outcome measures for the current study.

Objective cognitive outcome measures

Two different cognitive tasks were run. Stimulus presentation, response monitoring and timing were controlled by E-prime software (Psychology Software Tools Inc., Sharpsburg, Pennsylvania).

Psychomotor vigilance test (PVT) [17]. In this task, participants were asked to detect a visual stimulus, presented at random times. Because this is a visual task, participants were seated approximately 50 cm from a computer monitor. All stimuli were presented in black against a white background. A trial began with a fixation point ("+") presented in the center of the monitor. This was replaced by a 15 mm diameter circle lasting 1 s. The onset of the circle varied randomly between 2 s and 10 s (on average, every 6 s) after the onset of the fixation point. The participant was asked to press the left mouse button as quickly as possible after presentation of the circle. Feedback then informed the participant that a correct response had occurred and the actual reaction time (RT; in ms) was displayed. If participants failed to respond, a feedback message "no response was detected" was displayed. The feedback message also lasted 1 s after which the next trial was initiated with the presentation of the fixation point. The task lasted 10 min. Performance was measured according to: 1a) accuracy of responding; 1b) number of lapses (response occurring with a RT greater than 500 ms); and 2) mean and median RTs, and variability in individual participant's RTs.

Because it is known that performance improves after the first few trials, it is possible that improvements following therapy might be a confound of prior exposure to the task (participants had already been exposed to the task prior to therapy). Practice trials lasting about 1 min were therefore initially run at both pre and post-treatment sessions. This served two purposes. It assured that the participants did understand the instructions and nature of the task. Also, the practice sessions should have removed any improvement that might have been experienced during the actual testing.

Distraction task: This task also lasted about 10 min. Participants were presented with short and long duration auditory tones and asked to determine their duration. A total of 500 moderate intensity (70 dB SPL) auditory pure tones (1000 Hz) were presented binaurally through Sony MDR-V6 headphones. The duration of half the stimuli was 190 ms and for the other half, 310 ms. The short and long stimuli were presented in random order. A stimulus occurred every 1400 ms. Participants were asked to press one mouse button for short duration stimuli and a second button for long duration stimuli. A response had to occur within 1200 ms. This 1000 Hz "standard" stimulus was presented on 84% of trials. A small frequency change was however introduced on the remaining trials. A 950 Hz "deviant" was thus presented on 16% of trials. Standards and deviants occurred in random order with the restriction that a deviant be followed by at least three presentations of the standard. Performance was measured by accuracy of and speed of responding (RT). Accuracy and RT were collapsed across short and long duration trials because accuracy of detection of specific stimulus duration was not a concern in this study. Importantly, accuracy and RT were however measured separately for standard and deviant trials. Performance should deteriorate following presentation of the deviant if participants do switch attention to the processing of its irrelevant feature, its pitch.

Practice trials lasting about 1 min were also run in both pre and post-treatment sessions. Again, this served to assure that the participants did understand the nature of the task and should have removed any possible improvement after the first few trials.

Data Analyses

Subjective outcome measures

The effectiveness of treatment on the various measures was determined by using a one-tailed t-test, $\alpha=0.05$, because the interest was focused only on improvement with CBT-I. Thus, treatment was considered to be successful if post-treatment measures significantly improved from pre-treatment measures. Treatment was not considered to be successful if measures failed to change or if they were worse, regardless of whether they were statistically significant or not.

Total scores obtained on the ISI were analyzed using a paired-sample t-test to compare pre and post-treatment conditions. For the sleep diary data, means for the 2-week pre and post-treatment periods were computed for the SOL, WASO, and SE of each participant. Paired-sample t-tests were then run to compare pre and post-treatment conditions.

Objective cognitive outcome measures

Performance was measured in two ways, accuracy of responding and RT. These were analyzed separately. For each of the tasks, RTs were computed only on correct trials. There were too few errors to reliably analyze the error data. The participant's mean RT was computed for the PVT and the distraction task in the pre and post-treatment conditions. A problem with the use of the mean RT is that it can be skewed by extremely fast or low RTs [36]. For this reason, the participant's median RT was also computed. Some studies have indicated that sleep deprivation also increases variability of single participant RTs within a task [15]. For this reason, the standard deviation (SD) of individual participant's RT distribution was also used as a dependent measure.

For the PVT, the same dependent measures (accuracy and RT) were used. In addition, researchers often examine "lapses" in performance. The number of lapses, defined as RTs greater than 500 ms, was thus computed. Sleep deprivation is associated with a deterioration in PVT measures [20]. It was expected therefore that successful outcome would be associated with an improvement on the measures at post-treatment. This was tested statistically using paired-sample one-tailed t-tests, $\alpha=0.05$, on the various performance measures.

The distraction task is unusual in that it measures two different cognitive processes: 1) the ability to sustain attention in order to detect the duration of the stimuli; and 2) the ability to automatically detect potentially highly relevant stimulus change. Our initial total sleep deprivation study indicated that both processes were affected, whereas partial sleep deprivation did not affect the ability to detect the deviant stimulus. It was therefore expected that: 1) performance on the relevant duration detection, requiring sustained attention, would improve following treatment; and 2) individuals with insomnia would be less able to detect the deviant, and thus show less deterioration in performance prior to treatment and more deterioration following treatment. This was tested statistically using a two-way ANOVA, $\alpha=0.05$, with repeated measures on treatment (pre, post) and type of stimulus (standard, deviant) on each of the performance measures.

Results

Subjective outcome measures

Table 2 presents sleep diary data and ISI scores at pre and post-treatment.

Sleep diary

Sleep onset latency (SOL). The SOL group mean at pre-treatment was 35.3 min (SD=28.7 min) and decreased to 10.6 min (SD=4.0 min) at post-treatment. This reduction was not statistically significant, $t(4)=1.80$, $p=0.15$. It did however reflect a clinically significant gain as the post-treatment mean was below the recommended diagnostic threshold of >30 min. The lack of statistical significance was probably due to the fact that there was wide variability in SOL prior to treatment. Three of the individuals had a pre-treatment SOL score that would be considered within normal range, thus limiting the extent to which treatment could result in an improvement.

Wake after sleep onset (WASO). Pre-treatment WASO was above the threshold diagnostic criteria of >30 min for all participants. At post-treatment, 4 of the 5 participants had a WASO score lower than this threshold. The WASO group mean at pre-treatment was 87.2 min (SD=39.0 min) and significantly decreased to 36.8 min (SD=31.3 min) at post-treatment, $t(4)=4.55$, $p=0.01$; $d=2.03$. The post-treatment WASO mean was however above the threshold criteria, thus remaining in the clinical range.

Sleep efficiency (SE). Pre-treatment SE met the threshold diagnostic criteria of <85% for all participants. At post-treatment, the SE score improved and no longer met this threshold for 4 of the participants. The SE mean at pre-treatment was 73.3% (SD=12.1%) and significantly increased to 89.4% (SD=5.9%) at post-treatment, $t(4)=2.99$, $p=0.04$; $d=1.34$. This increase suggested a significant clinical gain as the post-treatment SE mean was above the threshold diagnostic criteria.

Insomnia severity index

Pre-treatment ISI score was above the suggested threshold score for clinical insomnia trials (threshold of 11) for all participants. At post-treatment, 3 of the 5 participants had achieved remission (ISI scores lower than 7) and the 2 remaining participants showed a marked improvement (ISI mean change score between pre and post-treatment equal or greater than 9 points). The mean ISI score at pre-treatment was 18.8 (SD=5.1) and significantly decreased to 5.0 (SD=4.4) at post-treatment, t(4)=5.36, p=0.006; d=2.4. This reduction also suggested a significant clinical gain; ISI pre-treatment mean scores fell in the "clinical insomnia of moderate severity" category (scores of 15 to 21) and declined to join the "no insomnia" category (scores 0 to 7) at post-treatment.

Participant	Sleep Diary Data						ISI	
	SOL		WASO		SE		Total score	
	Pre	Post	Pre	Post	Pre	Post	Pre	Post
1	85	9.3	123.9	30.4	53	89	25	2
2	15.7	15.5	134.7	90.8	72.5	80	18	9
3	18.2	12.9	55.7	24.3	83.5	92.5	23	10
4	33.9	4.9	54	9.4	77	95.8	13	4
5	23.8	10.4	67.5	29.3	80.5	89.5	15	0
Mean (SD)	35.3 (28.7)	10.6 (4.0)	87.2 (39.0)	36.8 (31.3)	73.3 (12.1)	89.4 (5.9)	18.8 (5.1)	5.0 (4.4)

Table 2: Individual participant pre and post-treatment sleep diary data and ISI scores.

Objective cognitive outcome measures

Psychomotor vigilance test

Table 3 presents the effects of treatment on accuracy and speed of responding during the PVT.

Accuracy

Accuracy improved for all 5 participants following treatment. A significant effect of treatment was found for accuracy of responding, t(4)=2.45, p=0.04; d=1.1. Accuracy increased by 1.8% at post-treatment.

Speed of responding

RT improved for all 5 participants following treatment. A significant effect of treatment was again observed. Post-treatment was associated with a significant 53 ms decrease in the mean speed of responding, t(4)=3.87, p=0.009; d=1.73. This could however be a reflection of a reduction in the number of extremely long RTs. Post-treatment was associated with a significant 7% decrease of number of lapses (i.e., response occurring within a RT>500 ms), t(4)=2.36, p=0.04; d=1.06. The variance around individual participant RTs was also smaller after treatment than prior to it, t(4)=2.28, p=0.04; d=1.02. However, pre and post-treatment median RTs (not affected by extremely long RTs) were also significantly reduced, t(4)=4.02, p=0.008; d=1.80.

Accuracy (in %)		Lapses (in %)		RT (in ms)					
Pre	Post	Pre	Post	Pre			Post		
M	M	M	M	M	Med	SD	M	Med	SD
0.98 (0.03)	0.99 (0.01)	0.13 (0.14)	0.06 (0.09)	390 (91)	376 (90)	95 (23)	337 (71)	320 (69)	77 (27)
M: Mean; Med: Median; SD: Standard Deviation; Pre: Pre-treatment; Post: Post-treatment									

Table 3: PVT: Accuracy, lapses and RT (SD in parentheses) at pre and post-treatment.

Distraction task

For this task, data is based only on 4 of the 5 participants. One participant did not complete the task and was therefore excluded from the analysis.

Table 4A presents the effects of treatment on the accuracy of and speed of responding to detection of the duration of the standard and deviant stimuli. In this analysis, only the standards occurring before the deviant were analyzed. The two standards occurring after the deviant were analyzed subsequently.

Accuracy

Accuracy improved for all 5 participants following treatment. An overall significant main effect of treatment was also found, F(1,3)=9.91, p=0.05; ηp^2=0.77. Accuracy of detection of stimulus duration significantly increased by 5.9% at post-treatment, regardless of the type of stimulus (standard or deviant). Although accuracy of detection decreased following presentation of the deviant, the main effect of type of stimulus did not attain significance, F(1,3)=3.45, p=0.16. The extent of the decrease in accuracy following presentation of the deviant was however similar to that observed in other studies with larger sample sizes. Importantly, the interaction between treatment and type of stimulus was also not found to be significant, F<1. There was thus little evidence that treatment had an effect on the switching of attention following the presentation of the deviant.

Participants at times failed to respond to the stimuli. Treatment did not however significantly alter the number of failures to respond, F<1. The main effect of type of auditory stimulus and the interaction between treatment and type of stimulus were also not significant, F(1,3)=1.57, p=0.30, and F(1,3)=0.58, p=0.50, respectively.

Speed of responding

RT improved for all 5 participants following treatment. However, there was no evidence of an increase in the speed of responding following treatment, the main effect of treatment not being significant for either the mean or median RT, F<1 in both cases, or the standard deviation of the individual mean RT, F(1,3)=5.34, p=0.10. Slower RTs to the deviant stimuli can be used as evidence that the presentation of the irrelevant feature distracted resources away from the processing of the relevant feature (duration). Speed of responding did not however differ between the standard and the deviant. The main effect of type of auditory stimulus did not attain significance for the mean, F<1, or the median, F(1,3)=5.05, p=0.11, or the standard deviation of the individual mean RT, F<1. Again, the interaction between treatment and type of stimulus was also not significant for the 3 measures of speed of responding, F<1 in all cases.

Type of auditory stimulus	Accuracy (%)		Failures to respond (in %)		RT (in ms)					
	Pre	Post	Pre	Post	Pre			Post		
	M	M	M	M	M	Med	SD	M	Med	SD
Standard before deviant	0.81 (0.17)	0.85 (0.13)	0.06 (0.05)	0.06 (0.07)	634 (84)	64 (83)	14 (64)	64 (71)	63 (79)	11 (50)
Deviant	0.72 (0.10)	0.79 (0.13)	0.08 (0.05)	0.06 (0.07)	646 (101)	64 (99)	13 (53)	64 (62)	65 (76)	11 (43)
M: Mean; Med: Median; SD: Standard Deviation; Pre: Pre-treatment; Post: Post-treatment										

Table 4A: Distraction task: Accuracy, failures to respond and RT (SD in parentheses) for standard and deviant stimuli at pre and post-treatment.

The deterioration in performance following presentation of the deviant can be used as evidence of a switching of attention and distraction. Recovery from distraction was therefore also examined. It was quantified by examining performance on the two standards occurring after the presentation of the deviant. The standard occurring immediately after the deviant can also be considered a "deviant" because its features are different from the preceding deviant. The features of the second subsequent standard however match those of the standard immediately preceding it. Recovery from distraction should thus result in an improvement in performance upon presentation of the standards following the deviant. Therefore, performance measures were compared for the deviant stimulus and the two subsequent standards. Table 4B presents the effects of treatment on the accuracy of detection and speed of responding to the stimuli (standard and deviant).

Type of auditory stimulus	Mean accuracy (in %)	
	Pre-treatment	Post-treatment
Deviant	0.72 (0.10)	0.79 (0.13)
Standard after deviant 1	0.82 (0.12)	0.84 (0.14)
Standard after deviant 2	0.65 (0.35)	0.80 (0.17)

Table 4B: Distraction task; Mean (SD in parentheses) accuracy measure of recovery from distraction at pre and post-treatment.

Accuracy

Accuracy improved for all 5 participants following treatment. An overall significant main effect of treatment was also observed, F(1,3)=10.59, p=0.05; ηp^2=0.78. Accuracy of detection of the stimulus duration significantly increased by 8.3% at post-treatment, regardless of the type of stimulus (i.e., whether a deviant or subsequent standard was presented). The main effect of stimulus type (standard vs deviant) approached significance, but was not found to be significant, F(2,6)=1.25, p=0.35, nor was the interaction between treatment and type of stimulus, F<1. Recovery from distraction was thus not affected by treatment.

In the initial RT analyses, there was little evidence that speed of responding to the deviant was different than that to the standard. Similarly, there was no significant difference in the number of failure to respond to the deviants compared to the standards. There was thus little evidence of distraction for these measures. For this reason, recovery from distraction was not subsequently analyzed for these failures to respond and for speed of responding.

Discussion

Subjective outcome measures

The present findings suggest that CBT-I was successful in improving the overall quantity and quality of sleep in the 5 participants, as assessed by the 3 sleep diary variables (SOL, WASO, SE) and the ISI score at post-treatment. Of note, some of the analyses on the subjective treatment outcome variables were not found to be significant, either statistically or clinically. This lack of significance should however be interpreted in a clinical and qualitative context. First, the type of insomnia experienced by participants was not homogenous, resulting in a relatively large amount of variability in the sleep diary data, and particularly for the SOL variable. Second, the extreme scores recorded for one participant may have skewed the results: underlying anxiety issues were revealed for this participant during treatment, and this comorbidity may have had an impact on the effects of the treatment. Nevertheless, subjective outcome sleep data indicated that the overall participant's level of functioning following CBT-I fell within or close to the normative range. Such individuals would thus no longer have been diagnosed as having insomnia.

It should of course be mentioned that whatever benefits of treatment were obtained might be due to a placebo effect. In this initial study, a placebo condition was not run. Again, the purpose of this study was to determine if the apparent beneficial effects of CBT-I on subjective sleep measures would also carry over to objective measures of performance on cognitive tasks.

Objective cognitive outcome measures

Changes were indeed observed between pre and post-treatment measures of cognitive performance. Two cognitive tasks were employed, both requiring sustained attention and vigilance for successful performance. The frequently employed PVT did reveal a lower accuracy of target detection, a slower RT to these targets, and more frequent lapses compared to post-treatment scores in our participants. Although the PVT results are statistically significant, caution should be heeded in its application as a clinical assessment tool. For an outcome tool to be meaningful, it must accurately measure the full spectrum of the construct, including its extremes [37]. This consideration is particularly relevant in the field of insomnia in which inter-individual variability associated with the effects of insomnia on cognitive functioning is suspected [38]. RT measures did reveal a wide range of individual scores and thus met this criterion. In addition, a rather substantial decrease in RT (53 ms) was also found at post-treatment. On the other hand, a high level of accuracy (mean=0.98) was apparent in all participants before treatment. This may lead to a ceiling effect. Thus, although accuracy did significantly improve with treatment, the difference (0.018) was small. The restricted range of possible scores on outcome measures may therefore overestimate the individual's cognitive functioning. In this context, a wider range of task difficulty may be required in order to accurately detect different levels of cognitive functioning, and to discern any meaningful change that has occurred as a result of treatment. The distraction task, although infrequently used in the sleep literature, did appear to meet this criterion. The initial level of accuracy was far from a ceiling level. Post-treatment accuracy on this task increased by almost 6%. A second purpose of this task was to examine changes in cognitive processing as a result of changing a feature of the frequently presented standard stimulus. Prior to treatment, the presentation of the deviant did result in a decrease in accuracy of detection of the duration of the stimulus. Although the effect was not statistically significant, the trend was similar to that found in many studies. Again, this deterioration in performance has been interpreted as a result of a switching of attention away from the task-at-hand (the detection of the duration of the stimulus), and towards the processing of a novel feature (the frequency of the deviant). This is beneficial in that a potentially highly relevant change, one that might be critical for survival, has been detected. On the other hand, it does lead to a deterioration in performance (i.e., as result of distraction). Regardless of the outcome of the switch of attention, treatment did not significantly affect this cognitive process. The present findings mirror those obtained with our initial partial sleep deprivation study. Processes related to the detection of stimulus duration were affected by sleep loss, while processes related to the switching of attention upon presentation of a novel stimulus were not affected. Thus insomnia does not seem to alter the ability to switch attention to a potentially more relevant stimulus.

There are however problems with the use of the distraction task. It does have the benefit of being sufficiently difficult to result in levels of accuracy well below a ceiling level. However, many cognitive tasks could be designed to meet this criterion. In addition, in the present study, although the extent of improvement with treatment was significant, the effect size, as measured by Cohen's d, was actually lower compared to the results of the PVT. The real advantage of the distraction task was that it was designed to examine additional cognitive processes, those associated with the switching of attention upon presentation of a novel stimulus. Such switching of attention was not affected by treatment. It is possible that the extent of stimulus change (only a 50 Hz difference between the deviant and the standard) was too small to result in a large switch of attention. A larger extent of change might be considered in future studies.

In summary, the findings from the present study employing a relatively small number of individuals with insomnia indicate that these individuals appear to be unable to sustain attention on two different vigilance tasks to allow for an optimal level of performance. The use of CBT-I appears to be able to alleviate many of the symptoms of insomnia, and also results in an improvement on these vigilance tasks. This study did, of course, have several limitations. Similar to other exploratory studies, the sample size was small and homogenous, and it was not a randomized control design, thus limiting the generalization of the results. Still, the effects of treatment must have been quite consistent because even with a small sample size, these effects were statistically significant. Future research should however attempt to replicate the present findings by using a randomized experimental design including a placebo group. Obviously, a larger sample size presenting a diversity of clinical and sociodemographic characteristics should be tested.

References

1. Morin CM, Jarrin DC (2013) Epidemiology of insomnia: Prevalence, course, risk factors, and public health burden. Sleep Med Clin 8: 281-297.
2. Ohayon MM (2002) Epidemiology of insomnia: What we know and what we still need to learn. Sleep Med Rev 6: 97-111.
3. APA (2013) Diagnostic and statistical manual of mental disorders. American Psychiatric Association, USA.
4. AASM (2014) International classification of sleep disorders. American Academy of Sleep Medicine, USA.
5. Daley M, Morin CM, LeBlanc M, Grégoire JP, Savard J (2009) The economic burden of insomnia: Direct and indirect costs for individuals with insomnia syndrome, insomnia symptoms, and good sleepers. Sleep 32: 55-64.
6. Léger D, Bayon V, Ohayon MM, Philip P, Ement P, et al. (2014) Insomnia and accidents: cross-sectional study (EQUINOX) on sleep-related home, work and car accidents in 5293 subjects with insomnia from 10 countries. J Sleep Res 23: 143-152.
7. Léger D, Guilleminault C, Bader G, Lévy E, Paillard M (2002) Medical and socio-professional impact of insomnia. Sleep 25: 621-625.
8. Simon GE, VonKorff M (1997) Prevalence, burden, and treatment of insomnia in primary care. Am J Psychiatry 154: 1417-1423.
9. Edinger JD, Bonnet MH, Bootzin RR, Doghramji K, Dorsey CM, et al. (2004) Derivation of research diagnostic criteria for insomnia: report of an American Academy of Sleep Medicine Work Group. Sleep 27: 1567-1596.
10. Riedel BW, Lichstein KL (2000) Insomnia and daytime functioning. Sleep Med Rev 4: 277-298.
11. Fulda S, Schulz H (2001) Cognitive dysfunction in sleep disorders. Sleep Med Rev 5: 423-445.

12. Shekleton JA, Rogers NL, Rajaratnam SM (2010) Searching for the daytime impairments of primary insomnia. Sleep Med Rev 14: 47-60.
13. Fortier-Brochu E, Beaulieu-Bonneau S, Ivers H, Morin CM (2012) Insomnia and daytime cognitive performance: a meta-analysis. Sleep Med Rev 16: 83-94.
14. Buysse DJ, Ancoli-Israel S, Edinger JD, Lichstein KL, Morin CM (2006) Recommendations for a standard research assessment of insomnia. Sleep 29: 1155-1173.
15. Killgore WD (2010) Effects of sleep deprivation on cognition. Prog Brain Res 185: 105-129.
16. Horne JA (1993) Human sleep, sleep loss and behaviour. Implications for the prefrontal cortex and psychiatric disorder. Br J Psychiatry 162: 413-419.
17. Doran SM, Van Dongen HPA, Dinges DF (2001) Sustained attention performance during sleep deprivation: Evidence of state instability. Arch Ital Biol 139: 253-267.
18. Lim J, Dinges DF (2010) A meta-analysis of the impact of short-term sleep deprivation on cognitive variables. Psychol Bull 136: 375-389.
19. Dinges DF, Powell JW (1985) Microcomputer analyses of performance on a portable, simple, visual RT task during sustained operations. Behav Res Methods Instrum Comput 17: 652-655.
20. Lim J, Dinges DF (2008) Sleep deprivation and vigilant attention. Ann N Y Acad Sci 1129: 305-322.
21. Dorrian J, Rogers NL, Dinges DF (2005) Psychomotor vigilance performance: Neurocognitive assay sensitive to sleep loss. In: Kushida CA, editor. Sleep deprivation: clinical issues, pharmacology and sleep loss effects. New York: Marcel Dekker, Inc., USA. pp. 39-70.
22. Schröger E, Wolff C (1998) Behavioral and electrophysiological effects of task- irrelevant sound change: A new distraction paradigm. Cognitive Brain Research 7: 71-87.
23. Lichstein KL, Durrence HH, Taylor DJ, Bush AJ, Riedel BW (2003) Quantitative criteria for insomnia. Behav Res Ther 4: 427-445.
24. Morin CM (1993) Insomnia: Psychological assessment and management. Guilford Press, New York, USA.
25. Lecrubier Y, Sheehan DV, Weiller E, Amorim P, Bonora I, et al. (1997) The Mini International Neuropsychiatric Interview (MINI). A short diagnostic structured interview: Reliability and validity according to the CIDI. Eur Psychiatry 12: 224-231.
26. Nasreddine ZS, Phillips NA, Bédirian V, Charbonneau S, Whitehead V, et al. (2005) The Montreal Cognitive Assessment, MoCA: a brief screening tool for mild cognitive impairment. J Am Geriatr Soc 53: 695-699.
27. Morin CM, Bootzin RR, Buysse DJ, Edinger JD, Espie CA, et al. (2006) Psychological and behavioral treatment of insomnia:update of the recent evidence (1998-2004). Sleep 29: 1398-1414.
28. Siebern AT, Manber R (2011) New developments in cognitive behavioral therapy as the first-line treatment of insomnia. Psychol Res Behav Manag 4: 21-28.
29. Sheehan DV, Lecrubier Y, Harnett-Sheehan K, Janavs J, Weiller E, et al. (1997) The validity of the Mini International Neuropsychiatric Interview (MINI) according to the SCID-P and its reliability. Eur Psychiatry 12: 232-241.
30. Sheehan DV, Lecrubier Y, Sheehan KH, Amorim P, Janavs J, et al. (1998) The Mini-International Neuropsychiatric Interview (M.I.N.I.): the development and validation of a structured diagnostic psychiatric interview for DSM-IV and ICD-10. J Clin Psychiatry 59: 22-33.
31. Currie SR (2006) Sleep dysfunction. Clinician's handbook of adult behavioral assessment. Academic Press, Burlington, USA.
32. Schutte-Rodin S, Broch L, Buysse D, Dorsey C, Sateia M (2008) Clinical guideline for the evaluation and management of chronic insomnia in adults. J Clin Sleep Med 4: 487-504.
33. Morin CM, Belleville G, Bélanger L, Ivers H (2011) The Insomnia Severity Index: psychometric indicators to detect insomnia cases and evaluate treatment response. Sleep 34: 601-608.
34. Bastien CH, Vallières A, Morin CM (2001) Validation of the insomnia severity index as an outcome measure for insomnia research. Sleep Med 2: 297-307.
35. Morin CM, Vallières A, Guay B, Ivers H, Savard J, et al. (2009) Cognitive behavioral therapy, singly and combined with medication, for persistent insomnia: a randomized controlled trial. JAMA 301: 2005-2015.
36. Howell DC (2014) Measures of central tendencies. In: Fundamental statistics for the behavioral sciences. 8th edn, Boston: Cengage Learning, USA.
37. Kraus DR, Seligman DA, Jordan JR (2005) Validation of a behavioral health treatment outcome and assessment tool designed for naturalistic settings: The Treatment Outcome Package. J Clin Psychol 61: 285-314.
38. Fortier-Brochu E, Morin CM (2014) Cognitive impairment in individuals with insomnia: clinical significance and correlates. Sleep 37: 1787-1798.

Validity and Reliability of Persian Version of the Occupational Impact of Sleep Questionnaire (OISQ-P)

Valiollah Akbari[1], **Abbas Hajian**[2*] **and Seyed Morteza Hosseini**[2]

[1]*Assistant Professor of Psychiatry, Medical Doctor, Department of Psychology, University of Medical Sciences, Qom, Iran*

[2]*General Practitioner, University of Medical Sciences, Qom, Iran*

[*]**Corresponding author:** Abbas Hajian, M.D, General Practitioner, University of Medical Sciences, Qom, Iran; E-mail: abbashajian@ymail.com

Abstract

Study objectives: To assess the validity and reliability of the Persian translated version of the Occupational Impact of Sleep Questionnaire (OISQ).

Design: This observational and case-control study performed in two stages along with about one to two-month period.

Setting: We used the Persian version of the Pittsburg Sleep Questionnaire Index (PSQI-P) as a valid and reliable scientific tool to differentiate cases and controls.

Participants: From 150 people - all had official works - eventually, 121 persons (81 female and 40 male) were eligible for participation.

Measurements and Results: The α-Cronbach's validity coefficient of translated OISQ was 0.786 at the level of 1% ($p<0.001$). The α-Cronbach's correlation coefficients for reliability were 0.972 and 0.976 in stage one and two, respectively. It was found that scoring ≤12 and ≥20 from OISQ-P were compatible with good sleeper and poor sleeper, respectively.

Conclusion: The Persian version of the OISQ was a valid and reliable questionnaire. It also could differentiate good and poor sleepers.

Keywords: OISQ-P; PSQI-P; Reliability; Screening tool; Sleep; Validity

Introduction

Sleep and its effects on daytime activity, level of intelligence, health, body fitness and life quality have demonstrated strong straight and bidirectional relations [1]. According to these wide interrelations, quality and quantity of doing works in different jobs are not exclusive. Inadequate sleep and/or undiagnosed sleep disturbances in, specifically, working population could lead to occur unintentional work accidents and even death [1]. Although, having normal sleep has specific definition for each person, but there are common and clear definitions of signs and symptoms contributing to diagnose different disorders.

In large communities with prominent working population is very important to have effective workers and advanced economy. Achieving these goals needs fast, easy, advantageous, accurate and scientific approach to screen target population, continuously. Screening methods always were beneficial approaches to distinguish healthy from the sufferer. Occupational Impact of Sleep Questionnaire (OISQ) is one of most popular self-rating questionnaires, evaluating the impact of sleep on diurnal working function. We planned to assess validity and reliability of a Persian translated version of this questionnaire.

Materials and Method

The study was done as an observational and case control in fall, 2013. Primary sample size involving 150 people, 52 (34.7%) men and 98 (65.3%) women, all with official works in different units under supervision of the University of Medical Sciences. All samples were chosen by simple random selecting method. We did our study in two stages along with a period of time between 30 and 60 days. We made two similar files containing three attached questionnaires, including Pittsburg's Sleep Questionnaire Index (PSQI), Occupational Impact of Sleep Questionnaire (OISQ) and Mini Sleep Questionnaire (MSQ), all in Persian, for each stage and each participant.

During first stage, we described goals and two-time process of fully filling triple questionnaires in each stage. Fortunately, all selected accepted to take part in study. We took a verbal consent from each one and promised to save data privacy. We gave a number to each participant in order to compare two stages results, personally. After finishing second stage 121 persons were eligible based on meeting all criteria, including having daily works, not to do nocturnal or shift works, no supervising child and/or old, no pregnancy for women and answering all questions in both stages.

Persian version of Pittsburg's sleep questionnaire index (PSQI-P)

The eighteen questions in a self-rating questionnaire with Likert answering system, first time translated into Persian by Moghaddam et al in March, 2012. The α-Cronbach's coefficient for reliability measured 0.77 among all 258 participants of that study [2]. They also reported sensitivity and specificity of their questionnaire in differentiating cases, and controls were 94% and 72% respectively [2]. Consequently, they proved their work had enough reliability to distinguish some sleep disorders such as primary insomnia, major depression and daytime over sleepiness.

The PSQI-P contains seven sections designing based on international classification of sleep disorders to find involved people in at least last four weeks [2,3]. These sections categorized as subjective sleep quality, sleep latency, sleep duration, sleep efficiency, sleep disturbances, daytime dysfunction and hypnotic medication use. Each part of these categories could score from zero to 3 points; as a result, a fully filled PSQI-P score rated from zero to 21 [2,3]. Classification of these seven sections into three major factors also performed.

Factor 1 which also named as sleep efficiency included sleep duration and sleep efficiency. Factor 2 (perceived sleep quality) included sleep latency, subjective sleep quality and hypnotic medication use. Factor 3 that also stated as daily disturbances included sleep disturbances and daytime dysfunction [2,3]. Scoring ≥ 5 in PSQI-P considered as low sleep quality or being a poor sleeper and scoring < 5 considered as being a good sleeper or having good sleep quality [2]. We applied PSQI-P as a reliable scientific tool in order to differentiate cases, and controls. Similarly, David and Morgan used this method to evaluate Dutch version of OISQ in 2008 [4]. The PSQI has been translated in many languages, including Spanish, Chinese, Hebrew, French, German and Japanese [3].

Occupational impact of sleep questionnaire (OISQ)

The English version of OISQ designed by David and Morgan firstly in 2005 and late was translated to Dutch version in 2008 by primary designers [4]. It was a self-rating 24 questions questionnaire, basically evaluating impacts of sleep on daytime working quality during last four weeks. Each question had 5 different qualitative answering items based on Likert answering system. The items included Never/Not applicable (0), a little bit of the time (1), Some of the time (2), Most of the time (3) and All of the time (4).

Thus, each fully filled questionnaire scores between zero and 96. The higher scores imply on higher probability of inadequate working dysfunction due to poor sleep quality and/or quantity [4]. In order to choose more true words transferring more accurate concept, we have a sequential process to translate the source English questionnaire into target language, Persian. Initially, three copies of source questionnaire forwarded to three medical students in different levels of graduation - whom spoke Persian as their mother tongue language- for making primary translations.

Then all three translated questionnaires were given to another medical student in order to synthetize the best primary questionnaire by choosing proper translated words for each line. After that, this preferred questionnaire posted to two different English language experts to translate it back into English, without mailing the source one. They made the work blindly. Eventually, we achieved to a general consensus on the final translated questionnaire after a meeting with three medical specialists and two English language experts. The α-Cronbach's coefficient for reliability in Dutch version reported 0.93 and cut points to differentiate good and poor sleeper were ≤ 10 and ≥ 20 respectively.

Data analysis

This study had eventually 121 eligible daytime office workers, who all were compatible with including criteria. We used the 18 version of Statistical Program of Social Sciences (SPSS). Mean and standard deviation was computed for each variable. To analyze α-Cronbach's coefficient for reliability and Guttman Split-half coefficient for internal consistency was done. We measured repeatability by performing Test re-test exam. Using this exam help us to check consistency of repeating OISQ-P since it was expected to not to change over time.

As this questionnaire needs at least four weeks interval to evaluate repeatability, we considered a period of 30-60 days interval between refilling the questionnaires. On the other hand, Test re-test exam is able to show method defects, as the data of test and re-test have wide difference, it shows something else except every considered one is missed.

Although, it is a proven psychological examination formula tests stable traits too. While sleep disorders in shift or night workers are stable problem, using Test re-test method help to be reassured of participants responds and not to have something missed or incompatible. Inter-item correlation measurement was done for validity value by examining OISQ and PSQI answers. We used ANOVA exam to define cut points of translated OISQ. We considered level of significant p less than 0.05. We also calculated equation of continuity of OISQ-P response rate and found the R-square for this equation.

Results

This study performed completely in two predicted stages. While from all 150 primary participants (98 women and 52 men), eventually 121 persons within 20 to 68 years of age with mean (±SD) age of 31.7 ± 9.5 matched with all inclusion criteria, mentioned above. Totally, 81 (67%) women by 20-62 years of age with mean (±SD) age of 29.7 ± 7.87 and 40 (33%) men by 24-68 years of age with mean (±SD) age of 35.8 ± 11.31 were eligible to take part in the study. Men were older than women (p<0.001, %95CI: 2.60-9.60).

Twenty nine (19.4%) of all removed due to incomplete answering (10, 6.7%), leaving study (7, 4.4%), pregnancy or supervising children (4, 2.7%) and others (2, 1.3%). According to analysis, we found no difference in time of getting slept (p=0.08), interval between going to bed until getting slept (p=0.97), time of awakening in the morning (p=0.69) and nocturnal sleep duration (p=0.49) between two genders. Thus, there was no significant subjective difference in quantitative parameters of nocturnal sleep between men and women. Probability values and some score findings reported in Table 1.

According to findings, there were four significant correlations. First, it showed direct relation between OISQ-P score and gender (p=0.029) with Pearson's correlation coefficient 0.173, implying on women experience the little impact of inadequate sleep quality on their working function.

Second, there was a positive direct correlation between Factor 1 (sleep efficiency) and age (p=0.03) with Pearson's correlation coefficient 0.171 which meant older people influenced more from sleep disturbances.

Third, we found strong correlation between Factor 3 (daily disturbances) and gender (p=0.008) with Pearson's correlation coefficient 0.231, implying on males were at risk of daily disturbances due to their sleep disorders. Fourth, there was a negative correlation coefficient (-0.208) between Factor 3 and age, that meant older people had the lesser sense of daily disturbances.

Variables	Stage one	Stage two
PSQI-P* score rate	1-16	1-16
OISQ-P** score rate	0-90	0-92
PSQI-P score mean (±SD)	7.13 ± 3.46	6.74 ± 3.27
OISQ-P score mean (±SD)	52.21 ± 22.84	54.79 ± 23.69
PSQI-P score and age	P=0.313	P=0.274
OISQ-P score and age	P=0.185	P=0.134
PSQI-P score and gender	P=0.130	P=0.290
OISQ-P score and gender	P=0.125	P=0.029
Factor 1 and age	P=0.283	P=0.030
Factor 1 and gender	P=0.434	P=0.450
Factor 2 and age	P=0.473	P=0.400
Factor 2 and gender	P=0.339	P=0.292
Factor 3 and age	P=0.011	P=0.128
Factor 3 and gender	P=0.008	P=0.187

Table 1: Probability values and some score findings. (*Persian version of Pittsburg's Sleep Questionnaire Index, **Persian version of Occupational Impact of Sleep Questionnaire).

Reliability analysis was performed by measuring α-Cronbach's coefficient. It showed a great internal consistency in our translated version of OISQ-P. It measured 0.972 and 0.976 in stage one and two respectively. We calculated this value for PSQI-P as 0.789 and 0.805 in initial and additional stages, respectively.

However, analysis of the Guttman Split-half coefficient as 0.906 in first stage and 0.925 in second one, again implied on reliability of our translated questionnaire OISQ-P. We found validity value of OISQ-P as 0.847 (p<0.001) and 0.786 (p<0.001), at the significant level of 1%, in primary and secondary stage, respectively.

Cut Points of OISQ-P

In order to find real cut points for translated questionnaire, we measured a mean of OISQ-P, MSQ-P and PISQ-P based on the latter subjective sleep quality answers. Table 2 shows measurement.

According to our findings, founded good sleepers, who had proper sleep quality, scored ≤12.7 and ≤12.63, whether poor sleepers scored ≥19.38 and ≥18.75 from OISQ-P in first and second stage, respectively. Figures 1 and 2 show graphs of this finding.

	Stage one				Stage two			
	MSQ-P*		PSQI-P**		MSQ-P		PSQI-P	
	mean	%95CI	mean	%95CI	mean	%95CI	Mean	%95CI
Good sleepers	21.47	19.28-23.65	3.93	03.55-04.31	21.33	19.24-23.43	3.92	03.55-04.28
Poor sleepers	29.74	27.89-31.57	9.03	08.36-09.69	28.9	27.05-30.76	8.59	07.93-09.25
ANOVA	F=32.06 , P<0.000		F=123.44 , P<0.000		F=28.213 , P<0.000		F=115.5 , P<0.000	

Table 2: Measurement of OISQ-P cut points. (*Persian version of Mini Sleep Questionnaire, **Persian version of Pittsburg's Sleep Questionnaire Index).

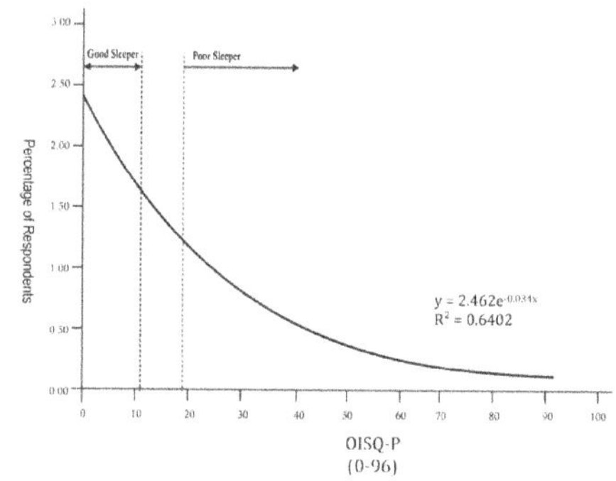

Figure 1: Graph of all scores from OISQ-P in first stage with cut points limits

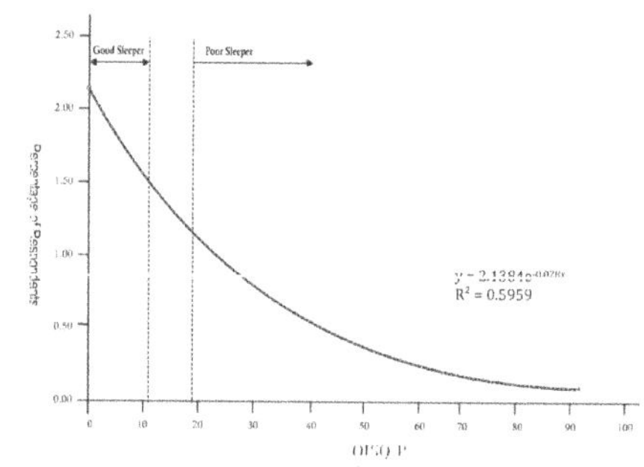

Figure 2: Graph of all scores from OISQ-P in second stage with cut points limits

Discussion

Sleep disorders had extensive multi aspects side effects in both human and animal [5-8]. Negative impacts from simple but bothering symptoms such as bruxism and increasing appetite up to life threatening one such as cardiovascular disease, coronary artery calcification, respiratory dysfunction, immune system dysfunction and even death due to road and work accidents, all heightened morbidity and mortality in at least in last two decades which complain of low sleep quality increased up to 33% among 20-59 years-old population in the united states [5-7,9]. Unfortunately, such complications would fail performance cycles for family and whole society by making disasters, passive working population, handicaps and other irreversible miserable outcomes. In this study, we tried to prepare a fast, easy and scientific screening tool in order to find how sleep influences on worker functions and who is a good or a poor sleeper. Data analysis showed strong values for reliability and validity of our translated Persian version of OISQ, fortunately. This prepared tool for all who speak or understand Persian is now available also to detect whose sleep is good or not. It is possible by counting a fully filled OISQ-P score. Anybody who scores ≥ 20 consider as a poor sleeper that means his or her sleeping quality worsened his or her working function and who scores ≤12 consider as a good sleeper with good working function in last four weeks.

Although, based on our study, older people daily functions influenced more negatively than younger because of sleep deficiency, but they suffered lesser from daily disturbance, which is compatible with another study [10]. The latter maybe due to its natural history of chronically event, getting consistent with gradually occurring daily disturbances lowers sense of bothering by that kind of disturbances and eventually would make it easier to ignore, in high probability. The fact that older people impact more from sleep efficiency maybe due to aging, other synchronous systemic diseases and/or drug complications -which did not include in our study as variables- affecting natural physiology of sleep. We found women experience daily disturbances much more than men; however, it doesn't impact on their working functions, subjectively. It may be due to kind of easier jobs they should do, which perform by lower stress and responsibility or their higher self-assurance level. Unfortunately, data showed a vicious cycle between using hypnotic medications and poor sleep quality subjectively. As sleep-influencing medications lead to imbalance in the normal sleep cycles, it would make real sleep disorder in somebody who was not involved before. It seems very important to attend because of increased prevalence of self-ordered sleep medications and complaints of lower sleep quality in last years, based on reports of other study [5,11].

Limitations

The process of translation from to any other language always would have some mistakes, as every language influenced deeply by bases and changes of history, culture and art. Therefore, we never claim our Persian translation transfers all concepts of its English version. Although, we had a previous model for performing the study,4 though OISQ is unable to detect all factors of PSQI except of sleep efficiency and especially sleep impacts on quality of daily working functions. Another limitation of study was absent from variables evaluating other factors, which could affect sleep characteristics as other basic systemic disorders.

Acknowledgement

This study was an adoption of the medical student's thesis who was the corresponding author for this study, too. This study was done under supervision of the department of psychiatry in the University of Medical Sciences, Qom, Iran.

References

1. Van Dongen HP, Belenky G (2009) Individual differences in vulnerability to sleep loss in the work environment. Ind Health 47: 518-526.
2. Farrahi Moghaddam J, Nakhaee N, Sheibani V, Garrusi B, Amirkafi A (2012) Reliability and validity of the Persian version of the Pittsburgh Sleep Quality Index (PSQI-P). Sleep Breath 16: 79-82.
3. Shochat T, Tzischinsky O, Oksenberg A, Peled R (2007) Validation of the Pittsburgh Sleep Quality Index Hebrew translation (PSQI-H) in a sleep clinic sample. Isr Med Assoc J 9: 853-856.
4. Verster JC, David B, Morgan K, Olivier B (2008) Validation of the Dutch Occupational Impact of Sleep Questionnaire (OISQ). Ind Health 46: 601-606.
5. Pressman MR, Mahowald MW, Sanders MH, Banser RC, Wilson KC. Definition and consequences of sleep deprivation.
6. White DP, Douglas NJ, Pickett CK, Zwillich CW, Weil JV (1983) Sleep deprivation and the control of ventilation. Am Rev Respir Dis 128: 984-986.
7. Schiffman PL, Trontell MC, Mazar MF, Edelman NH (1983) Sleep deprivation decreases ventilatory response to CO2 but not load compensation. Chest 84: 695-698.
8. King CR, Knutson KL, Rathouz PJ, Sidney S, Liu K, et al. (2008) Short sleep duration and incident coronary artery calcification. JAMA 300: 2859-2866.
9. Dahlgren A, Kecklund G, Akerstedt T (2005) Different levels of work-related stress and the effects on sleep, fatigue and cortisol. Scand J Work Environ Health 31: 277-285.
10. Ahlberg K, Jahkola A, Savolainen A, Könönen M, Partinen M, et al. (2008) Associations of reported bruxism with insomnia and insufficient sleep symptoms among media personnel with or without irregular shift work. Head Face Med 4: 4.
11. Walsh JK, Krystal AD, Amato DA, Rubens R, Caron J, et al. (2007) Nightly treatment of primary insomnia with eszopiclone for six months: effect on sleep, quality of life, and work limitations. Sleep 30: 959-968.

33

Can Auto-CPAP Determine Therapeutic CPAP Pressure in Children with OSA?

Rapee Opasatian, Aroonwan Preutthipan*

Division of Pediatric Pulmonology, Department of Pediatrics, and Sleep Disorder Center, Faculty of Medicine, Ramathibodi Hospital, Bangkok, Thailand

Abstract

Objective: In current standard practice the therapeutic pressure of CPAP is determined by manually titration under attended polysomnography (PSG). Since PSG is not easily accessible, auto-CPAP may be an attractive alternative. Our goal is to compare the pressure levels obtained from home auto-CPAP with overnight PSG titration in children with OSA.

Methods: We performed a prospective cohort study in 2-18 year-old children with OSA referred for CPAP titration under PSG. Children were instructed to use auto-CPAP devices at home for 8 weeks, either before or after PSG titration. One night PSG titration was performed following AASM clinical guidelines for the manual titration of positive airway pressure. Data from only those children who used auto-CPAP ≥ 4 hours per day, for >consecutive 7 days and percent days with device usage ≥ 80% were selected for analysis. Average device pressure ≤ 90% of time from auto-CPAP were obtained and compared with PSG titrating pressure.

Results: Eleven of 17 children were enrolled and completed the protocol (male 9/11, aged 9.6 ± 4.2 years, BMI 31.5 ± 10.0 kg/m^2). Three children refused to use auto-CPAP. Three children were non-adherence. Six of 11 children had already undergone adenotonsillectomy. There were no significant differences in the pressure levels obtained from home auto-CPAP and PSG titration (11.05 ± 3.68 vs. 11.18 ± 3.34 cm H_2O, p=0.84). However, when considering on actual values of the pressure, only 5/11 children had pressure differences <2 cm H_2O. Pressure levels obtained from auto-CPAP significantly differed from PSG titration in the group of children with history of adenotonsillectomy (p=0.036).

Conclusion: In children with OSA, the use of home auto-CPAP may not accurately determine the therapeutic CPAP pressure as compared with manually titration under attended PSG, especially in children who previously had adenotonsillectomy.

Keywords: Auto-titrating positive airway pressure; Positive airway pressure therapy; Obstructive sleep apnea; Children; Adenotonsillar hypertrophy; Polysomnography; Adenotonsillectomy.

Introduction

In adults, the treatment of choice for obstructive sleep apnea (OSA) is continuous positive airway pressure (CPAP) device, which functions by blowing air into the airway to overcome the critical closing pressure of the pharynx and maintain a patent pharyngeal airway during sleep [1]. Unlike adults, CPAP is considered in children only when OSA persists despite adenotonsillectomy or such surgery is contraindicated. The pressure level that each patient requires needs to be titrated individually under attended polysomnography, during which CPAP pressure is started at a low level and progressively increased to find the level at which the following obstructive respiratory events, including apneas, hypopneas, respiratory effort-related arousals, and snoring, are eliminated. The pressure required for resolution of events is often higher if the patient is supine, and may be higher in REM sleep when muscle tone is the lowest. Therefore, the final prescription should reflect the single fixed pressure required to treat the worst apnea in supine REM sleep [2]. To standardize CPAP titration technique, the American Academy of Sleep Medicine (AASM) have published a clinical guideline for the manual titration of CPAP pressure in OSA patients in 2008 [3].

Over the last two decades, auto-CPAP machines have developed and focused mainly for adult patients. The CPAP pressure was initially set up as a range: Lowest and highest pressure levels. The machines are programmed to adjust CPAP pressure automatically based on detection of apnea, hypopnea, flow limitation, snoring, pressure fluctuations or increased airway resistance. With the implement of auto-CPAP, the need for CPAP titration under polysomnography is supposedly decreased. A systematic review with meta-analyses on 24 randomized controlled trials comparing auto-CPAP with single fixed pressure CPAP in adults with OSA found that auto-CPAP improved compliance by 11 minutes per night and reduced the Epworth Sleepiness Scale by 0.5 points. Although statistically significant differences were found but clinical importance was unclear. Therefore the choice of therapy still depends on patient's preference or cost [4].

There have been relatively fewer studies of auto-CPAP use in children as compared to adults. In 2004, Polombini et al. demonstrated that auto-CPAP was safe and effective for children with OSA in an attended setting. It was also found to be useful for pressure titration [5]. In 2009, Marshall et al. demonstrated that auto-CPAP was feasible and safe to be used at home in children with sickle cell anemia, which resulted in improved sleep-related breathing disorders and at least one aspect of cognition [6].

All auto-CPAP devices have a slot in the machine allowing for a smart card to capture data. The data can be downloaded and viewed

***Corresponding author:** Preutthipan A, Division of Pediatric Pulmonology, Department of Pediatrics, and Sleep Disorder Center, Faculty of Medicine, Ramathibodi Hospital, Bangkok, Thailand, Email: aroonwan.pre@mahidol.ac.th

or printed out. Some machines report not only the patients' adherence but also the amount pressure the patients have received and express as an average pressure and as a percentile pressure. In 2017, Mihai et al. conducted a retrospective study in children comparing these downloaded pressure data with the CPAP pressure determined by PSG. They found that downloaded pressure from auto-CPAP report were usually below treatment pressure determined under PSG [7]. Since this study was a retrospective review and recruited CPAP-naïve children whose parents reported CPAP use of at least 1 to 2 hours a night, 39% of the children were found to be non-adherence as using auto-CPAP less than 90% of the time. Therefore downloaded pressure data may be confounded with the data from non-adherence children. We hypothesized that if the children were adherence to auto-CPAP, downloaded pressure data might be closed to the CPAP pressure determined by attended PSG titration. If so, instead of performing PSG titration, auto-CPAP could be started in a new patient right after diagnosis of OSA and the optimum CPAP pressure level could be obtained easily from downloaded data. For any cost reasons, the patient could transition to fixed pressure CPAP afterwards. So the objective of this prospective study was to compare the pressure level derived from auto-CPAP downloaded data with the CPAP pressure determined under attended PSG in children with OSA.

Materials and Methods

Subjects

The study was conducted prospectively from February 2016 to January 2017. We enrolled children aged 2 to 18 years old, diagnosed with OSA by PSG. They needed CPAP therapy and were willing to use auto-CPAP at home with acceptance from parents. Children with neuromuscular weakness and central hypoventilation were excluded. This study was approved by the Institutional Review Board (IRB) of Ramathibodi Hospital. All children and parents provided informed consent.

Methods

Polysomnographic studies

A standard attended PSG for titration of CPAP, was performed at Ramathibodi Hospital Sleep Disorder Center. We used PSG equipment (Grael system, Compumedics, Melbourne, Australia). The measured parameters included the recording of frontal, central and occipital electroencephalograms, left and right electrooculograms, submental and bilateral tibial electromyogram, electrocardiogram, nasal thermistor, nasal pressure, pulse oximetry, end tidal CO2, thoracic and abdominal belt for respiratory effort monitoring, and infra-red camera. Signals were recorded with Compumedics® (Compumedics Ltd, Abbotsford, Australia) and scored following the American Academy of Sleep Medicine (AASM) criteria [8]. Apneas were defined as a drop in peak signal excursion by ≥ 90% of pre-event baseline using oronasal thermal sensor. Obstructive apnea defined by criteria of apnea for at least duration of 2 breaths during baseline breathing and associated with presence of respiratory effort. Hypopneas were defined as a peak signal excursions drop by ≥ 30% of pre-event baseline using nasal pressure and the duration lasts for ≥ 2 breaths and ≥ 3% oxygen desaturation from pre-event baseline of the event associated with arousal. Children were accompanied by parents throughout the night. The studies were conducted by two skillful clinical sleep technicians experienced with children. One night PSG titration was performed following AASM clinical guidelines for the manual titration of positive airway pressure [3], with the goal to eliminate all obstructive apneas and hypopneas and minimize arousals and snoring.

Auto-CPAP studies

All patients were instructed to use auto-CPAP devices (System One REMstar Auto, Philips Respironics Inc, Murrysville, Pennsylvania, United States). This device detects upper airway resistance by flow limitation. It measures changes in airflow by an internal pneumotachograph to identify respiratory events. If flow decreases by 40% to 80% for at least 10 sec, the event is labeled a hypopnea; a decrease in flow by more than 80% for at least 10 sec is labeled an apnea [9,10]. The device starts off at the minimum pressure set point for five minutes. At this minimum pressure setting, the patient is awake and the upper airway is patent and upper airway resistance is low. As the patient falls asleep the upper airway begins to collapse thus increasing the resistance. The device then delivers proper pressure until there is no flow limitation [11].

Auto-CPAP was assigned to be used at home for 2 weeks either before or after PSG titration. The period in between the use of auto-CPAP at home and PSG titration was less than 8 weeks. The study flow diagram is shown in Figure 1. Auto-CPAP pressure were adjusted to 4-15 cm H_2O in children aged <12 years, and 4-20 cm H_2O in children aged >12 years. Mask fitting was completed by our clinical sleep technicians. We let the patients select their own masks according to their preference to optimize acceptability and comfort. Another important aim of mask fitting was to minimize leaks. The patient came back to our sleep clinic after two weeks of home auto-CPAP. The data from auto-CPAP were downloaded using EncorePro Basic (Philips Respironics Inc, Murrysville, Pennsylvania, United States). The pressure parameter taken from the standard report was "average device pressure ≤ 90% of time", at which the device spent 90% of the session time at or below this pressure. Adherence data were also downloaded. Data from only those who used auto-CPAP ≥ 4 hours per day, for >consecutive 7 days and percent days with device usage ≥ 80% were selected for analysis. Average device pressure ≤ 90% of time from auto-CPAP was compared with PSG titrating pressure.

Statistical analysis

Data were analyzed using SPSS version 20. Descriptive statistics include mean, standard deviation, and median values. The data are expressed as the mean+SD for continuous variables or numbers and percentages for categorical variables. Continuous variables were compared using paired Student t test or the Mann-Whitney test. Categorical variables were compared using the $\lambda 2$ test or the Fisher's exact test. Relationship between two continuous variables was assessed using Pearson's correlation coefficient. A p value of <0.05 was considered statistically significant.

Results

Seventeen OSA patients who needed CPAP therapy were invited

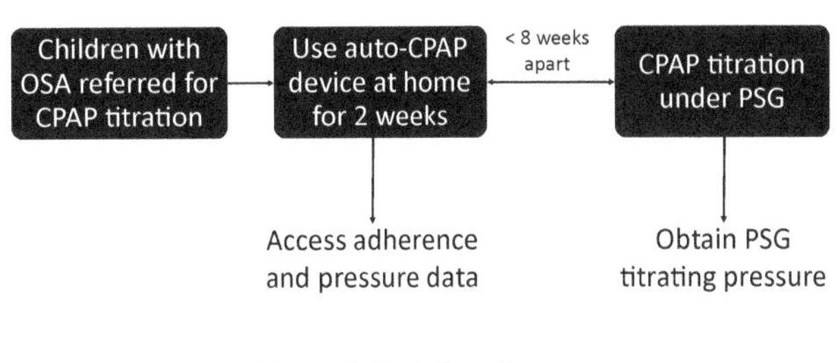

Figure 1: Study flow diagram.

to participate to the study. Three patients refused to use auto-CPAP at home. Another three patients who failed to meet the criteria of CPAP adherence were excluded. Informed consent was obtained from all individual participant included in the study. Data from 11 patients were analyzed in this study. Of the remaining 11 patients, 9 (82%) were male. Demographic data are shown in Table 1. Six (55%) were obese. Mean body mass index z-score was above 2.0. Five (45%) presented with enuresis. Nine (82%) had severe OSA as apnea hypopnea index >10 events/h. All of our patients had been treated with intranasal corticosteroids and leukotriene inhibitor. Six (55%) had undergone adenotonsillectomy.

Average device pressure ≤ 90% of time derived from auto-CPAP was 11.05+3.68 cmH_2O, and PSG titrating pressure was 11.18+3.34 cm H_2O. There was no statistically significant difference between these two pressure variables (p value=0.84). However, when considering on actual values of the pressure as shown in Figure 2, 6 (55%) patients had pressure differences >2 cm H_2O as shown in Figure 3, 3 (27%) had pressure differences >4 cm H_2O. PSG pressure was higher than auto-CPAP pressure in 5 patients and lower in 6 patients. The largest difference was 9.3 cm H_2O found in the last patient as shown in Figure 3.

Of 6 patients with history of adenotonsillectomy, 5 (83%) had pressure differences >2 cmH2O. In contrast to 5 patients without history of adenotonsillectomy, there was only 1 (20%) patient having pressure differences >2 cmH_2O. Fisher's exact test showed a statistically significant difference between these two percentages (p value=0.036). No other conditions of the patients (including age, sex, body mass index, OSA severity, allergic rhinitis, Prader Willi Syndrome) were found to be associated with the pressure differences >2 cm H_2O.

Figure 4a shows no correlation between PSG pressure and auto-CPAP pressure in patients with history of adenotonsillectomy (r=0.03, p value=0.518) in contrast to the patients without history of adenotonsillectomy, in whom PSG pressure correlates well with auto-CPAP pressure (r=0.91, p value=0.035) as shown in Figure 4b.

No patients reported adverse events from auto-CPAP.

Discussion

This pilot study indicates that although auto-CPAP devices are safe to be used in children, they cannot be used to determine the optimal CPAP pressure requirement or replace CPAP titration under PSG. The actual pressure levels derived from auto-CPAP differed from PSG pressure greater than 2 cmH_2O in more than half of the patients. Auto-CPAP pressure levels were found to be either higher or lower than PSG pressure. And the pressure difference was as high as 9 cm H_2O in one patient. The findings of this study suggest that a manual CPAP titration under attended PSG is still essential to determine the most effective pressure for fixed-pressure CPAP in children.

Most of the studies with similar objectives comparing the pressure levels derived from auto-CPAP with PSG titrating pressure have been conducted in adults. The results were not consistent. Luo et al. found that automatic titration pressure derived from REM star Auto was

Demographic data		
Sex (male), n	9	
Age (mean ± SD, range), year	9.6 ± 4.2, 4-17	
Body weight (range), Kg	12.6-122	
BMI (mean ± SD, range), Kg/m²	31.5 ± 10.0, 14.9-45.9	
BMI Z-score (mean ± SD)	3.8 ± 2.4	
Weight for height (mean ± SD), %	184.5 ± 62.1	
Clinical manifestation		
Snoring	100%	
Abnormal breathing during sleep	64%	
Enuresis	45%	
Excessive daytime sleepiness	27%	
Underlying diseases		
Adenotonsillar hypertrophy	73%	
Allergic rhinitis	45%	
Obesity (%W/H>140)	55%	
Morbid obesity (%W/H>200)	27%	
Prader-Willi syndrome	18%	
OSA severity		
AHI range	5.7-135.7	
Moderate OSA (AHI 5-10)	18%	
Severe OSA (AHI>10)	82%	
Previous OSA treatment		
Intranasal corticosteroids	100%	
Leukotriene inhibitor	100%	
Adenotonsillectomy	54.50%	
Auto-CPAP pressure (mean ± SD), cmH_2O	11.05 ± 3.68	p value=0.84*
Attended PSG pressure (mean ± SD), cmH_2O	11.18 ± 3.34	

*Comparison between auto-CPAP pressure and attended PSG pressure

BMI: body mass index, W/H: weight for height, OSA: obstructive sleep apnea, AHI: apnea- hypopnea index, CPAP: continuous positive airway pressure, PSG: polysomnography

Table 1: Demographic data of participants (n = 11).

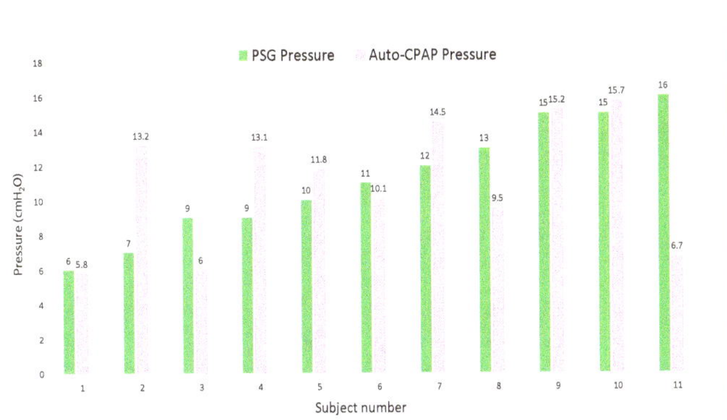

Figure 2: Comparison of pressure levels obtained from polysomnographic titration and auto-CPAP.

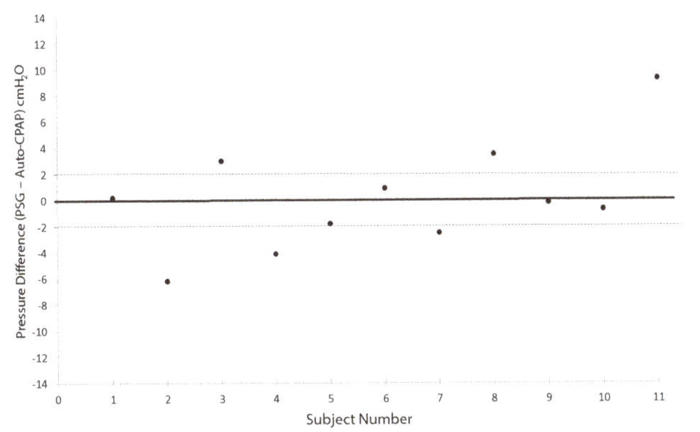

Figure 3: Pressure difference (PSG pressure – auto-CPAP pressure) of each patient in cmH_2O.

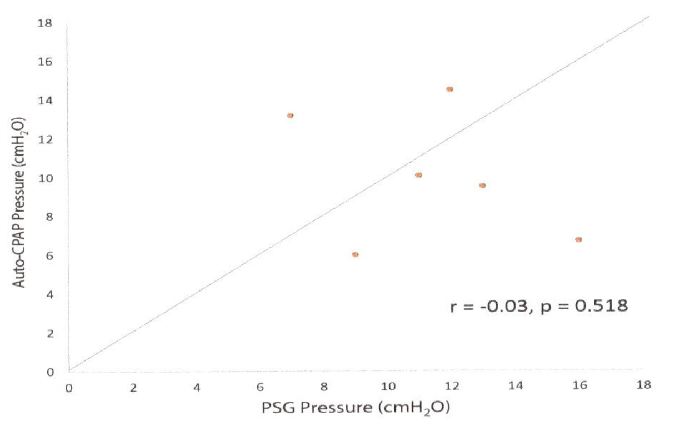

Figure 4a: Poor correlation between PSG and auto-CPAP pressure in patients with history of adenotonsillectomy (n = 6).

significantly higher than that derived from manual titration under PSG [12]. Choi et al. reported no significant differences in pressure level between full-night manual titration and auto-adjusting titration [13]. Lloberes et al. found that daytime auto-CPAP titration yielded a higher treatment pressure than PSG titration but the clinical outcomes were similar [14].

So far very few studies on auto-CPAP have been conducted in children. Mihai et al. conducted a retrospective study comparing treatment pressure derived from auto-CPAP and those from overnight PSG titration. They found that average device pressure < 90% of time

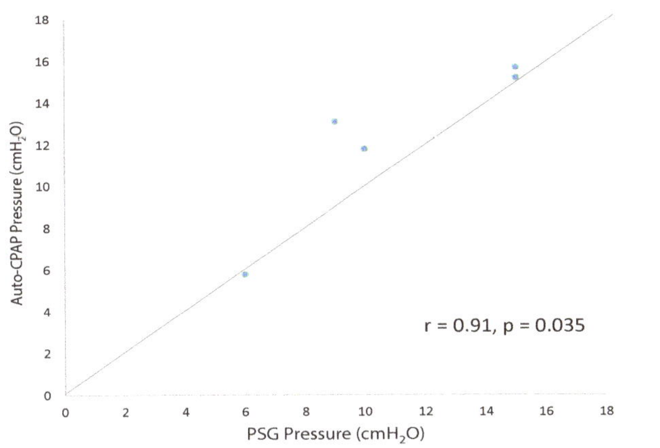

Figure 4b: Strong correlation between PSG and auto-CPAP pressure in patients without history of adenotonsillectomy (n = 5).

downloaded from auto-CPAP did not statistically differ from PSG pressure. However the pressure difference falling within 2 cm H_2O were noted only in 69% of cases. The magnitude of difference ranged from 8 cm H_2O under PSG pressure to 3 cm H_2O over PSG pressure [7]. The results of Mihai's study were compatible with our current study. In addition to the results and recruiting children as subjects, the similarity between ours and Mihai's study was the use of REMstar Auto as a single auto-CPAP device at home, not in the sleep laboratory. We also selected average device pressure <90% of time as a representative of auto-CPAP pressure. Dissimilar factors that strengthened of our study were the prospective study design and non-adherence subjects were excluded. We selected patients only those who used auto-CPAP ≥ 4 hours per day, for >consecutive 7 days and percent days with device usage ≥ 80% in comparison with Mihai's study that included patients who used at least 1 to 2 hours a night. One limitation of our study was a smaller sample size that may explain why the differences in pressure levels derived from the two techniques could not be demonstrated.

Our study confirmed that auto-CPAP devices were well tolerated and safe to be applied in children with no adverse effects reported. Only 3 out of 14 recruited children failed to meet the criteria of CPAP adherence. The youngest age of our adherence patients was found to be 4 years with the body weight of 12.6 Kg. This indirect evidence confirmed the usefulness of auto-CPAP in children with OSA as reported by Palombini et al, Marshall et al. and Mihai et al. Unfortunately we did not collect data of the polysomnographic parameters, oxygen saturation or the quality of life that might be improved after auto-CPAP therapy [5-7].

One interesting finding was the effect of adenotonsillectomy to the pressure difference. In children with no history of adenotonsillectomy the pressure determined by auto-CPAP correlated well with PSG titration pressure. However, in children who had undergone adenotonsillectomy there was no significant correlation. The effect of adenotonsillectomy on the function of auto-CPAP devices have never been described before. In adults, upper airway surgical treatment was found to have some benefits by reducing nasal CPAP pressure levels [15,16]. In children, adenotonsillectomy also reduces CPAP requirement most likely due to alleviation of upper airway obstruction [17]. However it is unknown why auto-CPAP devices function differently in patients with and without history of adenotonsillectomy. It is likely that there may be some changes in the pattern of air flow through the upper airway surrounded by surgical scar resulting in the changing pattern of auto-CPAP response. Further studies on this issue are needed to confirm and explain this finding.

It should be noted that we used the same auto-CPAP device in all children. Our results cannot be applied to other brands of auto-CPAP since different devices used different proprietary algorithms to adjust pressure and the performance of one device should not be assumed to be equivalent to that of another [18]. Isetta et al. conducted a bench test to assess how 7 available auto-CPAP devices respond to a simulated OSA patient. They found wide variations in mean and maximum pressure, and also the time to reach maximum pressure [19]. Therefore the pressure derived from each brand of auto-CPAP may not be the same.

In conclusion, although auto-CPAP is safe to be used at home in children, it cannot replace the role of PSG titration in determining the most effective fixed pressure level of long-term CPAP therapy in children with OSA.

Limitation

Although the number of subjects is only 11, we still see the difference of pressure levels greater than 2 cm H_2O in more than half of the patients. We use 2 cm H_2O as a cutoff of pressure difference because this is important in clinical practice. The magnitude of pressure difference in one patient is as high as 9 cm H_2O which may cause harmful effect clinically. Therefore the pressure level obtained from auto-CPAP cannot be used to replace the pressure derived from polysomnography. Auto-CPAP pressure levels were either higher or lower than PSG pressure. So it would be too difficult to predict optimal pressure from auto-CPAP.

Acknowledgements

We thank Teeradej Kuptanon, Wanaporn Anantaseree, Pravit Jetanachai, Anchalee Leejakpai, Vijittra Hongtong and Ramathibodi Hospital Sleep Disorder Center for all their support. Moreover, our special thanks go to children and parents who kindly participated in this project.

Conflict of interest

The authors declare that they have no conflict of interest.

Funding

No funding was received for this research.

References

1. Huang J, Pinto SJ, Yuan H, Katz ES, Karamessinis LR, et al. (2012) Upper airway collapsibility and genioglossus activity in adolescents during sleep. Sleep 35: 1345-1352.
2. Halbower A (2018) CPAP for pediatric obstructive sleep apnea. In: Chervin R, Hoppin A, editors. UpToDate. UpToDate, Waltham, MA.
3. Kushida CA, Chediak A, Berry RB, Brown LK, Gozal D, et al. (2008) Clinical guidelines for the manual titration of positive airway pressure in patients with obstructive sleep apnea. J Clin Sleep Med 4: 157-171.
4. Ip S, D'Ambrosio C, Patel K, Obadan N, Kitsios GD, et al. (2012) Auto-titrating versus fixed continuous positive airway pressure for the treatment of obstructive sleep apnea: A systematic review with meta-analyses. Syst Rev 1: 20.
5. Palombini L, Pelayo R, Guilleminault C (2004) Efficacy of automated continuous positive airway pressure in children with sleep-related breathing disorders in an attended setting. Pediatrics 113: e412-e417.
6. Marshall MJ, Bucks RS, Hogan AM, Hambleton IR, Height SE, et al. (2009) Auto-adjusting positive airway pressure in children with sickle cell anemia: Results of a phase I randomized controlled trial. Haematologica 94: 1006-1010.
7. Mihai R, Vandeleur M, Pecoraro S, Davey M, Nixon G (2017) Autotitrating CPAP as a tool for CPAP initiation for Children. J Clin Sleep Med 13: 713.
8. Berry RB, Budhiraja R, Gottlieb DJ, Gozal D, Iber C, et al. (2012) Rules for scoring respiratory events in sleep: Update of the 2007 AASM manual for the scoring of sleep and associated events. deliberations of the sleep apnea definitions task force of the american academy of sleep medicine. J Clin Sleep Med 8: 597-619.
9. Gagnadoux F, Pevernagie D, Jennum P, Lon N, Loiodice C, et al. (2017) Validation of the system one remstar auto A-flex for obstructive sleep apnea treatment and detection of residual apnea-hypopnea index: A european randomized trial. J Clin Sleep Med 13: 283-290.
10. Li QY, Berry RB, Goetting MG, Staley B, Soto-Calderon H, et al. (2015) Detection of upper airway status and respiratory events by a current generation positive airway pressure device. Sleep 38: 597-605.
11. Morgenthaler TI, Aurora RN, Brown T, Zak R, Alessi C, et al. (2008) Practice parameters for the use of autotitrating continuous positive airway pressure devices for titrating pressures and treating adult patients with obstructive sleep apnea syndrome: An update for 2007. Sleep 31: 141-147.
12. Luo J, Xiao S, Qiu Z, Song N, Luo Y (2013) Comparison of manual versus automatic continuous positive airway pressure titration and the development of a predictive equation for therapeutic continuous positive airway pressure in chinese patients with obstructive sleep apnoea. Respirology 18: 528-533.
13. Choi JH, Jun YJ, Oh JI, Jung JY, Hwang GH, et al. (2013) Optimal level of continuous positive airway pressure: Auto-adjusting titration versus titration with a predictive equation. Ann Otol Rhinol Laryngol 122: 339-343.
14. Lloberes P, Rodriguez B, Roca A, Sagales MT, de la Calzada MD, et al. (2004) Comparison of conventional nighttime with automatic or manual daytime CPAP titration in unselected sleep apnea patients: Study of the usefulness of daytime titration studies. Respir Med 98: 619-625.
15. Zonato AI, Bittencourt LRA, Martinho FL, Gregório LC, Tufik S (2006) Upper airway surgery: The effect on nasal continuous positive airway pressure titration on obstructive sleep apnea patients. Eur Arch Otorhinolaryngol 263: 481-486.
16. Ayers CM, Lohia S, Nguyen SA, Gillespie MB (2016) The effect of upper airway surgery on continuous positive airway pressure levels and adherence: A systematic review and meta-analysis. ORL J Otorhinolaryngol Relat Spec 78: 119-25.
17. Shine NP, Lannigan FJ, Coates HL, Wilson A (2006) Adenotonsillectomy for obstructive sleep apnea in obese children: Effects on respiratory parameters and clinical outcome. Arch Otorhinolaryngol 132: 1123-1127.
18. Zhu K, Roisman G, Aouf S, Escourrou P (2015) All APAPs are not equivalent for the treatment of Sleep Disordered Breathing: A bench evaluation of eleven commercially available devices. J Clin Sleep Med 11: 725-734.
19. Isetta V, Navajas D, Montserrat JM, Farre R (2015) Comparative assessment of several automatic CPAP devices' responses: A bench test study. ERJ Open Res 1: 00031.

Association of Short Sleep Duration with Psychological Conditions in Cancer Survivors: From the Korea National Health and Nutrition Examination Survey

Hyung-Suk Yoon[1,2,3], Jae Jeong Yang[2,3], Hwi-Won Lee[1,2] and Daehee Kang[1,2,4,*]

[1]Department of Biomedical Sciences, Seoul National University Graduate School, Seoul, Republic of Korea

[2]Department of Preventive Medicine, Seoul National University College of Medicine, Seoul, Republic of Korea

[3]Institute of Environmental Medicine, Seoul National University Medical Research Center, Seoul, Republic of Korea

[4]Cancer Research Institute, Seoul National University, Seoul, Republic of Korea

[*]**Corresponding author:** Daehee Kang, Department of Preventive Medicine, Seoul National University College of Medicine, Seoul, Republic of Korea, E-mail: dhkang@snu.ac.kr

Abstract

Background: Cancer survivors experience various psychological complications. This study aims to explore the concurrent association between short sleep duration and poor psychological conditions among adult cancer survivors in Korea.

Methods: Cross-sectional study using data from the fourth and fifth Korea National Health and Nutrition Examination Surveys (2007-2012) included 1,042 cancer survivors and 33,867 non-cancer controls. Psychological conditions (i.e., severe distress, depression, suicidal ideation and suicide attempt) were compared between cancer survivors and non-cancer controls. Based on logistic regression models controlling for age and sex, associations between short sleep duration and psychological status were evaluated among cancer survivors.

Results: Cancer survivors exhibited higher estimated proportions of depression, suicidal ideation, and suicide attempt than non-cancer controls. Short sleep duration was found to have a significantly increased likelihood for poor psychological outcomes such as severe distress, depression, and suicidal ideation in cancer survivors (OR=2.21, 95% CI 1.28-3.81; OR=3.14, 95% CI 1.47-6.72, and OR=2.32, 95% CI 1.70-3.78, respectively).

Conclusions: Our findings indicate that short sleep duration can place cancer survivors at a higher risk of adverse psychological conditions. Interventions focused on improving both sleep behavior and psychological stability among cancer survivors are needed.

Keywords: Short sleep; Psychological conditions; Cancer survivorship

Introduction

Currently, about 32.6 million people live with cancer worldwide [1]. Following the global phenomenon, Korea has a cancer prevalence of about 1.2 million cases, and a significant number of individuals with cancer have either been undergoing or completed treatment [2]. Emerging evidence has indicated that cancer survivors are particularly prone to sleep problems, i.e., symptoms of insomnia and sleep disturbance, with a greater prevalence rate than the general population [3,4]. These cancer-related sleep problems appear to impede survivors' daily life and are easily linked to an increased risk for physical and psychological complications [5]. Furthermore, in symptom clusters accompanied with cancer diagnosis, sleep problems and psychological disorders can concurrently occur among cancer survivors [5,6]. Their synergic effects may result and affect survivors' health outcome.

Despite its prevalence and importance, sleep problems of cancer survivors are not yet fully investigated: a large proportion still remains unknown. Few studies focused on the association of decreased sleep quantity with psychological complications among cancer survivors. This study thus aims to explore the concurrent relationship between short sleep duration and psychological conditions among adult cancer survivors from a nationwide population-based sample in Korea.

Method and Material

Study population

This study is based on the nationwide population-based sample from the Fourth and Fifth Korea National Health and Nutrition Examination Survey (KNHANES IV and V, 2007-2012). Described elsewhere in detail, the KNHANES is a nationally representative survey to investigate the health and nutritional status of Koreans [4,7]. Brief information on the KNHANES is summarized as follows: since 1998, this ongoing surveillance system has been carried out every year; non-institutionalized civilians aged one and over are selected by using a multi-stage clustered probability sampling design; and three component surveys-the Health Interview, the Health Examination, and the Nutrition Surveys are conducted by well-trained medical staff [7]. Among the 63,301 respondents who were targeted for KNHANES IV and V, about 79.6% participated in surveys [4], from an initial study samples totaling from KNHANES IV and V cycles, people who were under 19 years of age or those with missing information on the history of cancer diagnosis, sleep duration, and psychological conditions (i.e., severe distress, self-reported prevalence of depression, suicidal ideation, and suicide attempt) were excluded. A final total of 34,909 subjects, including 1,042 cancer survivors and 33,867 non-cancer controls, were selected for analyses.

Variable collection

Information on individual characteristics including cancer history, sleep duration, and psychological conditions were collected based on the interview-based questionnaire survey according to the KNHANES protocol.

Cancer history: All study subjects were asked if they have ever been diagnosed with cancer or a malignancy of any kind by a doctor. Cancer survivors who concurred with the question further responded to sub-questions regarding the specific cancer type and the age at cancer diagnosis. In the case for survivors with multiple cancer diagnoses, the first cancer diagnosis was considered for the definition of the primary outcome.

Sleep duration: Average sleep duration was assessed with a single, open-ended question: 'How many hours of sleep do you usually get each day?' Short sleep duration referred to subjects who usually slept for less than 5 hours per day.

Psychological conditions: Mental health status was assessed by the domains of severe distress, depression, suicidal ideation, and suicide attempt. Severe stress group included subjects who reported their daily life stress level to be severe or high. Depression was evaluated based on the subjects' self-report on whether or not they 'currently suffer[ed] from depression'. Suicidal ideation and attempt was defined by the following questions: 'Have you ever thought about killing yourself during the past year?' and 'Have you ever attempted to commit suicide during the past year?'

Statistical analysis

In accordance with a stratified multi-stage clustered probability sampling method, to yield unbiased national estimates, data were weighted as described in the statistical analysis for the KNHANES. Based on the survey procedures available through SAS version 9.4 (SAS Institute, Cary, North Carolina), all analyses were conducted by using survey weightings to estimate the statistics. Using chi-squared test, estimated proportions and standard errors were calculated to compare the psychological conditions between cancer survivors and non-cancer controls. Associations between short sleep duration and psychological conditions were evaluated among cancer survivors: logistic regression analyses were performed and odds ratios (ORs) and 95% confidence intervals (CIs) were estimated accounting for sex and age.

Results and Discussion

Cancer survivors were more likely to be women and older compared to non-cancer controls ($p<0.001$). Among the cancer survivors, gastric cancer was the most common type and the mean survival time after cancer diagnosis was 7.7 ± 0.3 years (Data not shown).

Estimated proportions of depression and suicidal ideation were significantly higher in cancer survivors: 4.8% vs. 2.8% for depression and 22.5% vs. 14.9% for suicidal ideation ($p<0.001$). Suicide attempt, although marginally significant, was also higher in cancer survivors compared to non-cancer controls (1.6% vs. 0.8%, $p=0.062$; Figure 1).

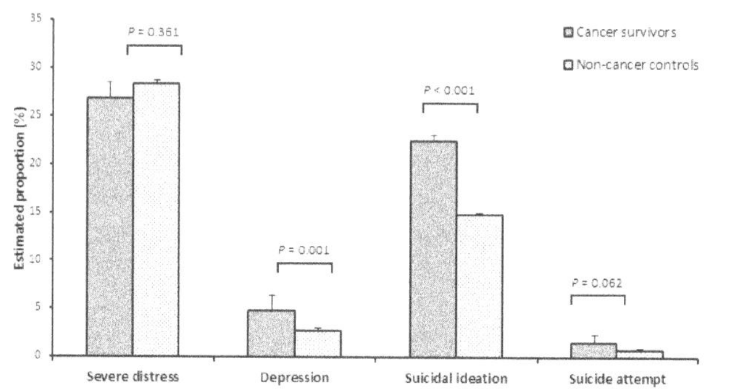

Figure 1: Comparison of psychological conditions between cancer survivors and non-cancer controls.

Short sleep duration exhibited a higher likelihood of poor psychological conditions among cancer survivors. Accounting for sex and age, cancer survivors who slept for less than 5 hours per day had a significantly increased odds of severe distress (OR=2.21, 95% CI 1.28-3.81), depression (OR=3.14, 95% CI 1.47-6.72), and suicidal ideation (OR=2.32, 95% CI 1.70-3.78; Table 1).

	Severe distress	Depression	Suicidal ideation	Suicide attempt
	OR (95% CI) a	OR (95% CI) a	OR (95% CI) a	OR (95% CI) a
Sleep duration (hours/day)				
5-9 hours	1 (reference)	1 (reference)	1 (reference)	1 (reference)
< 5 hours	2.21 (1.28-3.81)	3.14 (1.47-6.72)	2.32 (1.70-3.78)	2.91 (0.81-10.5)

Table 1: Association between short sleep duration and psychological conditions among cancer survivors.

In our study, adult cancer survivors appeared to be vulnerable to psychological complications such as severe distress, depression, and suicidal behaviors compared to the general population in Korea. This is in line with the previous findings [8-10]. Adding to the evidence, our results present the possibility that short sleep duration can act as a trigger to induce poor psychological conditions among cancer survivors. Given the high prevalence of short sleep in cancer survivors, it is presumed that more people will face psychological defects throughout their days fighting cancer, which may progress to morbid outcomes as well as poor prognosis.

Concurrent relationship between sleep problems and psychological symptoms in cancer survivors can be explained by the negative feedback loop with inflammatory responses; thus, understanding the inflammatory dynamics associated with cancer-related sleep problems and psychological outcomes is imperative to enhance survivors' health status [11]. Though this study is notable in that it is based on a large-scale, nationally representative data, considering the study limitations (i.e., cross-sectional design using self-reported information), further studies will help to elucidate the chronological changes of sleep-related health outcomes in post-cancer trajectories.

Conclusion

Cancer survivorship does not mean disease-free status: these survivors may face disease- and treatment-related complications in both physical and/or psychological aspects. Furthermore, we now know that a substantial number of cancer survivors suffer from sleep disturbance, which may inflict negative consequence on mental health. Thus, greater emphasis in terms of public health and prevention is needed to develop concomitant, multimodal interventions aimed at improving both sleep behaviors and psychological stability in cancer survivors.

References

1. International Agency for Research on Cancer. GLOBOCAN 2012: Estimated cancer incidence, mortality and prevalence worldwide in 2012.
2. Jung KW, Won YJ, Kong HJ, Oh CM, Cho H, et al. (2015) Cancer statistics in Korea: incidence, mortality, survival, and prevalence in 2012. Cancer Res Treat 47: 127-141.
3. Savard J, Morin CM (2001) Insomnia in the context of cancer: a review of a neglected problem. J Clin Oncol 19: 895-908.
4. Yoon HS, Yang JJ, Song M, Lee HW, Lee Y, et al. (2015) Short sleep duration and its correlates among cancer survivors in Korea: the Korea National Health and Nutrition Examination Surveys. Asian Pac J Cancer Prev 16: 4705-4710.
5. Garland SN, Johnson JA, Savard J, Gehrman P, Perlis M, et al. (2014) Sleeping well with cancer: a systematic review of cognitive behavioral therapy for insomnia in cancer patients. Neuropsychiatr Dis Treat 10: 1113-1124.
6. Irwin MR (2013) Depression and insomnia in cancer: prevalence, risk factors, and effects on cancer outcomes. Curr Psychiatry Rep 15: 404.
7. Kweon S, Kim Y, Jang MJ, Kim Y, Kim K, et al. (2014) Data resource profile: the Korea National Health and Nutrition Examination Survey (KNHANES). Int J Epidemiol 43: 69-77.
8. Dalton SO, Laursen TM, Ross L, Mortensen PB, Johansen C (2009) Risk for hospitalization with depression after a cancer diagnosis: a nationwide, population-based study of cancer patients in Denmark from 1973 to 2003. J Clin Oncol 27: 1440-1445.
9. Ahn E, Shin DW, Cho SI, Park S, Won YJ, et al. (2010) Suicide rates and risk factors among Korean cancer patients, 1993-2005. Cancer Epidemiol Biomarkers Prev 19: 2097-2105.
10. Recklitis CJ, Diller LR, Li X, Najita J, Robison LL, et al. (2010) Suicide ideation in adult survivors of childhood cancer: a report from the Childhood Cancer Survivor Study. J Clin Oncol 28: 655-661.
11. Irwin MR, Olmstead RE, Ganz PA, Haque R (2013) Sleep disturbance, inflammation and depression risk in cancer survivors. Brain Behav Immun 30: S58-67.

A Profile of Sleep Architecture and Sleep Disorders in Adults with Chronic Traumatic Brain Injury

Catherine Wiseman-Hakes[1,2*], **Brian J. Murray**[3], **Tatyana Mollayeva**[1,2], **Judith Gargaro**[2,4], **and Angela Colantonio**[1,2,5]

[1]*Rehabilitation Sciences Institute, University of Toronto, Toronto, Ontario, Canada*

[2]*Toronto Rehabilitation Institute- University Health Network, Toronto, Ontario, Canada*

[3]*Division of Neurology, Department of Medicine, Sunnybrook Health Sciences Centre, University of Toronto, Toronto, Ontario, Canada*

[4]*ABI Behaviour Services, West Park Health Care Centre, Toronto, Ontario, Canada*

[5]*Department of Occupational Therapy and Occupational Science, University of Toronto, Toronto, Ontario, Canada*

[*]**Corresponding author:** Catherine Wiseman-Hakes, 1Rehabilitation Sciences Institute, University of Toronto, Toronto, Ontario, Canada;
E-mail: catherinew.hakes@utoronto.ca

Abstract

The primary acceleration-deceleration mechanism of traumatic brain injury (TBI) leaves the brain structures that regulate sleep and wakefulness vulnerable to pathological changes, and there are external secondary factors experienced post-injury that can contribute to the development of difficulties initiating or maintaining sleep, early morning awakening, and/or dissatisfaction with sleep.

Patients with TBI are at risk for developing chronic sleep-wake disturbances, and complaints of insomnia and hypersomnia are commonly reported. The objective of this study was to examine sleep architecture and explore the presence and types of sleep disorders in adults with chronic TBI.

Method: Participants (N=13, mean time post injury 4.5 years) underwent polysomnography and the Maintenance of Wakefulness Test. Polysomnographic findings were compared to age and sex normative data. Sleep disorders were diagnosed according to the criteria of the International Classification of Sleep Disorders, 2nd edition.

Results: Compared to normative data, 92% had abnormal sleep architecture with increased N1 ($p=.002$), reductions in REM sleep ($p=0.017$) and total sleep time, and poor sleep efficiency. All were diagnosed with a treatable sleep disorder according to the ICSD-2.

Conclusion: These exploratory findings add to a growing body of evidence that TBI is associated with a high prevalence of sleep disorders which underlie alterations in sleep architecture including increased arousability, greater amounts of transitional sleep stages, and altered REM latency and duration.

These results highlight the importance of regular screening and assessment of sleep-wake disorders early in the rehabilitation stage for this population in order to prevent the development of chronic sleep disorders.

Keywords Sleep; Sleep disorders; Traumatic brain injury; Polysomnography; Sleep architecture

Introduction

The primary acceleration-deceleration mechanism of traumatic brain injury (TBI) leaves the brain structures that regulate sleep, wakefulness and arousal vulnerable to pathological changes [1]. In addition to the TBI, there are external secondary factors experienced by many individuals post-injury that may contribute to the development of disturbed sleep over time such as changes in, or reductions in, activity, mobility, and lifestyle.

These may result in alterations to the sleep-wake schedule, mood and/or weight due to reduced mobility and activity. All of these can contribute to the development or exacerbation of pre-existing sleep disturbances.

Accordingly, patients with TBI have been found to be at high risk for developing chronic sleep-wake disturbances (SWDs) [2] and up to 70% are reported to have complaints of insomnia and hypersomnia across the continuum of recovery [3-7]. Symptoms of insomnia, including difficulty falling asleep, staying asleep, difficulties with early awakening, as well as fragmented sleep are reported in 50-70% of those with TBI [8-13].

A recent meta-analysis and review further highlights the incidence of sleep disturbances after TBI [6]. For those with moderate-severe TBI, evidence from polysomnography (PSG) studies suggests that excessive daytime sleepiness (EDS) and post-traumatic hypersomnia or post-traumatic pleiosomnia, specifically an increased sleep tendency per 24 hours, are most typically reported [14-17].

Studies involving polysomnography (PSG), an objective measure of sleep, report that 50% of those with moderate-severe TBI present with treatable sleep disorders other than insomnia, such as obstructive and central sleep apnea, restless leg syndrome (RLS), periodic leg movement disorder (PLMD), post-traumatic hypersomnia and circadian rhythm abnormalities [9,18-20].

Sleep disturbances have been found to begin in the early acute stage of injury and a recent PSG evaluation conducted in an acute care trauma centre found that compared to patients with orthopaedic and or spinal cord traumatic injuries, acute TBI patients showed a significantly longer duration of nocturnal sleep and earlier night-time sleep onset [21].

During the inpatient rehabilitation stage of recovery, results from actigraphy have identified that 67% of participants had a sleep-wake cycle disturbance, co-existing with self-report of difficulty with initiating and maintaining sleep. Other studies using self-report measures have also reported sleep disruptions amongst those in an inpatient rehabilitation setting [22, 23].

In the chronic stage of TBI (>1 year), preliminary polysomnographic findings have identified changes in sleep architecture, in comparison to the general population.

They include decreased sleep efficiency (amount of time asleep divided by amount of time in bed) [24]; increased percentage of stage 1 sleep [9]; reduced percentage of both slow wave sleep [24, 25], and REM sleep [25]; as well as increased awakenings and number of arousals [25]. However, there has been a lack in formal diagnoses of underlying sleep disorders which may be contributing to these findings.

Despite the increasing awareness regarding post-traumatic sleep and wake disturbances, sleep is not routinely assessed amongst this population.

Many patients, therefore, may go undiagnosed and thus are ineffectively managed or not treated. Moreover, given that this increased awareness is a relatively recent trend, there is a paucity of information regarding the sleep of individuals in the chronic stage post injury.

The aims of this study are as follows: 1.To objectively examines sleep architecture via overnight PSG in a sample of adults with chronic TBI; 2.To diagnose any underlying sleep disorders that result in symptoms of insomnia or hypersomnia and disturbed sleep architecture.

We hypothesized that we would find alterations in sleep architecture as previously reported [9, 24, 25] in comparison to age norms. We further hypothesized that some participants would have underlying sleep disorders that caused their symptoms of insomnia or hypersomnia.

Materials and Method

The study was approved by the local research ethics review boards. This cross-sectional study was conducted in accordance with the Strengthening the Reporting of Observational studies in Epidemiology (STROBE) statement for case-control studies [26]. This study was part of a longitudinal study examining the impact of treatment for sleep and arousal disorders on outcomes for adults with chronic traumatic brain injury. The findings specific to outcomes are published elsewhere [5].

Setting and participant recruitment

Participants were assessed in the Sleep Disorders Clinic and Brain Sciences Program at a teaching hospital affiliated with the University of Toronto.

Participants were recruited over a 2-year period from across Southern Ontario by means of clinicians working in major rehabilitation centres in Toronto, community-based rehabilitation practitioners, and an announcement on the Brain Injury Association of Canada website. Follow-up and clinical care was provided to all participants in the study.

Participants

Eligible participants had to meet the following criteria: 1. Be between the ages of 18-60 years; 2. Have a diagnosis of moderate-severe traumatic brain injury or mild traumatic brain injury with persistent symptoms; 3. During the initial interview, have self-reported post-traumatic sleep and/or wake disturbance (e.g., excessive daytime sleepiness), with dissatisfaction with sleep such that it was a cause of significant distress and/or a score of 15 or greater on the Insomnia Severity Index (ISI), which represents "Clinical Insomnia" (see Measures), those with night-time sleep problems, or a score of 8-14 which represents "Sub-threshold Insomnia" or those with adequate or excessive night time sleep and excessive daytime sleepiness [27]; 4. Be able to speak and read English; and 5. Provide informed written consent to participate. (See table 1)

Individuals were excluded from the study if they: 1. had a history of psychosis; 2. were actively using substances such as alcohol or non-prescription drugs; 3. had pre-injury sleep disturbances as determined during the initial assessment; 4. had ingested alcohol and/or caffeine in the 24-hour period previous to the PSG appointment. The sample size is consistent with that used in previous studies of TBI (range N=7-14 subjects with TBI per study) [5, 9, 21, 25, 28].

All eligible participants completed the Insomnia Severity Index (ISI) [27], and participated in the Diagnostic Interview for Insomnia [27], and provided a list of current medications.

Following a comprehensive clinical evaluation of sleep and wakefulness by a neurologist who was also a diplomate of the American Board of Sleep Medicine, an Epworth Sleepiness Scale (ESS) score was also obtained [29].

Where indicated, participants were referred for blood work to evaluate endocrine function, ferritin levels, and vitamin B12 to disentangle possible alterations in endocrine function, in particular, full or partial hypo-pituitarism, which is common following TBI, as well as assess other common medical contributors to sleep-wake disorders [30].

Overnight polysomnography (PSG) was performed followed by a Maintenance of Wakefulness Test (MWT) the following day where clinically indicated [31]. The PSG and MWT test were scored by a registered PSG technologist.

ID	Age	Sex	TBI Severity	Time Post injury (years)	Onset of Sleep disturbance	Sleep Architecture	ESS	Insomnia Severity Index	Prescribed Medications
1	18	F	Severe	2	Post-injury	Normal	13	17 (moderate)	Quetiapine
2	19	M	Severe	1	Post-injury	Abnormal	7	22 (severe)	None
3	21	M	Moderate	4.5	Post-injury	Abnormal	13	17 (moderate)	Escitalopram
4	28	F	Severe	2	Post-injury	Abnormal	16	26 (severe)	Trazadone Zopiclone Sertraline Doxycycline Acetominophen Codeine
5	29	M	Severe	22	Post-injury	Abnormal	15	14 (sub-threshold)	Bupropion Risperidone Desvenlafaxine
6	31	M	Severe	1	Post-injury	Abnormal	14	17 (moderate)	Modafinil Bupropion Escitalopram
7	32	M	mTBI with persistent symptoms	2	Post-injury	Abnormal	15	21 (moderate)	None
8	37	F	Severe	2	Post-injury	Abnormal	8	13 (sub-threshold)	Synthroid Clopidogrel Escitalopram Atorvastatin Propranolol
9	47	M	mTBI with persistent symptoms	2	Pre-existing mild OSA, exacerbated post-injury	Abnormal	15	22 (severe)	Topiramate Methlyphenidate Duloxetine Meloxicam Tramadol Pregabalin Puprenorphine
10	49	M	Severe	1	Post-injury	Abnormal	14	25 (severe)	Citalopram Nortriptyline Amplodipine Metroprolol
11	53	F	Severe	3	Post-injury	Abnormal	15	23 (severe)	Lamotrigine
12	55	F	Severe	18	Post-injury	Abnormal	12	17 (moderate)	None
13	58	F	Severe	1.5	Post-injury	Abnormal	6	10 (sub-threshold)	Metoprolol Amiodarone Fluoxetine Atrovastin Levothyroxine Warfarin

Table 1: Participant demographics and characteristics, TBI=Traumatic Brain Injury.

Variables of interest

The following variables were examined: insomnia severity, excessive daytime sleepiness (by self-report standardized measures); sleep onset latency (SOL), total sleep time (TST), sleep efficiency (SE), arousal index (the number of spontaneous arousals per hour; SAI), Wake After Sleep Onset (WASO), percentage of stage N1 sleep, percentage of stage N2 sleep, percentage of stage N3 sleep, Rapid Eye Movement (REM) latency, REM percentage of total sleep (as measured by PSG), apnea hypopnea index (AHI), lowest oxygen saturation (lowest SaO2) and periodic limb movement index (PLMI); normality of sleep architecture and the ability to remain awake while resisting the desire to sleep during the day (as measured by a MWT).

Study measures

Insomnia Severity Index (ISI) [27]. This index is designed to be both a brief screening measure of insomnia and an outcomes measure for use in treatment research. Its reliability and validity have been established and it has also been found to sensitive to change following pharmacologic and/or behavioral intervention for primary insomnia

Polysomnography: All PSGs were recorded on digital equipment (Compumedics, Australia) using standard recording and scoring methods [32]. During each study, monitoring of the following took place: Electroencephalogram (EEG), electro-oculogram (EOG), surface electromyography (EMG), respiratory measures (abdominal and thoracic effort [measured with respiratory inductive plethysmography belts], nasal/oral pressure [measured with a nasal/oral pressure transducer], nasal/oral flow [measured with a thermistor]), oxygen saturation, and a 2-lead ECG.

Expanded EEG or EMG montages were used if nocturnal seizures or parasomnias were suspected. All studies were videotaped and audiovisual recordings were time-synchronized to the remainder of the data. Sleep was manually scored according to the American Academy of Sleep Medicine [AASM] criteria [32]. Sleep disorder diagnoses were made after clinical assessment according to the International Classification of Sleep Disorders (ICSD-2) [33].

Maintenance of wakefulness test (MWT) [31]: This test involves giving the participant four opportunities to maintain wakefulness during the day at 9am, 11am, 1pm, 3pm, for 40 minutes each time. They are placed in a slightly reclined position, in a dimly lit room, with the instructions "Please sit quietly and try to remain awake". The latency to sleep onset was recorded.

The MWT was used to quantify EDS, as well as to provide an indicator of future risk of accidents [31, 34]. Patients with TBI are typically administered the Multiple Sleep Latency Test (MSLT) [35]; however the MWT may identify different aspects of alertness for those with severe TBI [36]. Furthermore, EDS impairs function and puts patients at risk of sustaining further injury [34].

Epworth sleepiness scale (ESS) [29]: This 8-question scale was designed to evaluate daytime sleepiness, and asks the respondent the likelihood that he/she would fall asleep under various scenarios.

This questionnaire was administered as part of the routine clinical evaluation of sleep. Most rested individuals have a score under 10. The reliability and validity of the ESS has been well established [37].

Analysis

Sleep was manually scored according to the American Academy of Sleep Medicine [AASM] criteria [32]. The following variables were derived: total sleep time, sleep efficiency (amount of time asleep as compared to amount of time in bed),arousal index (per hour), percentages of each sleep stage and REM latency (time to first REM period).

Variables were compared to age and sex-based normative data [38]. Sleep disorders were diagnosed following clinical assessment according to the ICSD-2 [33].

Statistical analysis

Descriptive statistics are reported using means and standard deviations. Paired t-tests were used to compare sleep architecture variables to matched published age and sex normative values. Significance was set at $p \leq 0.05$. All analysis was performed with SPSS version 22.

Sleep disorder diagnoses

The ICSD-2 classification was used that lists 84 sleep disorders under 7 major categories, including: 1- insomnias; 2 - sleep-related breathing disorders (SRBD); 3 - hypersomnias; 4 - circadian rhythms sleep disorders; 5 - parasomnias; 6 - sleep-related movement disorders; and 7 - other sleep disorders and isolated symptoms [38].

Results

Sleep study results and PSG parameters

Table 2 provides the sleep parameters of the 13 participants. We documented reductions in total sleep time (mean=343.8 minutes ± 92.6), reduced sleep efficiency (mean=74.9 ± 15.7) and increased incidence of wake after sleep onset (mean=73.9 ± 53.7). Further, all severe TBI participants exhibited sleep fragmentation (multiple arousals or awakenings); increased arousal index (mean=13.28 ± 7.7) as well as alterations in sleep staging in comparison to published age and sex norms.

We further identified increased stage N1 (p=0.002), which indicates transitions in state, and alterations in REM percentage (p=0.017) and or REM onset latency (Table 2) compared to normative values of same age and sex [38]. All the insomnia group participants who completed the ESS (4 out of 5) were excessively sleepy with a mean score of 12.53 ± 3.4.

Two of five participants who underwent MWT had abnormal findings (criterion: one epoch of sleep considered as failure due to risk of driving accident). Of the three participants with sleep-related breathing disorder (SRBD), two (66.7%) had abnormal MWT findings. Of the three with relatively "normal" (i.e., considered as mildly abnormal) polysomnographic data, two were unable to maintain alertness as per MWT and one had MWT findings considered normal with modafinil taken at the time of assessment. For this individual a modafinil washout was tried however he was unable to function without the medication.

ID	Sex	Stage N1 % (Norm) * p=0.002	Stage N2 % (Norm)	Stage N3 % (Norm)	REM Latency Latency Norm=90-120 Mins	REM (Mins) %age (Norm) *p=0.017	Total SleepTime (Mins)	Sleep Effic (%)	Wake After Sleep Onset (Mins)	Arousal Index	AHI	Lowest SaO2 (%)	PLMI	ESS	MWT Latency (Mins)	Sleep Diagnosis ICDS-II
1	F	3 (3.74)	50 (49.3)	27 (23.43)	29.5	20 (22.12)	457	95	12.5	3	0.1	96	0	13	8.13	HS
2	M	9.2 (3.74)	52.4 (57.8)	19.3 (23.04)	128.5	19.1 (22.12)	390	88	18.5	18.7	0.2	93	0	7	Not performed	MD and OSA
3	M	19.7 (4.18)	36.8 (45.54)	19.7 (21.09)	252.2	23.8 (28)	294	61.5	121	7.3	0.2	91	1.4	13	18.3	Insom
4	F	4.5 (4.18)	43 (52.7)	41.8 (17.69)	87.5	10.7 (25.23)	201	50.8	88.5	6.9	0.3	93	2.4	16	Not performed	Insom
5	M	10.3 (4.17)	71.2 (56.89)	12.9 (12.46)	251	5.6 (23.47)	329	87.3	35	21.7	1.1	90	11.8	15	Not performed	MD
6	M	10 (4.17)	58.9 (56.89)	21.1 (12.46)	286	10.7 (23.47)	505	73	58	11	2.6	92	3.3	14	Normal with (modafinil)	HS
7	M	9.9 (4.17)	58.2 (56.89)	3.7 (12.46)	83	27.6 (23.47)	326	91.6	30	6.6	0.1	92	2.7	15	23.8	HS
8	F	16.3 (4.17)	57 (53.77)	26.7 (14)	No REM	Absent (22.15)	260	65	63	14.3	0	93	16.6	8	Normal	CRSD and MD
9	M	11 (5.64)	59.7 (54.75)	19.2 (8.85)	121	10.1 (22.85)	462	88.2	59	9.6	20.1	78	0	15	8.1	OSA, CSA and Insom
10	M	33.2 (5.64)	50.8 (54.75)	3.9 (8.85)	119.5	12.1 (22.85)	280	53.4	198	16	1.5	97	31.2	14	Normal	MD, OSA
11	F	7.3 (4.85)	51 (57.8)	19.9 (10.63)	117	21.8 (21.77)	389	90	36	6.2	4.2	88	0	15	14.4	HS and OSA
12	F	25.3 (4.85)	49.6 (57.8)	5.1 (10.83)	66	20 (21.77)	237	60.5	127.5	24.1	3.5	88	0	12	Normal	OSA
13	F	30.4 (4.85)	40.1 (57.8)	0.4 (10.63)	70	29.1 (21.77)	339	70.3	114	27.3	53.1	79	0	6	26	OSA

Table 2: Age and sex-related norms from Williams, R.L., Karacan, I., and Hursch, C.J. (1974). Electroencephalography (LEG) of Human Sleep: Clinical Applications. Chichester, Sussex: John Wiley.

AHI=Apnea/Hypopnea Index, SaO2=Oxygen Saturation, PLMI=Periodic Limb Movement Index, HS=Hypersomnia, Insom=Insomnia, CRSD=Circadian Rhythm Sleep Disorder, MD=Movement Disorders (PLMD, RLS), SA=Sleep Apnea (Obstructive or Central), OSD=Other Sleep Disorders

Note: In this sample 70% (N=9) have a diagnosis in the insomnia family: 23% (N=3) insomnia, 8% (N=1) CRSD, 31% (N=4) MD, 39% sleep-related breathing disorder (N=5); 31% (N=4) have a diagnosis of hypersomnia; 39% (N=5) have more than one diagnosed sleep disorder

Clinical findings: Diagnosis of sleep disorders

All participants were diagnosed with a treatable sleep disorder as per the ICDS-2 criteria and 5 of 13 (38.5%) had co-morbid sleep disorders. We refer the reader to Tables 1 and 2 for specifics. Among the sample, participants were diagnosed with sleep apnea (Obstructive Sleep Apnea (OSA) N=4 and Obstructive and Central Sleep Apnea (OSA and CSA) N=1) 39%; Hypersomnia (N=4) 31%; Sleep-related movement disorders (N=4) 31%, Circadian rhythm sleep disorder (N=1) 8%, Insomnia (N=3) 23%, and Other sleep disorder (N=2) 15.5%.

While the sleep diagnoses varied, all participants had a diagnosis of TBI, ten in the severe category, and one in moderate-severe and two in the mild category with persistent symptoms.

When sleep was considered according to individual sleep diagnosis, we identified that the group with SRBD, RLS and/ or PLMD displayed greater amounts of lighter stages of sleep of (i.e., stage 1).

Discussion

The aims of this study were to objectively examine sleep architecture via overnight PSG in a sample of adults with chronic TBI as compared to normative data by age and sex, and to describe any underlying sleep disorders that resulted in symptoms of insomnia or hypersomnia.

There are several key findings. Firstly, among the participants, twelve of thirteen had abnormal sleep architecture as compared to published age and sex norms. Specifically, increased stage N1 sleep, alterations in percentage of N3 stage and reduced REM percentage which are consistent with previously reported changes in sleep architecture in patients with TBI [9,24,25]. Secondly, all participants were diagnosed with a treatable sleep disorder based on alterations in sleep parameters upon completion of their assessment. Lastly and importantly, sixty percent (6 out of 10) were unable to maintain wakefulness during controlled conditions during the day.

Clinical implications

All participants reported symptoms of insomnia or hypersomnia with increased sleep need, and dissatisfaction with their sleep. Despite the fact that the participants ranged from 1 to 22 years post-injury, only 1 of 13 had undergone specialist investigation of sleep complaints shortly post-injury (at three months). However, all participants were diagnosed according to the ICSD-2, with a treatable sleep and/or wake disorder upon completion of all study investigations.

In this sample, the mean time post-injury was 4.5 years, and two participants were more than 15 years post-injury, yet both had been struggling with trauma-related onset of sleep disturbances.

Two participants, who were actively driving a motor vehicle at the onset of the study, reported severe daytime sleepiness with impaired alertness based on MWT, and subsequently had to stop driving until they were adequately treated. All participants reported that their sleep-wake disturbance had a negative impact on their mood and quality of life.

Thus these findings have implications for those providing clinical management of individuals with TBI. We suggest that routine screening of sleep, assessment of any identified sleep related issues as well as prevention and treatment efforts should be an integral part of any TBI rehabilitation program.

Limitations

Given the heterogeneity of the sample, we were unable to control for medications and therefore the sleep findings must also be considered in light of possible medication effects on sleep [39]. Seventy seven percent of the sample was taking multiple medications at the time of investigation, (see Table 1) some of which are known to enhance sleep, or to compromise or alter sleep. These include selective serotonin reuptake inhibitors (SSRIs) and serotonin–norepinephrine reuptake inhibitors (SNRIs), known to suppress REM and increase lighter stages of sleep [40, 41] and to cause symptoms of insomnia in a small number of (4 to 18%) of depressed samples. 'Atypical' anti-psychotic agents (e.g., quetiapine) have been reported to increase total sleep time and sleep efficiency.

Adverse effects of anti-psychotic agents however, may also include SRBD, RLS, and circadian rhythm disturbances [43,44]. Pregabalin, a medication used to treat neuropathic pain, has been shown to increase slow-wave sleep as a proportion of the total sleep period, reduce sleep-onset latency and reduce the number of awakenings in healthy volunteers [45,46]. Stimulants are recognized to create difficulties with initiating sleep thus increasing sleep onset latency, as well as being REM-suppressants [47]. Finally, modafinil, is reported to cause insomnia in placebo-controlled trials in some patients [48].

We further recognize that the sample was small, and therefore, the findings although comprehensive, are exploratory and thus may not be representative of the wider TBI population. We also recognize that the normative data is dated; however to our knowledge there are no more recent normative data available.

The majority of participants had severe TBI, and were symptomatic, reporting significant dissatisfaction with their sleep post-injury. All participants were placed on the sleep lab schedule and thus their PSG were not necessarily congruent with their circadian phase. Consequently, these results may not truly represent the habitual sleep-wake schedule of the participants and are not 'free running'.

Conclusion

This study adds to the understanding of persistent sleep disorders in a sample of adults with chronic TBI, utilizing both objective- and self-report measures. To our knowledge, it is the first study to both examine sleep architecture via PSG compared to published age and sex norms, and provide a diagnosis of sleep disorders according to the ICSD-2.

In addition, these findings highlight the heterogeneity and complexities of these multi-faceted disorders, including the possible confounds of medication, an important consideration for this population who are often prescribed multiple medications that may impact sleep. Our results also suggest that currently, significant delays occur in the identification, diagnosis and treatment of sleep disorders associated with TBI.

There is a need for greater awareness and understanding of sleep and sleep disturbances following TBI, streamlined referrals for assessment, and the development of practice guidelines. We recommend that patients with TBI of all severities be screened for disorders of sleep, wakefulness and arousal in the early stage of rehabilitation as this may pre-empt the development of chronic sleep disorders.

These results add to a small but growing body of evidence that sleep-wake disorders associated with TBI are complex and remain highly prevalent many years post-injury. Further research with larger samples and free-running PSG is needed.

Declaration of Interest

The authors report no conflicts of interest.

Acknowledgement

The study was funded through a doctoral fellowship in Clinical Research from the Canadian Institutes for Health Research, and a University of Toronto Open Fellowship to Dr. Wiseman-Hakes. Other support came from the Toronto Rehabilitation Institute who receives funding through the Ontario Ministry of Long Term Care. Support was also provided through the Ontario Work Study Program.

We gratefully acknowledge the involvement of Mr. Dana Jewell, chief sleep technologist at Sunnybrook Health Sciences Centre, and Ms. Richelle Bercasio, administrative assistant.

References

1. Werner C, Englehard K (2007) Pathophysiology of traumatic brain injury. Br J Anaesth 99: 4-9.
2. Gosselin N, Tellier M (2010) Patients with traumatic brain injury are at high risk of developing chronic sleep-wake disturbance. J Neurol Neurosurg Psychiatry 81: 1297.
3. Gardani M, Morfiri E, Thomson A, O'Neill B, McMillan TM (2015) Evaluation of sleep disorders in patients with severe traumatic brain injury during rehabilitation. Archives of Physical Medicine and Rehabilitation 96: 1691-7.
4. Duclos C, Dumont M, Wiseman-Hakes C, Arbour C, Mongrain V, et al. (2014) Sleep and wake disturbances following traumatic brain injury. Pathologie Biologie (Paris) 62: 252-61.
5. Wiseman-Hakes C, Murray B, Moineddin R, Rochon E, Cullen N, et al. (2013) Evaluating the impact of treatment for sleep/wake disorders on recovery of cognition and communication in adults with chronic TBI. Brain Injury 27: 1364–76.
6. Mathias JL, Alvaro PK (2012) Prevalence of sleep disturbances, disorders, and problems following traumatic brain injury: a meta-analysis. Sleep Medicine 13: 898-905.
7. Ponsford JL, Ziino C, Parcell D, Shekleton JA, Roper M, et al. (2012) Fatigue and sleep disturbance following traumatic brain injury: Their nature, causes and potential treatments. Journal of Head Trauma Rehabilitation 27: 224–33.
8. Hou L, Han X, Sheng P, Tong W, Li Z, et al. (2013) Risk factors associated with sleep disturbance following traumatic brain injury: clinical findings and questionnaire based study. PLoS ONE 8: e76087.
9. Ouellet MC, Morin CM. (2006) Subjective and objective measures of insomnia in the context of traumatic brain injury: A preliminary study. Sleep Medicine 7: 486–497.
10. Parcell DL, Ponsford JL, Rajaratnam SM, Redman JR (2006) Self-reported changes to nighttime sleep after traumatic brain injury. Archives of Physical Medicine and Rehabilitation 87: 278–285.
11. Ponsford JL, Parcell DL, Sinclair KL, Roper M, Rajaratnam SM (2013) Changes in sleep patterns following traumatic brain injury: a controlled study. Neurorehabil Neural Repair 27: 613-621.
12. Rao V, Spiro J, Vaishnavi S, Rastogi P, Mielke M, et al. (2008) Prevalence and types of sleep disturbances acutely after traumatic brain injury. Brain Injury. 22: 381-386.
13. Wiseman-Hakes C, Colantonio A, Gargaro J (2009) Sleep and wake disorders following traumatic brain injury: A systematic review. Critical Reviews in Physical and Rehabilitation Medicine. 21: 317–374.
14. Baumann CR (2012) Traumatic brain injury and disturbed sleep and wakefulness. Neuromolecular Medicine14: 205-212.
15. Castriotta RJ, Atanasov S, Wilde MC, Masel BE, Lai JM, et.al. (2009) Treatment of sleep disorders after traumatic brain injury. Journal of Clinical Sleep Medicine 5: 137–144.
16. Sommerauer M, Valko PO, Werth E, Baumann CR (2013) Excessive sleep need following traumatic brain injury: a case–control study of 36 patients. Journal of Sleep Research 22: 634-639.
17. Watson NF, Dikmen S, Machamer J, Doherty M, Temkin N (2007) Hypersomnia following traumatic brain injury. Journal of Clinical Sleep Medicine 3: 363–368.
18. Baumann CR, Werth E, Stocker R, Ludwig S, Bassetti CL (2007) Sleep-wake disturbances 6 months after traumatic brain injury: A prospective study. Brain 130: 1873–1883.
19. Castriotta RJ, Murthy JN (2011) Sleep disorders in patients with traumatic brain injury: A review. CNS Drugs 25:175–185.
20. Verma A, Anand V, Verma NP (2007) Sleep disorders in chronic traumatic brain injury. Journal of Clinical Sleep Medicine 3: 357–362.
21. Wiseman-Hakes C, Duclos C, Blais H, Dumont M, Bernard F, et al. (2015) Sleep in the Acute Phase of Severe Traumatic Brain Injury: A Snapshot of Polysomnography. Neurorehabilitation and Neural Repair. Epub ahead of print.
22. Makley MJ, English J, Drubach DA, Kreuz AJ, Celnik PA, et.al (2008) Prevalence of sleep disturbance in closed head injury patients in a rehabilitation unit. Neurorehabil Neural Repair 22: 341-347.
23. Nakase-Richardson R, Sherer M, Barnett SD, Yablon SA, Evans CC, et. al. (2013) Prospective evaluation of the nature, course, and impact of acute sleep abnormality after traumatic brain injury. Arch Phys Med Rehabil 94: 875-882.
24. Shekleton JA, Parcell DL, Redman JR, Ponsford JL, Rajaratnam SMW (2010) Sleep disturbance and melatonin levels following traumatic brain injury. Neurology 74: 1732–1738.
25. Parcell DL, Ponsford JL, Redman JR, Rajaratnam SM (2008) Poor sleep quality and changes in objectively recorded sleep after traumatic brain injury: A preliminary study. Archives of Physical Medicine and Rehabilitation 89: 843–850.
26. von Elm E, Altman DG, Egger M, Pocock SJ, Gotzsche PC, Vandenbroucke JP (2007) The Strengthening the Reporting of Observational Studies in Epidemiology (STROBE) statement: guidelines for reporting observational studies. Lancet 370: 1453-1457.
27. Morin CM (1993) Insomnia: Psychological assessment and management. New York: Guilford Press.
28. Duclos C, Dumont M, Blais H, Paquet J, Laflamme E, et al. (2013) Rest-Activity Cycle Disturbances in the Acute Phase of Moderate to Severe Traumatic Brain Injury. Neurorehabil Neural Repair 28: 472-482.
29. Johns MW. (1991) A new method for measuring daytime sleepiness: The Epworth sleepiness scale. Sleep 14: 540–545.
30. Bushnik T, Englander J, Katznelson L (2007) Fatigue after TBI: Association with neuroendocrine abnormalities. Brain Injury 21: 559–566.
31. Doghramji K, Mitler MM, Sangal RB, Shapiro C, Taylor S, et al. (1997) A normative study of the maintenance of wakefulness test (MWT). Electroencephalography and Clinical Neurophysiology 103: 554–562.
32. Iber C, Ancoli-Israel S, Chesson A Jr, Quan SF (2007) The AASM manual for the scoring of sleep and associated events: Rules, terminology and technical specifications. Westchester, IL: American Academy of Sleep Medicine.
33. Williams RL, Karacan I, Hursch CJ (1974) Electroencephalography (LEG) of Human Sleep: Clinical Applications. Chichester, Sussex: John Wiley.
34. American Academy of Sleep Medicine (2005) International Classification of Sleep Disorders, 2nd ed.: Diagnostic and coding manual. Westchester.
35. Coelho FM, Narayansingh M, Murray BJ (2011) Testing sleepiness and vigilance in the sleep laboratory. Current Opinion in Pulmonary Medicine 17: 406–411.
36. Carskadon MA, Dement WC, Mitler MM, Roth T, Westbrook PR et.al. (1986) Guidelines for the Multiple Sleep Latency Test (MSLT): a standard measure of sleepiness. Sleep 9: 519-524.
37. Baumann CR, Stocker R, Imhof HG, Trentz O, Hersberger M et.al. (2005) Hypocretin-1 (orexin A) deficiency in acute traumatic brain injury. Neurology 65: 147–149.
38. Johns MW (1992) Reliability and factor analysis of the Epworth sleepiness scale. Sleep 15: 376–381.
39. Mollayeva T, Shapiro C (2013) Medication Effects. Kushida C, editor. In: Encyclopedia of Sleep. Elsevier Academic Press 330-337.
40. Black K, Shea C, Dursun S, Kutcher S (2000) Selective serotonin reuptake inhibitor discontinuation syndrome: proposed diagnostic criteria. J. Psychiatr Neurosci 25: 255-261.
41. Brown D (2006) The effect of medication on sleep. Respiratory care clinics of North America 12: 81-99.
42. Hensel J, Pillmann F (2008) Late-life somnabulism after therapy with metoprolol. Clin Neuropharmacol 31: 248-250.
43. DeMartinis N, Winokur A (2007) Effects of psychiatric medications on sleep and sleep disorders. CNS and Neurological disorders 6: 17-29.
44. Thase M (2000) Treatment issues related to sleep and depression. J Clin Psychiatry 61: 46-50.
45. Bazil C (2008) Nocturnal seizures and the effects of anticonvulsants on sleep. Current Neurol Neurosci Rep 8: 149-54.

46. Hindmarch I, Dawson J, Stanley N (2005) A double-blind study in healthy volunteers to assess the effects on sleep of pregabalin compared with alprazolam and placebo. Sleep 28: 187-193.
47. Adler C, Caviness J, Hentz J, Lind M, Tiede J (2003) Randomized trial of modafinil for treating subjective daytime sleepiness in patients with parkinson's disease. Movement Disorders 18: 287-293.
48. Wiseman-Hakes C, Victor JC, Brandys C, Murray BJ (2011) Impact of post-traumatic hypersomnia on functional recovery of cognition and communication. Brain Injury 25: 1256-1265.

An Oxygen Therapy Prevents Ventricular Arrhythmia in Patients with Diastolic Heart Failure and Sleep Apnea

Daisuke Tezuka[1], **Jun-ichi Suzuki**[1,2*] **and Mitsuaki Isobe**[1]

[1]*Department of Cardiovascular Medicine, Graduate School of Medicine and Dentistry, Tokyo Medical and Dental University, Japan*

[2]*Department of Advanced Clinical Science and Therapeutics, Graduate School of Medicine, The University of Tokyo, Japan*

***Corresponding author:** Jun-ichi Suzuki, Department of Advanced Clinical Science and Therapeutics, Graduate School of Medicine, The University of Tokyo, 7-3-1 Hongo, Bunkyo-ku, Tokyo 113-8655, Japan, E-mail: junichisuzuki-circ@umin.ac.jp

Abstract

The background and purpose

Diastolic and systolic heart failure (DHF and SHF) are the different clinical subsets. Because many heart failure patients have sleep apnea syndrome (SAS), oxygen supply improves the patient's prognosis. Thus, the purpose of this study was to compare the effects of oxygen treatment for premature ventricular contractions (PVCs) suppression in patients between DHF and SHF.

Methods and subjects

Patients with heart failure (BNP>80 pg/ml), SAS (AHI> 5) and frequent PVCs (>30/h) were admitted to the hospital for at least 2 consecutive nights. On the first night, the respiratory and Holter monitoring was performed without nasal oxygen treatment; the same monitor with nasal oxygen therapy (3 L/min) was performed on the second night.

Essential results

The DHF patients (more than 40% of LVEF, n=7) showed a significant decline of PVC numbers (63.1 ± 33.0% post/pre) compared to those (119.8 ± 45.3% post/pre, p<0.05) of the SHF patients (less than 40% of LVEF, n=8) by the oxygen treatment. The DHF patients also showed higher SDNN (253.0 ± 260.0 ms) levels compared to those of SHF patients (52.9 ± 22.4 ms, p<0.05). However, AHI and BNP levels were compatible between the two groups.

The principal conclusion

The oxygen treatment may be useful for prevention of ventricular arrhythmia in patients with DHF and SAS.

Keywords: Diastolic dysfunction; Premature ventricular contractions; Brain natriuretic peptide

Introduction

Diastolic heart failure (DHF) and systolic heart failure (SHF) are the different clinical subsets of chronic heart failure (CHF) that are most commonly encountered in clinical practice. Although the clinically overt DHF and SHF appear to be separated by distinctive morphologic and functional changes, clinical characteristics are similar [1]. Although the left ventricle is not dilated and the ejection fraction is preserved in DHF, it is dilated and the ejection fraction is reduced in SHF. The neurohormonal abnormalities including brain natriuretic peptide (BNP) in DHF and SHF are similar. Although ventricular arrhythmia is known to be major causes of poor prognosis in both SHF and DHF patients [2], the management and treatment of DHF has not yet been elucidated.

Sleep-related periodic breathing is known to occur in patients with CHF [3]. These breathing disorders are associated with arterial oxyhemoglobin desaturation and excessive arousals, resulting in sympathetic activation and arrhythmias [4]. Although home oxygen therapy [5], improved clinical conditions of sleep apnea syndrome (SAS) in CHF patients, few studies of SAS in DHF with ventricular arrhythmias have been reported. Thus, studies with detailed findings and laboratory examinations for arrhythmia in SAS and DHF are needed.

Methods

Patients

Fifty patients with CHF admitted to the Department of Cardiovascular Medicine of the Tokyo Medical and Dental University Hospital were candidates for the study. The patients were enrolled from January 2004 to December 2005. Patients <80 years of age were eligible if they met the following criteria: at least one episode of cardiac decompensation; and stable condition while receiving cardiac medication. This study was approved by the ethics committee in

Tokyo Medical and Dental University. Written informed consent was obtained from all participants. The patients were admitted to the hospital for at least 2 consecutive nights for this study. The following tests were also obtained: complete blood count, serum electrolytes, blood urea nitrogen, serum creatinine, brain natriuletic peptide (BNP), echocardiography, and chest X-ray.

Sleep study

Holter electrocardiogram and respiratory monitoring were performed using the Morpheus C system (Teijin Pharma Co. Tokyo, Japan) [6]. For each subject, the overnight sleep study was recorded between 9:30 PM and 5:30 AM. On the first night, the respiratory and Holter monitoring was performed without nasal oxygen treatment; the same monitor with nasal oxygen therapy (3 L/min) was performed on the second night. The data were automatically calculated the apnea hypopnea index (AHI) and the oxygen desaturation index (ODI); patients who had a score of 5 or more on the AHI were diagnosed as SAS [7].

Holter monitoring

All patients underwent Holter recording with 3-channel real-time recorders. For each patient, the total number of premature ventricular contractions (PVCs) was recorded. Heart rate variability (HRV) was assessed, both in time and frequency domains, on the Holter recordings after full revision of the electrocardiogram and editing of beats when indicated. Time-domain HRV variables included the mean of all R-R intervals for the entire recording; the standard deviation of all R-R intervals (SDNN) was measured [6,7].

Other studies

Left ventricular ejection fractions (LVEF) were calculated using echocardiogram by standard techniques. Chest X-ray and arterial blood samples were obtained according to strict criteria as previously reported [8].

Statistical analysis

We used the Wilcoxon rank-sum test to assess significant differences between the groups, since the data were not normally distributed. A value of $p<0.05$ was considered significant. Values are reported as mean ± SD.

Results

In this study, 37 of 50 patients were diagnosed with SAS (AHI > 5) and CHF (BNP >80 pg/ml); we analyzed arrhythmia in these 37 patients. According to our defined thresholds, there were 15 patients who had frequent PVCs (more than 30 PVCs/hour). The 15 patients with frequent PVCs in CHF and SAS were further divided into two groups. The 'SHF (n=8)' group included patients who had impaired LV systolic function (less than 40% of LVEF), frequent PVCs and SAS. The "DHF (n=7)" group included patients who had preserved LV systolic function (more than 40% of LVEF) and frequent PVCs and SAS. Between the two groups, average LVEF was statistically different; the SHF group showed a lower level (26.4 ± 6.9%) compared to that of the DHF group (56.4 ± 11.7%, $p<0.05$ vs. SHF). All other factors were statistically comparable between the two groups (Table 1).

The DHF patients showed a significant decline of PVC numbers (63.1 ± 33.0% post/pre) compared to that of the patients in the SHF group (119.8 ± 45.3 % post/pre, $p<0.05$) by the oxygen treatment. The DHF patients also showed higher SDNN (253.0 ± 260.0 ms) levels compared to the patients in the SHF group (52.9 ± 22.4 ms, $p<0.05$). All other factors including NYHA grading, background diseases, beta blocker treatment, ODI, AHI and BNP levels were statistically comparable between the two groups (Table 1).

Group	DHF	SHF	P
Patient Number	7	8	
Sex (M/F)	5/2	5/3	
Age	70.1 ± 7.5	63.3 ± 5.1	NS
NYHA class	2.6 ± 0.5	2.6 ± 0.7	NS
BNP (pg/mL)	678 ± 671	737 ± 838	NS
CTR in X-p (%)	61.2 ± 9.4	59.7 ± 7.9	NS
LVEF in UCG (%)	56.4 ± 11.7	26.4 ± 6.9	<.05
PVCs (%post/pre)	63.1 ± 33.0	119.8 ± 45.3	<.05
SDNN (no Oxygen)	253.0 ± 260.0	52.9 ± 22.4	<.05
SDNN(with Oxygen)	111.7 ± 24.1	79.8 ± 16.5	NS
AHI	27.2 ± 23.9	14.9 ± 12.5	NS
ODI	29.6 ± 24.0	20.0 ± 10.8	NS
Beta blocker Tx.	4/7	4/8	NS
Causes of CHF			

DCM	3	3	
Ischemic	3	4	
Valve	1	1	

Table 1: SHF or DHF patients with frequent PVCs and SAS

Discussion

In this paper, we have clearly shown that the oxygen treatment suppressed PVC numbers in the DHF patients compared to the SHF group. In our previous study, we confirmed that oxygen treatment to prevent PVCs is effective in patients with higher BNP levels, greater LVEF, and higher SDNN [9]. It has also been reported that asymptomatic DHF patients have a higher incidence of all-case mortality adjusted for age, sex, and LVEF. The diastolic dysfunction was associated with an increased risk of mortality [10]. However, the overall mortality of symptomatic patients with DHF or SHF is similar [11]. In SHF, the rate of sudden death is significantly higher compared to the general population. However, incidence of sudden cardiac death decreases with the increased severity of systolic heart failure [12]. These results suggest that the risk of mortality in DHF patients may be related to arrhythmia.

The pathophysiology of ventricular arrhythmia in DHF patients with SAS is complex and not completely understood. It has been shown that the frequency and severity of arrhythmia can increase in SAS patients [13]. Firstly, we clarified the difference of SDNN between the SHF and the DHF group in this study. This result demonstrated that the impairment of cardiac autonomic function in DHF patients with SAS might be a trigger for ventricular arrhythmia. Nasal oxygen therapy may be effective for the suppression of ventricular arrhythmia through the improvement of cardiac autonomic function. It has been reported that an altered autonomic balance has been suggested as a possible pathogenetic factor, and autonomic dysfunction is implicated in the subsequent development of heart failure patients with SAS [14]. From our results, nasal oxygen therapy may be effective to suppress PVCs in DHF patients with SAS when the patients have impaired autonomic function.

Secondly, we have also revealed that the DHF group showed comparable BNP levels to the SHF group. Recently, it was reported that plasma BNP level and cardiac autonomic function are closely related to prognosis in patients with heart failure. Plasma BNP levels are also known to be a strong predictor for mortality in heart failure patients. Thus, BNP levels are statistically related to cardiac sympathetic nerve innervations [15]. In this study, comparable BNP levels with preserved LVEF might be a condition of insufficient treatments of conservative therapies. It has been well known that conservative treatments of DHF improve the prognosis of the patients. However, these drugs cannot be used in some cases because of hypotension, bradycardia, and/or systemic adverse effects. Therefore, this oxygen therapy, an alternative treatment for DHF, should be considered to use in DHF patients with such conditions.

In conclusion, the oxygen treatment may be useful for prevention of ventricular arrhythmia in patients with DHF and SAS.

References

1. Chatterjee K, Massie B (2007) Systolic and diastolic heart failure: differences and similarities. J Card Fail 13: 569-576.
2. Cohn JN (1996) The management of chronic heart failure. N Engl J Med 335: 490-498.
3. Bradley TD, Floras JS (1996) Pathophysiologic and therapeutic implications of sleep apnea in congestive heart failure. J Card Fail 2: 223-240.
4. Somers VK, Dyken ME, Clary MP, Abboud FM (1995) Sympathetic neural mechanisms in obstructive sleep apnea. J Clin Invest 96: 1897-1904.
5. Sasayama S, Izumi T, Seino Y, Ueshima K, Asanoi H, et al. (2006) Effects of nocturnal oxygen therapy on outcome measures in patients with chronic heart failure and cheyne-Stokes respiration. Circ J 70: 1-7.
6. Pittman SD, MacDonald MM, Fogel RB, Malhotra A, Todros K, et al. (2004) Assessment of automated scoring of polysomnographic recordings in a population with suspected sleep-disordered breathing. Sleep 27: 1394-403.
7. van de Borne P, Oren R, Abouassaly C, Anderson E, Somers VK (1998) Effect of Cheyne-Stokes respiration on muscle sympathetic nerve activity in severe congestive heart failure secondary to ischemic or idiopathic dilated cardiomyopathy. Am J Cardiol 81: 432-436.
8. Javaheri S, Ahmed M, Parker TJ, Brown CR (1999) Effects of nasal O2 on sleep-related disordered breathing in ambulatory patients with stable heart failure. Sleep 22: 1101-1106.
9. Suzuki J, Ishihara T, Sakurai K, Inagaki H, Kawabata M, et al. (2006) Oxygen therapy prevents ventricular arrhythmias in patients with congestive heart failure and sleep apnea. Circ J 70: 1142-1147.
10. Mc Murray JV, Pfeffer M (2005) Heart failure. Lancet 365: 1877-1889.
11. Owan TE, Hodge DO, Herges RM, Jacobsen SJ, Roger VL, et al. (2006) Trends in prevalence and outcome of heart failure with preserved ejection fraction. N Engl J Med 355: 251-259.
12. MERIT-HF Investigators (1999) Effect of metoprolol CR/XL in chronic heart failure: Metoprolol CR/XL Randomised Intervention Trial in Congestive Heart Failure (MERIT-HF). Lancet 353: 2001-2007.
13. Molnar J, Zhang F, Weiss J, Ehlert FA, Rosenthal JE (1996) Diurnal pattern of QTc interval: how long is prolonged? Possible relation to circadian triggers of cardiovascular events. J Am Coll Cardiol 27: 76-83.
14. Narkiewicz K, Montano N, Cogliati C, van de Borne PJ, Dyken ME, et al. (1998) Altered cardiovascular variability in obstructive sleep apnea. Circulation 98: 1071-1077.
15. Kyuma M, Nakata T, Hashimoto A, Nagao K, Sasao H, et al. (2004) Incremental prognostic implications of brain natriuretic peptide, cardiac sympathetic nerve innervation, and noncardiac disorders in patients with heart failure. J Nucl Med 45: 155-163.

Permissions

All chapters in this book were first published in JSD&T, by OMICS International; hereby published with permission under the Creative Commons Attribution License or equivalent. Every chapter published in this book has been scrutinized by our experts. Their significance has been extensively debated. The topics covered herein carry significant findings which will fuel the growth of the discipline. They may even be implemented as practical applications or may be referred to as a beginning point for another development.

The contributors of this book come from diverse backgrounds, making this book a truly international effort. This book will bring forth new frontiers with its revolutionizing research information and detailed analysis of the nascent developments around the world.

We would like to thank all the contributing authors for lending their expertise to make the book truly unique. They have played a crucial role in the development of this book. Without their invaluable contributions this book wouldn't have been possible. They have made vital efforts to compile up to date information on the varied aspects of this subject to make this book a valuable addition to the collection of many professionals and students.

This book was conceptualized with the vision of imparting up-to-date information and advanced data in this field. To ensure the same, a matchless editorial board was set up. Every individual on the board went through rigorous rounds of assessment to prove their worth. After which they invested a large part of their time researching and compiling the most relevant data for our readers.

The editorial board has been involved in producing this book since its inception. They have spent rigorous hours researching and exploring the diverse topics which have resulted in the successful publishing of this book. They have passed on their knowledge of decades through this book. To expedite this challenging task, the publisher supported the team at every step. A small team of assistant editors was also appointed to further simplify the editing procedure and attain best results for the readers.

Apart from the editorial board, the designing team has also invested a significant amount of their time in understanding the subject and creating the most relevant covers. They scrutinized every image to scout for the most suitable representation of the subject and create an appropriate cover for the book.

The publishing team has been an ardent support to the editorial, designing and production team. Their endless efforts to recruit the best for this project, has resulted in the accomplishment of this book. They are a veteran in the field of academics and their pool of knowledge is as vast as their experience in printing. Their expertise and guidance has proved useful at every step. Their uncompromising quality standards have made this book an exceptional effort. Their encouragement from time to time has been an inspiration for everyone.

The publisher and the editorial board hope that this book will prove to be a valuable piece of knowledge for researchers, students, practitioners and scholars across the globe.

List of Contributors

Yi-jun Ge and Gui-hai Chen
Department of Neurology, the First People's Hospital of Chenzhou, China

Lan Xia
Department of Neurology, the Second Affiliated Hospital of Anhui Medical University, China

Theodore R Roy Belfor
OrthoSmile Inc. 54 so. Jefferson Avenue, Catskill, NY 12414, USA

Mena Yacoub
Department of Cardiology, Northside Hospital at Tampa Bay Heart Institute, St. Petersburg, Florida, USA

Irini Youssef, Moro O Salifu and Samy I McFarlane
Department of Medicine, State University of New York Downstate Medical Center, Brooklyn, New York, USA

Fang Wang
Department of Neurology, the First Affiliated Hospital of Anhui Medical University, China

Keisuke Hosokawa, Tsuguo Nishijima, Tetsuya Kizawa, Fumiyo Endo and Shigeru Sakurai
Division of Behavioral Sleep Medicine, Iwate Medical University, School of Medicine, Morioka, Japan

Tulay Ozer and Gokhan Duygulu
Kocaeli Derince Education and Research Hospital, Clinic of Radiology, Turkey

Rabia Terzi
Kocaeli Derince Education and Research Hospital, Clinic of Physical Medicine and Rehabilitation, Turkey

Zahide Yilmaz
Kocaeli Derince Education and Research Hospital, Clinic of Neurology, Turkey

Zafarullah Beigh and Omar Mohammad Shafi
Department of Otorhinolaryngology, Government Medical College, Srinagar, India

Raja Salman Khursheed
Department of Otorhinolaryngology, Zain and Alsabah Hospital, Kuwait

Rafiq Ahmad Pampori
Department of Otorhinolaryngology, Government Medical College, Srinagar, India
Government Medical College, Srinagar, India

Natasha J Williams and Girardin Jean-Louis
Center for Healthful Behavior Change, Division of Health and Behavior, Department of Population Health NYU School of Medicine, New York, USA

Mirnova E Ceïde
Montefiore Medical Center, Department of Psychiatry and Behavioral Science, Bronx, New York

Abishek Pandey
Department of Medicine, State University of New York-Downstate Medical Center, Brooklyn, New York, USA

Ricardo Osorio
Department of Psychiatry NYU School of Medicine, New York, New York, USA

Mary Mittelman
Department of Psychiatry and Department of Rehailitation Medicine, NYU School of Medicine, New York, USA

Samy I McFarlane
Department of Medicine, Division of Endocrinology State University of New York-Downstate Medical Center, Brooklyn, New York, USA

Xue Zhao
Department of Otolaryngology-Head and Neck Surgery, University of Michigan, Ann Arbor, MI, USA

Woravipa Ayudhaya
Department of Neurology, Sleep Disorders Center, University of Michigan, Ann Arbor, MI, USA

Fauziya Hassan
Department of Pediatrics and Communicable Diseases, Sleep Disorders Center, University of Michigan, Ann Arbor, MI, USA

Jeffrey J Stanley
Department of Neurology and Otolaryngology-Head and Neck Surgery, Sleep Disorders Center, University of Michigan, Ann Arbor, MI, USA

Marcela Smurra and Veronica Eguiguren
Hospital Tornú, Argentina

Susana Blanco
Faculty of Engineering, University of Belgrano-CONICET, Argentina

Cecilia DiRisio
Dosimetry Laboratory and Medical Technology, Faculty of Engineering, University of Belgrano, Argentina

Lílian KCR and Virgínia FMT
Physiotherapist, Master´s Student. Evidence-based Healthcare Program, Federal University of São Paulo (UNIFESP), Brazil

Cristiane K
Affiliate Professor. Department of Rheumatology, Federal University of São Paulo (UNIFESP), Brazil

Branca DBS
Assistant Professor. Department of Rheumatology, Santa Casa de Misericórdia, São Paulo, Brazil

Marco TM
Associate Professor. Department of Sports, Federal University of Minas Gerais (UFMG), Brazil

Seoyoun Kim, Hyojae Kim, Min Jeong Kim, Jaehong Park, Joohee Kim, Yesol Min, Tae Kyung Kim, Younggyun Lee, Jinhee IM and Sohee Kim
Korea International High School in Jeju, Daejeong-eup, Seogwipo-si, Jeju-do, Korea

Azizi Seixas, Dorice Vieira and Girardin Jean-Louis
Center for Healthful Behavior Change (CHBC), Division of Health and Behavior, Department of Population Health, New York University Medical Center, New York, NY 10016, USA

April J Rogers
Center for Healthful Behavior Change (CHBC), Division of Health and Behavior, Department of Population Health, New York University Medical Center, New York, NY 10016, USA
Department of Health Service Administration, St. John's University, Queens, NY 11439, USA

Kevin Xia and Kyaw Soe
Department of Medicine, Jersey Shore University Medical Center, Neptune, NJ 07753, USA

Felix Sogade
Department of Cardiology, Health Service of Central Georgia, Macon, Georgia 31201, USA

Barbara Hutchinson
President of Chesapeake Cardiac Care, Annapolis, Maryland, 21401, USA

Samy I McFarlane
Department of Medicine, Division of Endocrinology, State University of New York
Downstate Medical Center, Brooklyn, NY 11203, USA

Sajedeh Behtaj
Alborz Science and Research Branch, Islamic Azad University, Iran

Giovanni Mansueto, Sara Palmieri and Carlo Faravelli
Department of Health Sciences, Psychology and Psychiatry Unit, University of Florence, Florence, Italy

Bert H Jacobson and Taylor P Monaghan
School of Applied Health and Educational Psychology, Health and Human Performance, Oklahoma State University, USA

Palaniappan K
University of Newcastle, Singapore

Thenappan A
White Memorial Medical Center, Los Angeles, USA

Yumi Hirata
Division of Sleep Medicine, Graduate School of Comprehensive Human Sciences, University of Tsukuba, Japan

Makoto Satoh
International Institute for Integrative Sleep Medicine, University of Tsukuba, Japan
Ibaraki Prefectural Center for Sleep Medicine and Sciences, Japan

Yuji Yamaguchi and Masako Kato
Sleep Disorders Center at Fukuoka, Fukuoka Urasoe Clinic, Japan

Ajele Kenni Wojujutari, Oladejo Teslim Alabi and Olasupo Matthew
Department of Psychology, Obafemi Awolowo University, Ile-Ife, Osun State, Nigeria

Nermin Almomani and Amal Alakkam
Family Medicine Consultant, NGHA-Riyadh, Saudi Arabia

Imad Abdulmajeed
Public Health Specialist, NGHA-Riyadh, Saudi Arabia

Saeed Ur Rahman
Community Medicine Dept. DED, NGHA-Riyadh, Saudi Arabia

Samuel Reisman
Department of Medicine, Suny Downstate School of Medicine, USA

Reena Chittora, Durgesh Sharma and Maheep Bhatnagar
Department of Zoology, Mohan Lal Sukhadia University, Udaipur, India

Biswas RSR and Fazlee Kibria Chowdhury Md
Department of Medicine, Chattagram Maa O Shishu Hospital Medical College, Agrabad, Chittagong, Bangladesh

Rahman MH
Department of Medicine, Chittagong Medical College, Chittagong, Bangladesh

Felix Liao
7115 Leesburg Pike, Suite 310, Falla Church, VA 22043, USA

G Dave Singh
BioModeling Solutions, Inc., 17933 NW Evergreen Parkway, Suite 280, Beaverton, OR 97006, USA

Ferguson G and Ware MA
Alan Edwards Pain Management Unit, McGill University Health Centre, Montreal, Quebec, Canada

Akiko Noda
Chubu University Graduate School of Life and Health Sciences, Kasugai, Japan

Masahiro Miyaji
Geaduate School of Information Science and Technology, Aichi Prefectural University, Aichi, Japan

Yuki Wakuda
The University of Tokyo, Tokyo, Japan
YRP Ubiquitous Networking Laboratory, Tokyo, Japan

Yuki Hara
Department of Medical Technology, Nagoya University Graduate School of Medicine, Japan

Fumihiko Yasuma
Department of Medicine, National Hospital Organization Suzuka National Hospital, Suzuka, Japan

Toshio Fukuda
Depertment of Micro-Nano Systems Engineering, Graduate School of Engineering, Nagoya University, Nagoya, Japan

Kunihiro Iwamoto and Norio Ozaki
Department of Psychiatry, Nagoya University Graduate School of Medicine, Nagoya, Japan

Diana M Rosenthal, Ferdinand Zizi and Girardin Jean Louis
Department of Population Health, Center for Healthful Behavior Change, NYU School of Medicine, NY, USA

Donaldson F Conserve
Department of Health Promotion, Arnold School of Public Health, Education, and Behavior, University of South Carolina, Columbia, SC, USA

Dodley Severe and Michaele A Gedeon
University of the Aristide Foundation, Haiti, USA

Georges Casimir
Department of Psychiatry, SUNY Downstate Medical Center, Brooklyn, NY, USA

Samy I McFarlane
Department of Endocrinology, SUNY Downstate Medical Center, Brooklyn, NY, USA

Diana M Rosenthal, Ferdinand Zizi and Girardin Jean Louis
Department of Population Health, Center for Healthful Behavior Change, NYU School of Medicine, NY, USA

Donaldson F Conserve
Department of Health Promotion, Arnold School of Public Health, Education, and Behavior, University of South Carolina, Columbia, SC, USA

Dodley Severe and Michaele A Gedeon
University of the Aristide Foundation, Haiti, USA

Georges Casimir
Department of Psychiatry, SUNY Downstate Medical Center, Brooklyn, NY, USA

Samy I McFarlane
Department of Endocrinology, SUNY Downstate Medical Center, Brooklyn, NY, USA

Fructuoso Ayala-Guerrero
School of Psychology, National Autonomous University of Mexico, Mexico

Indira J Arreguín-González
Unit of Physical Medicine and Rehabilitation Centre Region, UMAE Lomas Verdes, Mexican Social Security Institute, Mexico

Carlos Raúl Castillo-Montoya
Autonomous Metropolitan University (UAM) Iztapalapa, Mexico

Sílvia HM Pucci and M Graça Pereira
School of Psychology, University of Minho, Braga, Portugal

Alethea N Hill
College of Nursing, Adult Health Nursing Department, University of South Alabama, USA

Natasha J Williams, Idoko Salifu and Girardin Jean-Louis
Center for Healthful Behavior Change, Division of Health and Behavior, Department of Population Health, NYU Langone Medical Center, USA

Chimene Castor and Jenna Gibilaro
Department of Nutritional Sciences, Howard University, USA

Samy I McFarlane
Department of Medicine, Division of Endocrinology, SUNY Downstate Medical Center, USA

Albert J Safi and Nancy A Hodgson
The Johns Hopkins University School of Nursing, Maryland, USA

Khem Ballaho
Freelance Clinical & Business Consultant, USA

Gosselin D, Campbell K and De Koninck J
School of Psychology, University of Ottawa, Canada

Grenier J
School of Psychology, University of Ottawa, Canada
Montfort Hospital, Ottawa, Canada

Valiollah Akbari
Assistant Professor of Psychiatry, Medical Doctor, Department of Psychology, University of Medical Sciences, Qom, Iran

Abbas Hajian and Seyed Morteza Hosseini
General Practitioner, University of Medical Sciences, Qom, Iran

Rapee Opasatian and Aroonwan Preutthipan
Division of Pediatric Pulmonology, Department of Pediatrics, and Sleep Disorder Center, Faculty of Medicine, Ramathibodi Hospital, Bangkok, Thailand

Hyung-Suk Yoon
Department of Biomedical Sciences, Seoul National University Graduate School, Seoul, Republic of Korea
Department of Preventive Medicine, Seoul National University College of Medicine, Seoul, Republic of Korea
Institute of Environmental Medicine, Seoul National University Medical Research Center, Seoul, Republic of Korea

Jae Jeong Yang
Department of Preventive Medicine, Seoul National University College of Medicine, Seoul, Republic of Korea
Institute of Environmental Medicine, Seoul National University Medical Research Center, Seoul, Republic of Korea

Hwi-Won Lee
Department of Biomedical Sciences, Seoul National University Graduate School, Seoul, Republic of Korea
Department of Preventive Medicine, Seoul National University College of Medicine, Seoul, Republic of Korea

Daehee Kang
Department of Biomedical Sciences, Seoul National University Graduate School, Seoul, Republic of Korea
Department of Preventive Medicine, Seoul National University College of Medicine, Seoul, Republic of Korea
Cancer Research Institute, Seoul National University, Seoul, Republic of Korea

Catherine Wiseman-Hakes and Tatyana Mollayeva
Rehabilitation Sciences Institute, University of Toronto, Toronto, Ontario, Canada
Toronto Rehabilitation Institute- University Health Network, Toronto, Ontario, Canada

Brian J. Murray
Division of Neurology, Department of Medicine, Sunnybrook Health Sciences Centre, University of Toronto, Toronto, Ontario, Canada

Judith Gargaro
Toronto Rehabilitation Institute- University Health Network, Toronto, Ontario, Canada
ABI Behaviour Services, West Park Health Care Centre, Toronto, Ontario, Canada

Angela Colantonio
Rehabilitation Sciences Institute, University of Toronto, Toronto, Ontario, Canada
Toronto Rehabilitation Institute- University Health Network, Toronto, Ontario, Canada
Department of Occupational Therapy and Occupational Science, University of Toronto, Toronto, Ontario, Canada

Daisuke Tezuka and Mitsuaki Isobe
Department of Cardiovascular Medicine, Graduate School of Medicine and Dentistry, Tokyo Medical and Dental University, Japan

Jun-ichi Suzuki
Department of Cardiovascular Medicine, Graduate School of Medicine and Dentistry, Tokyo Medical and Dental University, Japan
Department of Advanced Clinical Science and Therapeutics, Graduate School of Medicine, The University of Tokyo, Japan

Index

www.ingramcontent.com/pod-product-compliance
Lightning Source LLC
LaVergne TN
LVHW060610210926
848485LV00005B/1395
9781639270965